VETERINARY SCIENCES AND MEDICINE

MAMMARY GLANDS

ANATOMY, DEVELOPMENT AND DISEASES

Veterinary Sciences and Medicine

Additional books in this series can be found on Nova's website
under the Series tab.

Additional e-books in this series can be found on Nova's website
under the e-book tab.

VETERINARY SCIENCES AND MEDICINE

MAMMARY GLANDS

ANATOMY, DEVELOPMENT AND DISEASES

EDMUND B. RUCKER
EDITOR

New York

Additional color graphics may be available in the e-book version of this book.

Library of Congress Cataloging-in-Publication Data

ISBN: 978-1-62948-853-0
LCCN: 2013956181

Published by Nova Science Publishers, Inc. † New York

Contents

Preface		**vii**
Chapter I	Post-Pubertal Mammary Gland Development: Morphology and Mechanisms *Amber N. Hale and Edmund B. Rucker III*	**1**
Chapter II	Mammary Gland Micro-Environment: From Stem Cells to Functional Mammary Glands *Hai-Jun Huang, Xia Peng, Li Zhou, Shun Lu, Min Xiang, Yun-Guo Qian, Qi-Shuang Gao and Si-Wen Jiang*	**33**
Chapter III	Environmental Chemicals and Mammary Gland Development *Erin Pias Hines and Jennifer L. Rayner*	**45**
Chapter IV	Epigenetic Contributions to Mammary Gland Development and Breast Cancer Risk *Kurt B. Hodges, Dana Bazzoun, Kimberly M. McDole, Rabih Talhouk and Sophie A. Lelièvre*	**63**
Chapter V	Neoplastic Diseases of the Canine Mammary Gland *Maria Isabel Carvalho, Teresa Raposo, Helena Rodrigues, Isabel Pires, Justina Prada and Felisbina L. Queiroga*	**113**

Chapter VI	Infection of the Lactating Mammary Gland: Current Status on the Molecular Biology of Mastitis *Koen Breyne and Evelyne Meyer*	**141**
Chapter VII	Mastitis Resistance *Mayumi Sugimoto*	**173**
Chapter VIII	Indicators of the Mammary Gland Health Status in Dairy Animals *Aneta Brodziak, Jolanta Król, Piotr Stanek and Zygmunt Litwińczuk*	**193**
Chapter IX	Effect of Lipopolysaccharide on Cell Populations in the Bovine Mammary Gland *Petr Slama, Zdenek Havlicek and Jiri Skladanka*	**235**
Editor Contact Information		**251**
Index		**253**

Preface

"Mammary Glands: Anatomy, Development and Diseases" is a compilation of manuscripts that encompass a breadth of information from different species in including rodents, dogs, cows, goats, and sheep. The book progresses through distinct and differing themes, but adheres to a guiding principle that the dynamic mammary gland is formed and maintained through a complex series of developmental processes, and that genes and the environment greatly influence its long-term function and health.

The first chapter, "*Post-Pubertal Mammary Gland Development: Morphology and Mechanisms*," begins by discussing some of the classical anatomical features and developmental stages in the mammary gland. Using a mouse model, they initially discuss fetal and pre-pubertal (i.e., virgin) development before moving on to pregnancy, lactation, and involution. Important signaling pathways and mechanisms are covered at each stage, including: the Msx family, Lef1, estrogen, estrogen receptor, progesterone, progesterone receptor, RANKL, RANK, JAK, STATs, prolactin, C/EBP, apoptosis, and autophagy. This chapter highlights the molecular mechanisms that direct development and remodeling in this dynamic organ. The second chapter, *"Mammary Gland Micro-environment: From Stem Cells to Functional Mammary Gland,"* promotes a stem cell-based approach that could potentially be in the future as a type of therapy to repopulate the mammary gland with disease-free cell populations after surgical removal of cancerous tissue. They detail the use of genetically modified ES cells that express an enhanced green fluorescent protein as a cell marker to track the lineage of these cells once injected into a mouse mammary gland. Using a high dose cell regime, they find that these transplanted cells persist after 15 weeks and contribute to the formation of new epithelial cells. The next chapter,

"*Environmental Chemicals and Mammary Gland Development*," details the effects of various chemicals on the mammary gland of laboratory animals based on the age of exposure during development. Environment chemicals discussed include: atrazine, DDT, polybrominated diphenylethers (PBDEs), perfluorooctanoic acid (PFOA), 2,3,7,8-tetrachlorodibenzodioxin (TCDD) and bisphenol A. Ultimately, the mammary gland is sensitive to these chemical agents, which could give rise to alterations in normal development, puberty, lactation, and susceptibility to breast cancer. The following chapter, "*Epigenetic Contributions to Mammary Gland Development and Breast Cancer Risk*," details the role of epigenetic mechanisms in the control of mammary gland cell phenotype. They discuss how epigenetics regulates mammary stem cell potential for differentiation and impacts the mammary epithelial architecture, as well as the contribution of the extracellular matrix in the differentiate process. Finally, they reveal the integration of nutrition and epigenetics in the context of normal development and breast cancer risk. The subsequent chapter, "*Neoplastic Diseases of the Canine Mammary Gland*," presents a clinically relevant model, canine mammary tumors, and the progress made in this field. They initially cover canine mammary anatomy, development, blood supply and lymph drainage, then move into a discussion of canine mammary tumors. The focus is on predisposing factors, aetiology, diagnosis and clinical management, prognostic factors, and treatment strategies.

The last series of chapters are focused on mastitis as a disease that affects mammals and greatly impacts the dairy livestock industry. The first chapter in this set, "*Infection of the Lactating Mammary Gland: Current Status on the Molecular Biology of Mastitis*," gives a good backdrop of mastitis as an inflammatory disease and covers the impact on immune cells such as lymphocytes, macrophages, and neutrophils. They cover the pros and cons of mastitis models, examining *in vitro* infection models and also *in vivo* pathogen-infection mouse mammary glands.

The next chapter, "*Mastitis Resistance*," examines genes in the cow genome that provide resistance to mastitis, forebrain embryonic zinc finger-like (FEZL) and insulin-like growth factor 1 receptor (IGF1R). They detail the downstrean genetic mechanisms regulated by these genes, and suggest that these pathways could be regulated to control innate immunity and serve as a potential tool for preventing mastitis. The following chapter, "*Indicators of the Mammary Gland Health Status in Dairy Animals*," details the symptoms and types of mastitis, its incidence, projected economic losses, and the effect on milk quality. A good part of the chapter is devoted towards addressing indicators of mammary gland health to detect mastitis. These include: somatic cell count, polymorphonuclear leukocytes, blood serum albumin, N-acetyl-β-D-glucosaminidasem L-lactate dehydrogenase, lactose, electrical conductivity, lactoferrin, lysozyme, lactoperoxidase, immunoglobulins, α-lactalbumin, cytokines, growth factors, as well as genetic markers. The final chapter, "*Effect of Lipopolysaccharide on Cell Populations in the Bovine Mammary Gland*," examines how lipopolysaccharide, a component of gram-negative bacteria, has the ability to induce an inflammatory response in the bovine mammary gland. This approach provides an important model to profile how neutrophils, lymphocytes and macrophages respond in an infected bovine mammary gland in order to improve prevention and treatment strategies for mastitis.

In: Mammary Glands
Editor: Edmund B. Rucker
ISBN: 978-1-62948-853-0

Chapter I

Post-Pubertal Mammary Gland Development: Morphology and Mechanisms

Amber N. Hale* and Edmund B. Rucker III
Department of Biology, University of Kentucky, Lexington, KY, US

Abstract

The mammary gland is a unique secretory organ that undergoes the majority of its development in the postnatally during puberty and in response to pregnancy. The mammary gland is primarily composed of mammary stroma, consisting of adipose and loose connective tissue, and mammary ductal epithelia. The post-pubertal development of the mammary gland is classically divided into 4 stages: mature virgin, pregnancy, lactation, and involution. In the mature virgin gland, mitotically active terminal end buds are present but the ductal tree, an arboreal structure of branching ducts, has extended to, but has not yet invaded the mammary fat pad. Upon recognition of pregnancy, ovarian hormones stimulate the proliferation and differentiation of the gland, which prompts the ductal tree to invade the fat pad and undergo branching morphogenesis. After parturition, the gland must produce

* Corresponding author: Tel.: 1.859.257.1807. Email address: Amber.Hale@uky.edu (A. N. Hale).

copious quantities of milk to support the growing litter. When the pups are weaned from the dam, the gland must return to a resting, virgin-like state. Gland remodeling after weaning, termed involution, occurs in two stages and is indispensable in removing epithelial tissue via apoptosis that is no longer needed after lactation. This chapter will focus on the molecular mechanisms that direct development and remodeling in this dynamic organ.

Abbreviations

Bmp, bone morphogenic protein; E, embryonic; E2, estrogen; ECM, extracellular matrix; ER, estrogen receptor; ERE, estrogen responsive element; FGF, fibroblast growth factor; GAS, γ- interferon activation sites; IL, interleukin; JAK, Janus kinase; LIF, leukemia inhibitory factor; MMP, metalloproteinase; Msx, homeobox, msh-like ; P4, progesterone; PR, progesterone receptor; PRL, prolactin; PRLR, prolactin receptor; PThrP, parathyroid hormone related peptide; RANK, receptor activator of nuclear factor κβ; RANKL, RANK ligand; STAT, signal transducers and activators of transcription; Tbx, T-box protein; TEB, terminal end bud; TED, terminal end duct; Th, T helper; TUNEL, Terminal deoxynucleotidyl transferase dUTP nick end labeling; WAP, whey acidic protein

Introduction

Interest in the mammary gland, the defining characteristic of the class Mammalia, has stretched across centuries. The primary function of the mammary gland across mammals is the nourishment of young; however additional functions, such as the transmission of immune factors to infants, are important in many species. It has been postulated that mammary glands arose evolutionarily from modified apocrine glands recently in evolutionary history, approximately 125-190 million years ago [1]. Obtaining evidence for these theories has been technically challenging, since the soft tissue of mammary glands is not well preserved in the fossil record. However, we can gain insight from Monotremata, an order of ancient egg laying mammals that represents an interesting link to the reptilian past. The platypus and echidna are extant egg laying species that have functional mammary glands that undergo a true lactation phase. This lends support to the postulation that early apocrine secretions served some beneficial role to protect and/or nourish eggs via semi-permeable shells, thus selecting for the retention of these glands [1]. While the evolutionary origin of the mammary gland is still being investigated and debated, developmental and molecular biologists have made astounding progress in elucidating the mechanisms controlling the development of the mammary gland in its current incarnation.

The mature mammary gland is an arboreal structure with ductal branches extending from a nipple area, colonizing a mammary fat pad, and finally branching and terminating into alveolar units. Mammary gland development is divided into four stages that align with the overall growth, sexual maturation and reproductive-associated changes of mammals, which are: embryonic, pre-pubertal, pubertal, and post-pubertal.

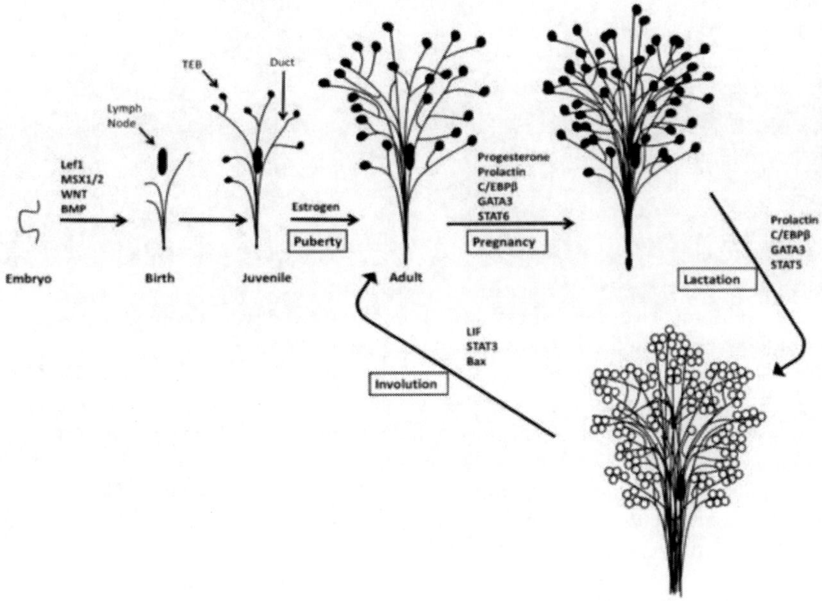

Figure 1. Schematic overview of mouse mammary gland development and major influencing factors. Mammary gland development is typically divided into embryonic, perinatal, puberty and adult stages. After sexual maturity pregnancy induced changes drive the terminal differentiation of the gland. These stages are pictured; pregnancy, lactation and involution. Many of the influential molecules discussed in this chapter are included in the figure above the developmental stage/process to which they are integral. Major developmental stages are depicted schematically; stage labels are below mammary glands and process labels are below arrows.

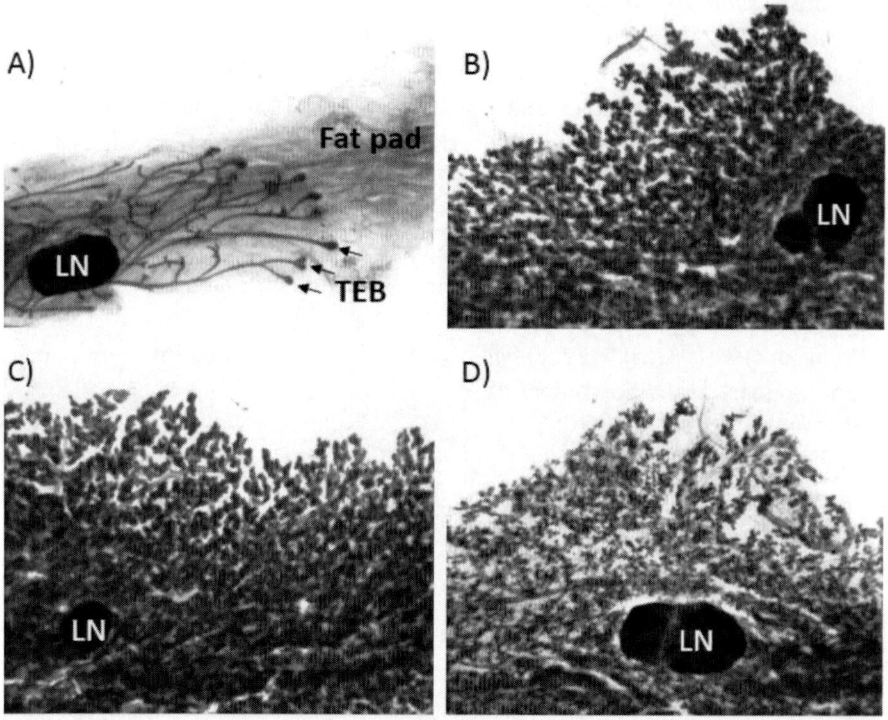

Figure 2. Anatomic overview of mouse mammary gland development at four stages. Whole-mounts were taken of mouse mammary glands at four distinct developmental stages: A) virgin 5-week-old glands; B) pregnancy day 14; C) lactation day 1; and D) involution. Epithelial cells stain with the dye carmine alum, whereas the surrounding fat pad is cleared. Notice in the virgin gland the formation of the ductal tree, as the epithelia migrate into the surrounding fat pad. Representative terminal end buds (TEBs) are shown with arrows. Lymph nodes (LN) are shown for orientation in all figures. Images were taken on an Olympus SZ-PT using 6.7X magnification and the imaging software QCapture Pro 6.0.

The initiation of mammary development in embryos occurs during gestation with the establishment of the anlagen; however, the majority of development occurs in the adult animal. Branching and elongation of the ductal epithelium ensues at the time of puberty, with the expansion of the alveolar epithelium proceeding in response to pregnancy. However, terminal differentiation is not achieved until lactation. This periodic developmental profile is unique amongst tissues and lends the mammary gland as an excellent model to study branching morphogenesis and other developmental paradigms in an adult animal. Furthermore, the accessory nature of the mammary gland is ideal since it allows researchers to make otherwise deleterious mutations in this relatively large, and easily accessible tissue. Classically, post-pubertal development has been separated into four main stages: virgin, pregnant, lactation, and involution (schematically represented in Figure 1 and whole mounts in Figure 2). These stages will be discussed individually following a description of embryonic and pre-pubertal development.

Fetal Development and Pre-Pubertal Development

Although the focus of this chapter is post-pubertal development, it would be incomplete without a brief overview of embryonic and pre-pubertal mammary development. In the interest of continuity, the mouse will be the primary focus of this chapter and only major developmental discrepancies will be addressed. In most studied mammalian species mammary lines, ridges of multi-layer ectoderm become visible on the ventral surface of the embryo running parallel to the anterior-posterior axis of the embryo between the limbs. The mammary lines, as anatomically evident structures, are controversial in the mouse; however, specific gene expression patterning corresponding to proposed mammary line location has been observed. *Wnt10b* can be detected in a restricted pattern and *Wnt6* in a broader area just antecedent to the anatomical detection of anlagen presence [2]. Histological analysis revealed a change in epithelia co-localizing with the *Wnt10b* expression, specifically a change to multi-layered cuboidal epithelia from the surrounding squamous epithelia. In addition, the mammary line also has a characteristic dense dermis below it [2]. In the mouse, the first visible surface feature of mammary development is five symmetrical pairs of mammary placodes at E11.5. Interestingly, unlike other models, the mouse placodes do not follow an anterior-posterior developmental pattern. Instead, they proceed pairwise in the order, numbered anterior-posterior: 3, 4, 1 and 5, then 2. Mammary placodes retain their expression of *Wnt10b*, *Wnt6*, fibroblast growth factor (*Fgf10*), and Lymphoid enhancer binding factor 1 (*Lef1*), a WNT pathway effector. *Lef1* $^{-/-}$ embryos fail to develop placodes by E13.5, a phenotype shared by overexpression of *Dkk1*, a WNT pathway inhibitor [3, 4]. Studies on placode development by Mailleux et al. revealed distinct signaling dependence. The thoracic placodes (1, 2, and 3) and the number 5 inguinal placode are dependent on FGF10/FGFR2b while placode 4 is independent of these signals[5]. Of late, bone morphogenic protein 4 (*Bmp4*) and T-box protein 3 (*Tbx3*) have also been shown to work synergistically to determine positioning of the mammary buds. For a more detailed review of signaling pathways involved in morphogenesis and associated mutants see Refs. [6, 7].

After the buds become visible at E13.5, there is a brief resting phase during which very few cells are mitotically active. Beginning again at approximately E15.5 and persisting through gestation, each bud extends a small sprout and invades the mammary fat pad precursor. The sprouts are completed by the formation of a lumen and by E18.5 each duct has undergone branching and resembles a small ductal tree. The interaction of parathyroid hormone related peptide (PTHrP) and its receptor PTHR1 drives the rudimentary ductal tree to branch. At the time of parturition, the immature mammary gland is comprised of approximately 10-15 small branches near the nipple.

Puberty

Mammary gland growth is isometric with the individual from approximately E18.5 until puberty, wherein the development will resume under the control of hormones. The ductal tree is primarily established during puberty under the control of circulating hormones. These circulating hormones bind to receptors located in the pituitary gland and throughout the female reproductive system to initiate changes in gene expression. Estrogen receptor (ER) and progesterone receptor (PR) are instrumental during this period and will be discussed in depth in sections that follow.

At approximately 3-4 weeks of age the ducts become capped with mitotically active, club-shaped structures termed terminal end buds (TEBs). TEBs are composed of inner "body" cells and outer, undifferentiated "cap" cells. The body cells differentiate into mammary epithelial cells. The cap cells ultimately differentiate into myoepithelial cells. The innermost layer of body cells undergoes apoptosis to form the hollow lumen. The programmed cell death rate in the presumed lumen is very high, with a rate far greater than that detected during involution when the entire gland undergoes remodeling [8]. TEB formation is dependent on the paracrine production of IGF-1 by stromal cells which respond to growth hormone, reviewed in [9]. The TEBs vary both among glands within an animal and between animals at the same time point. The number 2 and 3 glands have larger number and size of TEBs when compared to the number 4 inguinal mammary gland. The size difference of the TEBs is attributed to a larger number of cap cells rather than cell hypertrophy[10]. Circulating estrogen (E2) stimulates allometric ductal elongation via TEB proliferation which terminates when the TEBs reaches the limit of the fat pad. Concomitantly, secondary ductal branches are formed off of the primary ducts by TEB division. After expansion of the ductal tree during puberty, TEBs are permanently replaced by terminal end ducts (TEDs) which are not mitotically active. TEDs are then surrounded by stroma with the center cells undergoing apoptosis. The resultant structure is a single layer of epithelia cells resting on a basement membrane. The gland remains in this mature virgin state until stimulation by pregnancy.

Pregnancy and Lactation

Pregnancy hormones stimulate further branching of the ductal tree, the development of the lobuloalveolar compartment, and the terminal differentiation of the secretory epithelia. The ducts are composed of three major layers; the most apical is a single layer of cuboidal epithelial surrounding a hollow lumen, this layer is referred to as "luminal epithelia." Basal to the luminal epithelia, specialized myoepithelial cell layer encircles the luminal epithelia; these cells contain smooth muscle actin and assist with ductal contraction and movement of milk during lactation. Beyond the myoepithelial cells, a tough laminin-enriched basement membrane separates the epithelia and the surrounding connective tissue with a layer of extracellular matrix (ECM) proteins including proteoglycans and glycoproteins.

The epithelium of the alveoli is a single layer of squamous epithelium which is discontinuously surrounded by myoepithelial cells then finally a basement membrane. As pregnancy progresses, the myoepithelia becomes more discontinuous and the alveolar epithelium may contact the basement membrane directly. During late pregnancy, approximately pregnancy day 18.5, the alveolar epithelial cells produce milk proteins and lipids which are retained in the cells, causing them to appear more cuboidal or pyramidal due to the increased cytoplasmic volume. After the initiation of lactation, milk proteins and lipids are released into the alveolar lumen and the cells once again appear morphologically flattened. This is achieved in part by the contraction of the myoepithelial cells lining the alveoli in response to oxytocin. At this point, large milk fat droplets can be seen in the lumens. The alveoli continue to expand throughout lactation until the gland is completely filled. During the height of lactation, very few adipocytes can be visualized and the ratio of parenchyma to stroma is heavily weighted toward the parenchyma. The lactation phase will continue until the pups are weaned or gradually taper off as the pups begin to gain nourishment from other sources [11]. The pregnancy associated changes: ductal branching, lobuloalveolar development, proliferation, and differentiation are highly regulated processed. The signaling cascades responsible will be discussed at length in later sections.

Involution

Cessation of suckling, due to natural oracute weaning and milk stasis, results in the mammary gland remodeling to again resemble a resting, "virgin-like" state. Involution proceeds in two stages: the reversible stage and irreversible stage. The early, reversible stage is characterized by waves of apoptosis-mediated cell death. Transcriptional profiling studies have detected changes within hours of involution [12-14]. Histologically, secretory epithelia cells are sloughed and seen in alveoli in greater numbers during early involution than in any other stage. Many of these cells are terminal deoxynucleotidyl transferase dUTP nick end labeling (TUNEL) positive, a marker for apoptosis that detects DNA fragmentation [15]. It is estimated that during involution 80% of epithelial cells will die via apoptosis, a catastrophic event unparalleled in normal adult tissues. Many induced mutant mouse models generated exhibit involution phenotypes, see Radisky and Hartmann for review and references [16].

The second phase of involution is initiated approximately 72 hours post-lactation and is more drastic in nature. Once the gland has entered this phase, lactation cannot be re-initiated even if the pups are returned to the dam. The superfluous secretory alveoli collapse, the ECM is remodeled, and adipocytes increase in number. The irreversible phase is characterized by and dependent upon on a temporal increase in matrix metalloproteinase activity (MMPs) to stimulate ECM remodeling. Invasion of immune cells, primarily phagocytic cells such as macrophages, helps to clear cellular debris.

Autophagy most likely plays a role during mammary involution though at present this is poorly described in murine models. Autophagy, Greek for "self-eating," is a highly-conserved catabolic process initiated in response to cellular stress. In bovine, autophagy is observed morphologically and detected with molecular methods during involution. Additionally, pro-autophagic protein BECLIN1 has been shown to play an important role in mediating involution. It is clear that more work needs to be done to elucidate the role of autophagy during this stage in murine models [17-19].

Signaling Pathways

Msx Family

The class II homeobox, msh-like (Msx) genes, *Msx1*, *Msx2* and *Msx3*, are common to vertebrates and often define mesenchymal-epithelia interaction sites. *Msx3* expression is restricted to the dorsal neural tube[20], while *Msx1* and *Msx2* are more broadly expressed during embryogenesis. *Msx1* and *Msx2,* but not *Msx3*, are expressed at varying levels during every stage of mammary development except for pregnancy.

During embryonic development *Msx2* expression is detectable both in the epithelia and the mesenchymal cells, while after parturition expression is restricted to the mesenchymal cells in close proximity to mammary ducts. *Msx2* expression is dependent on reciprocal interactions with epithelial cells. In cleared fat pads *Msx2* is undetectable, indicating an essential epithelia interaction compartment for normal expression. *Msx2* expression, but not *Msx1*, is regulated by E2 and progesterone (P4), indirectly via the PR and directly as a transcriptional target respectively [21].

Msx2 is implicated in the regulation of branching, as the *in vitro* overexpression of *Msx2* is sufficient to drive branching. In addition, *in vivo* approximately one third of *Msx2* null mice have arrested embryonic mammary gland development with failed ductal branching [22]. *Msx1* null neonates do not exhibit a mammary defect, which is not surprising since homeobox genes typically exhibit high levels of functional redundancy [23]. However, double knockout *Msx1/2* mice fail to form mammary anlagen with a complete penetrance of the phenotype [22].

Mice that misexpress *Msx1* in the mammary gland exhibit a reduction in pregnancy-induced differentiation and an increase of *Cyclin D1* (*ccnd1*) expression, and an increase in cell proliferation. This model supports *in vitro* experiments with *Msx-1* overexpressing HC11 mammary epithelial cells which upregulate *ccnd1* expression and are unable to undergo functional differentiation in response to lactogenic hormones. The authors propose that

Msx1 prevents exit from the cell cycle, which drives an upregulation of *ccnd1* expression; ultimately, this proliferative cell fate prevents the terminal differentiation of the epithelial cells [24]. Although *ccnd1* is the only verified target of *Msx1* in the mammary gland identified to date, it can also be induced by *Msx2* most likely in response to hormonal signaling by E2 and P4. Interestingly, expression profiles of *Bmp2* and *Bmp4* closely resemble the profiles of *Msx1* and *Msx2*, respectively. It has been suggested that this indicates a regulatory relationship, though the nature of this relationship is yet to be determined owing to the early embryonic lethality of *Bmp2* and *Bmp4* null mice [25].

Lef1

Lef1 is a nuclear target of the Wnt signaling pathway. In the presence of Wnt signaling, dephosphorylated β-catenin enters the nucleus and engages *Lef1* to act as a transcriptional activator. Therefore, in the absence of Wnt signaling, *Lef1* is a transcriptional repressor. *Lef1* null neonates lack teeth, whiskers, and hair in addition to lacking mammary glands. Closer inspection of E13.5 embryos revealed a reduced number of mammary buds, indicating that the mammary rudiment develops improperly, arrests, and then regresses by the time of parturition. Since other visceral organs were unaffected, the defect seems to be specific to organs requiring epithelia of ectodermal origin to interact with surrounding mesenchyme [3].

Hormones

Through both endocrine ablation studies and targeted mouse transgenic models it has been elucidated that E2, P4, and prolactin (PRL) drive the pregnancy-induced growth and differentiation of the mature mammary gland. P4 is an ovarian hormone secreted by a temporary endocrine structure within the ovary, the corpus luteum. PRL is a peptide hormone that signals through PRL receptors (two isoforms, PRLRA and PRLRB).

Together, these hormones are responsible for initiating complex, and sometimes intersecting, gene pathways responsible for branching and alveologenesis during pregnancy. Transgenic mouse models have illuminated many of the signaling pathways that will be discussed in this chapter. For reference, a table has been included with a synopsis of the models discussed, see Figure 3.

	Genotype	Mammary phenotype	Ref
Embryo			
Lef1	*lef1* $^{-/-}$	No placode formation	[3]
Dkk1	K5-rtTA/tetO-Dkk1 (overexpression)	No placode formation	[4]
Msx1	*msx1* $^{-/-}$	No phenotype	[23]
Msx2	*msx2* $^{-/-}$	1/3 of embryos arrest mammary development before ductal branching/perinatal lethality	[22]
Msx1/Msx2	*msx1/msx2* $^{-/-}$	Anlagen fail to form	[22]
Puberty			
Esr1	ERα $^{-/-}$	No ductal side-branching or lobuloalveolar development	[26], [29]
	deleter-Cre;ERα $^{f/f}$	No data	[32]
	MMTV-tTA/tet-op-mERα	Toolbox/kinetics study	[34]
Esr2	ERβ $^{-/-}$	No phenotype	[29],[27]
	CMV-Cre;ERβ $^{f/f}$	No phenotype	[33]
Esr1/ Esr2	ERα $^{-/-}$; ERβ $^{-/-}$	same as ERα $^{-/-}$	[28]
Cebpb (C/EBPβ)	*cebpb* $^{-/-}$	Enlarged ducts/decreased side-branching	[58],[59]
Pregnancy/Lactation			
Msx1	(overexpression)	Reduction in differentiation/increase in proliferation	[24]
Pgr	PR $^{-/-}$	No ductal side-branching or lobuloalveolar development in response to hormonal stimulation	[38]
	PRA $^{-/-}$	No phenotype	[45]
	PRB $^{-/-}$	Reduced ductal side-branching and lobuloalveolar development	[46]
	ZP3-Cre;PR $^{f/f}$	Same as PR $^{-/-}$	[47]
	EIIa-Cre;PR $^{f/f}$	Same as PR $^{-/-}$	[48]
Cebpb (C/EBPβ)	*cebpb* $^{-/-}$	Reduced lobuloalveolar development in response to hormonal stimulation	[58], [59]
Ccnd1 (Cyclin D1)	*ccnd1* $^{-/-}$	Reduced lobuloalveolar development/ lactation failure	[53]
Stat6	*stat6* $^{-/-}$	Reduced lobuloalveolar development	[62]
Il4/Il13 (IL-4/IL-14)	*IL-4* $^{-/-}$;*IL-14* $^{-/-}$	Reduced lobuloalveolar development	[62]

Figure 3. (Continued)

	Genotype	Mammary phenotype	Ref
	WAP-rtTA-Cre;*gata*$^{f/f}$	Similar to MMTV-Cre;*gata*$^{f/f}$/ increased proliferation/cell death/ failure of lactation	[63]
	Keratin14-Cre;*gata*$^{f/f}$	Embryonic death, absent placodes in survivors	[64]
	WAP-Cre;*gata*$^{f/f}$	Reduced lobuloalveolar development/ defective lactation	[64]
Prl	PRL$^{-/-}$	Reduced lobuloalveolar development	[66]
Prlr	PRLR$^{-/-}$	Reduced ductal side-branching /lactation failure	[68],[67]
Jak2	*jak2*$^{-/-}$	No data -Embryonic lethal	[69],[70]
	MMTV-Cre;*jak2*$^{f/f}$	Defect in establishment of alveolar progenitor cells	[71]
	WAP-Cre;*jak2*$^{f/f}$	Reduced survival of secretory epithelia	[71]
Stat5a	*stat5a*$^{-/-}$	Defective lobuloalveolar development/lactation failure	[74]
Stat5b	*stat5b*$^{-/-}$	No phenotype	[76]
Stat5a/Stat5b	*stat5a*$^{-/-}$;*stat5a*$^{-/-}$	Transplant studies reveal failure of alveolar morphogenesis	[77], [78]
Stat1	*stat1*$^{-/-}$	No phenotype	[90]
Involution			
Stat3	*stat3*$^{-/-}$	No data -Embryonic lethal	[85]
	WAP-Cre;*stat3*$^{f/f}$	Delayed involution	[86]
	BLG-Cre;*stat3*$^{f/f}$	Delayed involution	[87]
Bcl-2	*bcl-2*$^{-/-}$	No phenotype	[91]
	WAP- *bcl-2* (overexpression)	Delayed involution	[92]
Bcl-x	*bcl-x*$^{-/-}$	No data -Embryonic lethal	[95]
	WAP-Cre; *bcl-x*$^{f/f}$	Accelerated involution	[96]
	MMTV-Cre; *bcl-x*$^{f/f}$	Accelerated involution	[96]
Bax	*bax*$^{-/-}$	Delayed involution	[98]
	WAP- *bax* (overexpression)	Lactation defect/forced involution	[100]

Figure 3. Transgenic mouse models and mammary phenotypes observed.

E2/ER

E2 is a steroid hormone with two characterized receptors, ERα and ERβ, which are members of the nuclear receptor superfamily. The canonical method of activation is: 1) ligand binding, 2) conformational change of receptor, 3) co-activator recruitment, and 4) dimerization and binding of receptor to estrogen responsive elements (EREs) in gene regulatory regions. Several ligand-independent, non-canonical pathways of ER activation have been described but are beyond the scope of this chapter. The expression patterns of the two ERs are distinct but overlapping, and ERα is the dominant receptor type expressed in the mammary gland. Three knockout mouse models have been generated to study the importance of ER in the overall growth and development of the organism. ERαKO, ERβKO, and ERα/ERβ double knockout (ERαERβKO) mouse models are all viable and progress to adulthood without defects [26-28]. ERαKO, ERβKO, and double knockout (ERαERβKO) do not show defects in embryonic or pre-pubertal mammary gland development, but after puberty females exhibit ovulation failure resulting in infertility or subfertility (ERβ). ERαKO mice do not undergo the expected ductal elongation and expansion during puberty. The ductal tree remains sparse with no lobuloalveolar development occurring [29]. Transplantation experiments of ERαKO epithelia into wild-type cleared fat pads developed without defect to puberty as expected, but failed to undergo any development in response to pregnancy. This effect is epithelia intrinsic since the converse experiment, ERαKO fat pad grafted into a wild-type host with wild-type mammary epithelial cells grows normally and responds to pregnancy hormones [30].

ERβKO females are sub-fertile, yet develop normal mammary glands and are able to undergo a normal lactation phase [27]. ERαERβKO mammary glands phenocopy ERαKO mammary glands, further underscoring the importance of ERα in this tissue. ER ablation causes defects in many reproductive tissues beyond the mammary gland and ovary, and are reviewed in Ref. [31].

The detection of residual expression from the ERαKO necessitated the generation of a true null allele. To address this, the Cre/LoxP system was used to generate an ERα floxed model for tissue-specific deletion strategies. Initially, a global Cre-mediated deletion was analyzed and the results phenocopied the ERαKO model [32]. An ERβ conditional knockout based on the Cre/LoxP system has also been generated using a similar targeting strategy as was used to generate the conditional ERαKO allele. LoxP sites were inserted flanking exon3 of the ERβ gene [33]. Exon three was chosen to ensure a true null allele and effectually reconcile conflicting reports of phenotypes of the ERβKO mice due to varying generation and housing conditions. In the context of the mammary gland, these models will be important to define the temporal requirement, if any, of ER in pregnancy-induced mammary gland development. Using any one of the current mammary directed Cre transgenic models, ER could be effectively attenuated at any point in the pregnancy cycle.

As a supplement to many of the previously mentioned loss-of-function models, an inducible, ERα model has also been generated using the tetracycline system. In this MMTV-tTA/tet-op-mERα model overexpressed ERα, and administration of doxycycline turns off expression of ERα [34]. These recent models, will be invaluable in further characterizing the role of ER in reproductive development and in oncogenesis when used combination with current cancer models.

P4/PR

P4 is a steroid hormone produced primarily in the ovary and adrenal gland of females. Its activity oscillates with the estrous cycle and is required for the establishment and maintenance of pregnancy. P4 is a ligand for the PR, a nuclear receptor superfamily member. Once the ligand is bound the ligand/receptor complex translocates to the nucleus and affects transcriptional activity of target genes either directly or indirectly. The PR has two receptor isoforms, PR alpha and beta (PRA/PRB), which are splice variants of the gene *Pgr* [35, 36]. The two receptors are structurally similar with the exception of an amino terminal extension of PRB [36, 37].

Since PR is under control of E2, a targeted approach to sort out the function of P4 independent of E2 was needed. The PR knockout mouse (PRKO) is viable and shows no overt defects through embryogenesis or adulthood. As expected, female mice are infertile, due to the well characterized role of P4 in establishment and maintenance of pregnancy. However, a surprising role for P4 in the mammary gland was revealed. PRKO females produced a rudimentary ductal structure, indicating the P4 was not essential for ductal elongation, but failed to proliferate and undergo normal lobuloalveolar development and ductal side-branching in response to hormonal stimulation [38]. This original characterization established a role for PR in normal mammary development and during pregnancy, but was insufficient to distinguish between systemic and local effects. To this end, several approaches have been taken to dissect the effect of PR in the mammary gland. Transplantation experiments wherein mammary epithelia from PRKO mice were transplanted into wild-type recipients and vice versa revealed that intrinsic PR expression was essential in the epithelia for ductal outgrowth in response to circulating hormones and for lobuloalveolar development during pregnancy [39-42]. A PR-LacZ reporter helped to clarify the PR expression in both spatial and developmental contexts. During development, the activity is restricted to the epithelia; however, at puberty the activity is high in the body cells of the TEBs and ductal luminal cells. The localization pattern changed in the adult where the activity is clustered around the terminal ductal side branches, and all activity is reduced toward the end of pregnancy at the time of terminal differentiation [43]. Interestingly, in the juvenile PR expression is uniform, but in the mature gland only sub-populations of mammary epithelial cells are PR positive, confirming earlier studies [44].

Isoform specific function was addressed elegantly with the generation of PRA and PRB-specific knockout alleles (PRAKO, PRKOB). The PRAKO did not show abnormal effects in the mammary gland, indicating that PRB was of greater importance in this tissue [45]. This was confirmed with the PRBKO model that exhibited reduced ductal side branching and lobuloalveolar development during pregnancy [46]. Importantly, this study also revealed an isoform specific activation of receptor activator of nuclear factor κβ ligand (RANKL) by PRB, the importance of RANKL in mammary morphogenesis will be addressed in another section focusing on receptor activator of nuclear factor κβ (RANK) signaling.

Two Cre-LoxP-based conditional PR knockout models have been produced allowing for greater spatial and temporal control of PR ablation. The models differ by targeting strategy, either exon 1 or exon 2 is flanked by LoxP sites, yet both produce homozygous null animals that phenocopy the original PRKO [47, 48]. Additionally, a knock-in of the reverse tetracycline-dependent transactivator (rtTA) at the PR locus (driven by the endogenous PR promoter) has been helpful in identifying target genes of PR signaling [49]. These mice ($PR^{rtTA/rtTA}$) phenocopy the PRKO model, and when treated with doxycycline PR promoter driven rtTA can induce expression of PR target genes in P4 responsive cells. This model combined with a reporter transgene allowed for the precise identification of PR responsive cells. In concordance with earlier studies, this model has confirmed the non-uniform pattern of PR expression in mature mammary epithelial cells, and has importantly clarified the role of RANKL as an effector of PR dependent side branching and alveologenesis [44, 49, 50]. These models will be useful in separating tissue intrinsic functions from systemic effects of PR deficiency and are applicable to many studies of reproductive biology beyond the mammary gland.

RANKL/RANK

RANK is present on mammary epithelial cells and when activated by its ligand, RANKL, is a mammary PR effector which is essential for mammary proliferation and morphogenesis during pregnancy [51]. In wild-type animals, RANKL is upregulated in response to P4 only in PR-positive cells, and PR-positive/RANKL cells cause proliferation in a paracrine fashion. This regulation was tested *in vivo* in a PRKO background with a conditional induction of RANKL targeted only to cells that would normally express ER, PR, and RANKL. With induction of RANKL by drug administration, the mammary defect observed in PRKO mice can be partially rescued [50]. This study highlighted the importance of the spatial organization of PR positive cells and showed that when RANKL was induced in PR-negative and PR-positive cells, the ductal outgrowth and alveolar development was disorganized. RANKL/RANK leads to nuclear factor κB (NFκB) dependent transcriptional activation of *ccnd1,* and disruption of RANKL or the components of this pathway result in a defect in alveolar proliferation [52]. These studies are supported by the *ccnd1* knockout mouse which has reduced lobuloalveolar development during pregnancy and fails to lactate [53].

Recent evidence has revealed that RANKL serves as an intersection point between P4 and PRL signaling. Srivastava et al. suggest that RANKL is induced by both P4 and PRL signaling and is dependent on Janus kinase 2 (JAK2)/ signal transducers and activators of transcription 5a (STAT5a) signaling [54]. Other points of intersection of P4 and PRL signaling and their potential consequences are reviewed in Ref. [55]. RANKL regulates CCAAT-enhancer binding protein (C/EBP), to which we will now turn our attention.

C/EBP

Of the six C/EBP transcription factor family members, C/EBPβ's three protein isoforms seem to be the most important for mammary gland development, though other family members are expressed [56]. C/EBPβ is expressed throughout mammary gland development but is lowest in the virgin, increases during pregnancy, is reduced modestly during lactation, and then is increased again during the reversible phase of involution [57]. Ablation of C/EBPβ causes defects in ductal outgrowth manifested by enlarged ducts and decreased branching [58, 59]. During pregnancy (transplantation or hormone supplementation experiments were required due to infertility of C/EBPβ$^{-/-}$

mice), ductal outgrowth occurred but lobuloalveolar development is negatively affected.

Another family member, C/EBPδ, has an important function in involution. The C/EBPδ knockout mice exhibit a delayed involution phase characterized by a delay in the appearance of apoptotic cells, indicating a role in early involution, a time when C/EBPδ expression is highest in wild-type glands. Expression analysis revealed a reduction in the levels of pro-apoptotic BAX and BAK, and an increase in anti-apoptotic Bcl-X. STAT3 is responsible for activating C/EBPδ at the initiation of involution. These results position C/EBPδ as a regulator of involution-induced cell death [60].

Cytokine Signaling, Stat6, and Alveolar Commitment

STAT6 is unique amongst STATs in the mammary gland as it is important early in gestation and is not directly downstream of PRL signaling (discussed below). Classically, *Stat6* has been characterized as a vital signaling molecule in the T helper (Th) cell lineage, specifically in the differentiation of Th2 cells. In this context, interleukin (IL) IL-4/IL-13 binds its cognate receptor leading to activation of JAK1 and TYK2 which in turn facilitate recruitment and activation of STAT6. STAT6 forms homodimers which translocate to the nucleus activating or repressing IL-4/IL-13 target genes including GATA binding protein, 3 (GATA3), a transcription factor, reviewed in Refs. [6, 61]. More recently, however, a new role for *Stat6* regulating mammary alveolar cell fate has emerged. In two transgenic models interrogating this pathway, concomitant IL-4/IL-13 knockout or *Stat6* knockout, resulted in curtailed alveolar development when compared to controls. Furthermore, in glands lacking SOCS5, a STAT6 inhibitor, accelerated development of the alveoli is observed [62].

Further support for this pathway's importance in mammary gland proliferation and differentiation is provided by two studies centering on GATA3, a transcription factor and target of IL-4/IL-13/STAT6 signaling. In mice with a conditional deletion of GATA3 before the onset of puberty and continuously thereafter (MMTV-Cre; *Gata3* $^{f/f}$), TEBs fail to develop punctually and the ductal epithelia does not invade the fat pad. At 8 weeks of age, a few TEBs are observed but these are unable to invade the fat pad. Additionally, the ducts that are present show a myriad of defects including structural defects and irregular ductal epithelia. Due to clonal expansion of GATA3-positive cells, the authors generated an acute, drug inducible *Gata3* model wherein the rtTA-cre is driven by the whey acidic protein (WAP) promoter (WAP-rtTA-Cre; *Gata3* $^{f/f}$). These mice were administered doxycycline at 12 weeks of age and the drug was given for 14 days. By the fifth day of drug administration, defects in luminal epithelia were observed, reminiscent of those observed in the MMTV-Cre; *Gata3* $^{f/f}$ model. Importantly, in the GATA3-deficient glands, luminal epithelia cells lost markers of differentiation and proliferated at a higher rate. Longer term deficiency led to cell death and defective lactation [63]. A second study also reports similar phenotypes for GATA3 loss in the pre-pubertal gland. Two additional models are included in this study, a model of GATA3 deficiency in the mammary primordia (keratin14-Cre; *Gata3* $^{f/f}$), and one that causes loss GATA3 during gestation (WAP-Cre; *Gata3* $^{f/f}$). Embryonic loss of GATA3 in the mammary primordia results in absent mammary placodes (one or more) and ablation of *Lef1* expression in the expected areas of placode formation, though any placodes formed in the mutant animals also expressed *Lef1*. Loss of GATA3 during gestation results in defective lobuloalveolar development and lactation [64]. These studies have indicated a clear role for GATA3 in formation of the mammary placodes in the embryo, ductal morphogenesis, maintenance of luminal cell differentiation in mature glands, pregnancy-stimulated lobuloalveolar development, and lactation. Based on these studies, the importance of the Th2 producing signaling pathway is important for mammary development, and adds more complexity to the tightly regulated PRL and P4 cell signaling that has been previously characterized.

PRL and Jak/Stat Signaling

PRL is a small peptide hormone produced primarily in the anterior pituitary, but may also be produced in other peripheral tissues. PRL historically has been characterized as a factor necessary for pregnancy-induced mammary alveolar development and lactation, for historical references see Ref. [65]. PRL binds to the PRLR to initiate Jak/Stat signaling. PRLR dimerization causes activation of Jak2. Jak2 phosphorylates three target STATs depending on the stage of mammary gland development: STAT1, STAT3 and STAT5. Canonically, phosphorylated STAT forms dimers and then translocates to the nucleus. Dimers bind conserved, palindromic sequences (TTCNNNGAA) termed γ-interferon activation sites (GAS), in gene promoter/regulatory regions to regulate the initiation of target gene activity.

PRL knockout mice (*Prl*$^{-/-}$) are viable, but females are infertile and mammary gland development is defective, manifesting with a fully developed ductal tree devoid of lobuloalveolar units. Since the females are infertile, stages beyond the mature virgin gland were not analyzed [66]. PRLR knockout mice fail to lactate and the glands appear poorly developed with few branches at maturity. Interestingly, multiparous females that are hemizygous for the PRLR knockout allele (*Prlr*$^{+/-}$) regain mammary function, indicating a response to repeated hormone stimulation [67, 68]. The next component in the cascade, Jak2, also has pleiotropic roles in both embryonic and post-natal development.

Since the traditional *Jak2* knockout mice (*Jak2* $^{-/-}$) die during embryogenesis due to defective hematopoiesis leading to severe anemia, a conditional knockout approach to study *Jak2* in the post-pubertal mammary gland was warranted [69, 70]. Wagner and colleagues developed a conditional deletion Jak2 model (*Jak2*$^{f/f}$), and using two Cre transgenic strains (MMTV-Cre and WAP-Cre) showed that JAK2 signaling is necessary for both development of alveolar progenitor cells in mature virgin glands, as well as maintenance and survival of the secretory epithelium in pregnant mice [71]. These functions are non-redundant and data indicates that STAT5 is activated only in a JAK2-dependent fashion.

The transcription factor STAT5 is produced by both *Stat5a* and *Stat5b*, two highly related genes derived from a recent gene duplication event [72]. In mammary tissue, *Stat5a* is the more abundant and is responsible for 70% of STAT5 present [73]. During late pregnancy and lactation, phosphorylated STAT5 increases precipitously, most likely due to its activation of β-casein and WAP, genes that increase dramatically in preparation for lactation. Knockout studies have revealed independent and overlapping roles of *Stat5a* and *Stat5b*. Mammary glands from Stat5a knockout females (*Stat5a* $^{-/-}$) fail to develop characteristic lobuloalveolar structure and exhibit a complete lactation failure during the first pregnancy [74]. It is important to note that even though *Stat5a* and *Stat5b* share 96% similarity, *Stat5b* does not compensate, indicating either an independent function or independent regulation [73]. After multiple rounds of pregnancy, lactation phase is sustained, which may be attributed to a late compensatory increase in *Stat5b* [75]. *Stat5b* knockout mice are viable and fertile, the mammary glands appear normal, and the primary reported defects are ablation of sexually dimorphic growth differences and liver-specific gene expression [76]. *Stat5a/b* double knockout mice are infertile due ovarian dysfunction, specifically defective corpus luteum formation. Owing to the aforementioned infertility phenotype, Teglund et al.

were unable to study the effects on mammary gland development but were able to conclude that either individually or cooperatively *Stat5a* and *Stat5b* mediate essentially all PRL and growth hormone dependent development [77]. In effort to investigate *Stat5a/b* null mammary development, *Stat5a/b* null glands were transplanted into wild-type recipients. These glands developed a ductal tree but did not undergo alveolar morphogenesis, indicating that STAT5 is necessary for the proliferation and differentiation of mammary alveoli [78].

The role of STAT3 in the mammary gland is best characterized as a harbinger of death, as phosphorylated STAT3 increases dramatically at the onset of involution (within 12 hours) and precedes the wave of post lactation apoptosis and alveolar collapse [79, 80]. The involution-associated cell death is dependent only on local factors such as mechanical stress due to milk stasis [80]. STAT3 activation is dependent on several secreted factors, namely leukemia inhibitory factor (LIF) [81, 82], serotonin [83] and TGF-β3 [84]. *Stat3* null animals die during early embryogenesis (E7.5), with the lethality attributed to a defect in visceral endoderm function [85]. Conditional deletion of *Stat3* in the mammary gland, driven by either WAP-Cre or β-lactoglobulin-Cre (BLG-Cre), both result in delayed involution and an extension of the reversible phase [86, 87].

Of late, the mechanism of cell death during early involution is being revisited due to the observed delay in TUNEL positivity of shed cells, and cell morphology that does not align with classical apoptotic condensation, fragmentation, and membrane blebbing. Recent work from the lab of Christine Watson suggests that the cell death is a STAT3-driven, cathepsin-dependent and executioner caspase-independent, lysosomal-mediated programmed cells death [88, 89]. This study necessitates re-evaluation of foundational literature and warrants further and more directed attention.

The level of STAT1 remains constant throughout the pregnancy cycle; however, active STAT1 is detected in the virgin gland and in the late involution gland. This pattern of pSTAT1 is a unique amongst STATs and the inverse of the pSTAT5 profile [80, 87]. No clear role has been defined for Stat1 in mammary development, and *Stat1* $^{-/-}$ mice are viable showing no overt developmental or mammary gland defects [90].

Cell Death Signaling

It is currently thought that of the cells that die during involution, the vast majority die by an apoptotic pathway. Apoptosis is a highly regulated, well described process wherein a cascade of intracellular signaling is initiated in response to an extrinsic or intrinsic signal. It is thought that a balance of pro-apoptotic and anti-apoptotic factors determines cell fate. The Bcl-2 protein family namesake, anti-apoptotic *Bcl-2,* is not expressed during lactation or early involution, but its expression increases in late (>10 days) involution. Based on this expression profile it is not surprising that *Bcl-2* knockout mice do not exhibit a gross mammary defect. Global ablation of *Bcl-2 (Bcl-2* $^{-/-}$) is not lethal, resulting in small, hypopigmented mice with polycystic kidney disease [91]. Overexpression of *Bcl-2* driven by the WAP promoter results in a delayed involution [92]. Studies have revealed that *Bcl-x* is expressed at higher levels than *Bcl-2* in many tissues during development and in the adult, including the mammary gland [93, 94]. The traditional knockout (*Bcl-x* $^{-/-}$) is not viable and dies embryonically due to excessive apoptosis of immature erythroid cells in the fetal liver [95].This model provided valuable information regarding the role of *Bcl-x* during development, but the embryonic lethality was prohibitive to study the role of *Bcl-x* in mature tissues. As a result two conditional, mammary specific *Bcl-x* knockout mouse models (WAP-Cre; *Bcl-x* $^{f/f}$, MMTV-Cre; *Bcl-x* $^{f/f}$) were generated. *Bcl-x* deficient mammary epithelia tissue exhibited an accelerated involution, a phenotype characterized by an increase in apoptosis, indicating that *Bcl-x* is necessary for cell survival during early involution [96].

Pro-apoptotic factors include Bcl-2 family members *Bax*, *Bad*, and *Bak* among others. *Bax* mRNA is highest at the lactation to involution transition and three splicing products are produced, however the protein level is unchanged [97]. *Bax* deficient mice intuitively exhibit hyperplasia in some cell lineages (B cells, thymocytes); however, counterintuitively males are infertile due to the absence of mature sperm and abnormal mammary development has also been reported [98, 99]. Loss of *Bax* delays involution, while overexpression of BAX in the mammary secretory epithelia in a WAP-Bax model results in a lactation defect as well as forced involution based on an increase in apoptotic cells and precocious *Stat3* activation [97, 100]. *Bak* and *Bad* are present throughout pregnancy and remain expressed highly through involution. It is hypothesized that the mammary gland is persistently poised to trigger involution and it is the balance of pro-apoptotic and anti-apoptotic factors determines lactation to involution transition [97, 101].

The nature of cell death signaling that occurs throughout the developmental cycle of the mature mammary gland is complex. In many cases canonical functions of proteins are observed, but many surprising roles have been elucidated using transgenic technologies.

Conclusion

The mammary gland is a dynamic organ that is reliant upon hormones, growth factors, and epithelial-stromal interactions to regulate well-established cell signaling pathways that orchestrate highly regulated developmental programs.

These events span from mid-gestation into adolescence and through adulthood, when terminal differentiation occurs within a cyclical pattern of growth and regression that is linked to reproduction. Due to the accessory nature of the gland, ease of accessibility, and transplantation potential, the mammary gland is a powerful model to characterize the genetics behind organ development and cell differentiation. In addition to its relevance in modeling normal development, the mammary gland is also essential in profiling breast cancer, neonate immunity, ageing and stem-cell based regeneration. The blossoming of mouse transgenic technologies over the past twenty years has led to breakthroughs in the understanding of the underlying mechanisms controlling mammary gland development. The early endocrine ablation studies that revealed the pituitary and ovarian control of mammary gland development eventually led to genetics-based approaches to further characterize these processes.

Genetic engineering has advanced from gain-of-function studies to knockout strategies, giving way to the current state of conditional (Cre/LoxP, Flp/FRT) and inducible (tet-on, tet-off) models. This increased specificity for inducing mutations has allowed researchers to investigate gene and signaling pathway contributions at restricted developmental stages. Although the genetic tools will continue to expand and increase the array if potential applications, technology is but a tool to address the basic biological questions that remain in the field. What is the nature of the crosstalk between the hormonal receptors? Which, if any, of the other immune cell lineage pathways are relevant for mammary cell lineage commitment? What are the specific regulatory mechanisms at work regulating the upregulation of target genes controlled by multiple transcription factors? How do microRNAs regulate the developmental program of the mammary gland? How do apoptosis and autophagy interact to promote regression during involution? How does the methylation state of DNA and histones impact development? These questions and many others will continue to propel this field in the coming years.

References

[1] Oftedal, OT, The mammary gland and its origin during synapsid evolution, *J Mammary Gland Biol Neoplasia*, 7 (2002) 225-252.

[2] Veltmaat, JM, Van Veelen, W, Thiery, JP, Bellusci, S, Identification of the mammary line in mouse by Wnt10b expression, *Dev Dyn*, 229 (2004) 349-356.

[3] Vangenderen, C, Okamura, RM, Farinas, I, Quo, RG, Parslow, TG, Bruhn, L, Grosschedl, R, Development of Several Organs That Require Inductive Epithelial-Mesenchymal Interactions Is Impaired in Lef-1-Deficient Mice, *Genes & Development*, 8 (1994) 2691-2703.

[4] Chu, EY, Hens, J, Andl, T, Kairo, A, Yamaguchi, TP, Brisken, C, Glick, A, Wysolmerski, JJ, Millar, SE, Canonical WNT signaling promotes mammary placode development and is essential for initiation of mammary gland morphogenesis, *Development*, 131 (2004) 4819-4829.

[5] Mailleux, AA, Spencer-Dene, B, Dillon, C, Ndiaye, D, Savona-Baron, C, Itoh, N, Kato, S, Dickson, C, Thiery, JP, Bellusci, S, Role of FGF10/FGFR2b signaling during mammary gland development in the mouse embryo, *Development*, 129 (2002) 53-60.

[6] Watson, CJ, Khaled, WT, Mammary development in the embryo and adult: a journey of morphogenesis and commitment, *Development*, 135 (2008) 995-1003.

[7] Robinson, GW, Cooperation of signalling pathways in embryonic mammary gland development, *Nat Rev Genet*, 8 (2007) 963-972.

[8] Humphreys, RC, Krajewska, M, Krnacik, S, Jaeger, R, Weiher, H, Krajewski, S, Reed, JC, Rosen, JM, Apoptosis in the terminal endbud of the murine mammary gland: a mechanism of ductal morphogenesis, *Development*, 122 (1996) 4013-4022.

[9] Kleinberg, DL, Feldman, M, Ruan, W, IGF-I: an essential factor in terminal end bud formation and ductal morphogenesis, *J Mammary Gland Biol Neoplasia*, 5 (2000) 7-17.

[10] Ball, SM, The development of the terminal end bud in the prepubertal-pubertal mouse mammary gland, *Anat Rec*, 250 (1998) 459-464.

[11] Richert, MM, Schwertfeger, KL, Ryder, JW, Anderson, SM, An atlas of mouse mammary gland development, *J Mammary Gland Biol Neoplasia*, 5 (2000) 227-241.

[12] Rudolph, MC, McManaman, JL, Hunter, L, Phang, T, Neville, MC, Functional development of the mammary gland: use of expression

profiling and trajectory clustering to reveal changes in gene expression during pregnancy, lactation, and involution, *J Mammary Gland Biol Neoplasia*, 8 (2003) 287-307.

[13] Stein, T, Morris, JS, Davies, CR, Weber-Hall, SJ, Duffy, MA, Heath, VJ, Bell, AK, Ferrier, RK, Sandilands, GP, Gusterson, BA, Involution of the mouse mammary gland is associated with an immune cascade and an acute-phase response, involving LBP, CD14 and STAT3, *Breast Cancer Res*, 6 (2004) R75-91.

[14] Clarkson, RW, Wayland, MT, Lee, J, Freeman, T, Watson, CJ, Gene expression profiling of mammary gland development reveals putative roles for death receptors and immune mediators in post-lactational regression, *Breast Cancer Res*, 6 (2004) R92-109.

[15] Watson, CJ, Involution: apoptosis and tissue remodelling that convert the mammary gland from milk factory to a quiescent organ, *Breast Cancer Res*, 8 (2006) 203.

[16] Radisky, DC, Hartmann, LC, Mammary involution and breast cancer risk: transgenic models and clinical studies, *J Mammary Gland Biol Neoplasia*, 14 (2009) 181-191.

[17] Zarzynska, J, Motyl, T, Apoptosis and autophagy in involuting bovine mammary gland, *J Physiol Pharmacol*, 59 Suppl 9 (2008) 275-288.

[18] Motyl, T, Gajkowska, B, Zarzynska, J, Gajewska, M, Lamparska-Przybysz, M, Apoptosis and autophagy in mammary gland remodeling and breast cancer chemotherapy, *J Physiol Pharmacol*, 57 Suppl 7 (2006) 17-32.

[19] Gajewska, M, Sobolewska, A, Kozlowski, M, Motyl, T, Role of autophagy in mammary gland development, *J Physiol Pharmacol*, 59 Suppl 9 (2008) 237-249.

[20] Shimeld, SM, McKay, IJ, Sharpe, PT, The murine homeobox gene Msx-3 shows highly restricted expression in the developing neural tube, *Mech Dev*, 55 (1996) 201-210.

[21] Satoh, K, Ginsburg, E, Vonderhaar, BK, Msx-1 and Msx-2 in mammary gland development, *J Mammary Gland Biol Neoplasia*, 9 (2004) 195-205.

[22] Satokata, I, Ma, L, Ohshima, H, Bei, M, Woo, I, Nishizawa, K, Maeda, T, Takano, Y, Uchiyama, M, Heaney, S, Peters, H, Tang, Z, Maxson, R, Maas, R, Msx2 deficiency in mice causes pleiotropic defects in bone growth and ectodermal organ formation, *Nat Genet*, 24 (2000) 391-395.

[23] Satokata, I, Maas, R, Msx1 deficient mice exhibit cleft palate and abnormalities of craniofacial and tooth development, *Nat Genet*, 6 (1994) 348-356.
[24] Hu, G, Lee, H, Price, SM, Shen, MM, Abate-Shen, C, Msx homeobox genes inhibit differentiation through upregulation of cyclin D1, *Development*, 128 (2001) 2373-2384.
[25] Phippard, DJ, Weber-Hall, SJ, Sharpe, PT, Naylor, MS, Jayatalake, H, Maas, R, Woo, I, Roberts-Clark, D, Francis-West, PH, Liu, YH, Maxson, R, Hill, RE, Dale, TC, Regulation of Msx-1, Msx-2, Bmp-2 and Bmp-4 during foetal and postnatal mammary gland development, *Development*, 122 (1996) 2729-2737.
[26] Lubahn, DB, Moyer, JS, Golding, TS, Couse, JF, Korach, KS, Smithies, O, Alteration of reproductive function but not prenatal sexual development after insertional disruption of the mouse estrogen receptor gene, *Proc Natl Acad Sci U S A*, 90 (1993) 11162-11166.
[27] Krege, JH, Hodgin, JB, Couse, JF, Enmark, E, Warner, M, Mahler, JF, Sar, M, Korach, KS, Gustafsson, JA, Smithies, O, Generation and reproductive phenotypes of mice lacking estrogen receptor beta, *Proc Natl Acad Sci U S A*, 95 (1998) 15677-15682.
[28] Dupont, S, Krust, A, Gansmuller, A, Dierich, A, Chambon, P, Mark, M, Effect of single and compound knockouts of estrogen receptors alpha (ERalpha) and beta (ERbeta) on mouse reproductive phenotypes, *Development*, 127 (2000) 4277-4291.
[29] Bocchinfuso, WP, Korach, KS, Mammary gland development and tumorigenesis in estrogen receptor knockout mice, *J Mammary Gland Biol Neoplasia*, 2 (1997) 323-334.
[30] Mallepell, S, Krust, A, Chambon, P, Brisken, C, Paracrine signaling through the epithelial estrogen receptor alpha is required for proliferation and morphogenesis in the mammary gland, *Proc Natl Acad Sci U S A*, 103 (2006) 2196-2201.
[31] Walker, VR, Korach, KS, Estrogen receptor knockout mice as a model for endocrine research, *ILAR J*, 45 (2004) 455-461.
[32] Antonson, P, Omoto, Y, Humire, P, Gustafsson, JA, Generation of ERalpha-floxed and knockout mice using the Cre/LoxP system, *Biochem Biophys Res Commun*, 424 (2012) 710-716.
[33] Antal, MC, Krust, A, Chambon, P, Mark, M, Sterility and absence of histopathological defects in nonreproductive organs of a mouse ERbeta-null mutant, *Proc Natl Acad Sci U S A*, 105 (2008) 2433-2438.

[34] Hruska, KS, Tilli, MT, Ren, S, Cotarla, I, Kwong, T, Li, M, Fondell, JD, Hewitt, JA, Koos, RD, Furth, PA, Flaws, JA, Conditional over-expression of estrogen receptor alpha in a transgenic mouse model, *Transgenic Res*, 11 (2002) 361-372.

[35] Schrader, WT, O'Malley, BW, Progesterone-binding components of chick oviduct. IV. Characterization of purified subunits, *J Biol Chem*, 247 (1972) 51-59.

[36] Conneely, OM, Sullivan, WP, Toft, DO, Birnbaumer, M, Cook, RG, Maxwell, BL, Zarucki-Schulz, T, Greene, GL, Schrader, WT, O'Malley, BW, Molecular cloning of the chicken progesterone receptor, *Science*, 233 (1986) 767-770.

[37] Jeltsch, JM, Krozowski, Z, Quirin-Stricker, C, Gronemeyer, H, Simpson, RJ, Garnier, JM, Krust, A, Jacob, F, Chambon, P, Cloning of the chicken progesterone receptor, *Proc Natl Acad Sci U S A*, 83 (1986) 5424-5428.

[38] Lydon, JP, DeMayo, FJ, Funk, CR, Mani, SK, Hughes, AR, Montgomery, CA, Jr., Shyamala, G, Conneely, OM, O'Malley, BW, Mice lacking progesterone receptor exhibit pleiotropic reproductive abnormalities, *Genes Dev*, 9 (1995) 2266-2278.

[39] Brisken, C, Park, S, Vass, T, Lydon, JP, O'Malley, BW, Weinberg, RA, A paracrine role for the epithelial progesterone receptor in mammary gland development, *Proc Natl Acad Sci U S A*, 95 (1998) 5076-5081.

[40] Conneely, OM, Mulac-Jericevic, B, Lydon, JP, Progesterone-dependent regulation of female reproductive activity by two distinct progesterone receptor isoforms, *Steroids*, 68 (2003) 771-778.

[41] Ismail, PM, Amato, P, Soyal, SM, DeMayo, FJ, Conneely, OM, O'Malley, BW, Lydon, JP, Progesterone involvement in breast development and tumorigenesis--as revealed by progesterone receptor "knockout" and "knockin" mouse models, *Steroids*, 68 (2003) 779-787.

[42] Soyal, S, Ismail, PM, Li, J, Mulac-Jericevic, B, Conneely, OM, Lydon, JP, Progesterone's role in mammary gland development and tumorigenesis as disclosed by experimental mouse genetics, *Breast Cancer Res*, 4 (2002) 191-196.

[43] Ismail, PM, Li, J, DeMayo, FJ, O'Malley, BW, Lydon, JP, A novel LacZ reporter mouse reveals complex regulation of the progesterone receptor promoter during mammary gland development, *Mol Endocrinol*, 16 (2002) 2475-2489.

[44] Seagroves, TN, Lydon, JP, Hovey, RC, Vonderhaar, BK, Rosen, JM, C/EBPbeta (CCAAT/enhancer binding protein) controls cell fate

determination during mammary gland development, *Mol Endocrinol*, 14 (2000) 359-368.

[45] Mulac-Jericevic, B, Mullinax, RA, DeMayo, FJ, Lydon, JP, Conneely, OM, Subgroup of reproductive functions of progesterone mediated by progesterone receptor-B isoform, *Science*, 289 (2000) 1751-1754.

[46] Mulac-Jericevic, B, Lydon, JP, DeMayo, FJ, Conneely, OM, Defective mammary gland morphogenesis in mice lacking the progesterone receptor B isoform, *Proc Natl Acad Sci U S A*, 100 (2003) 9744-9749.

[47] Fernandez-Valdivia, R, Jeong, J, Mukherjee, A, Soyal, SM, Li, J, Ying, Y, Demayo, FJ, Lydon, JP, A mouse model to dissect progesterone signaling in the female reproductive tract and mammary gland, *Genesis*, 48 (2010) 106-113.

[48] Hashimoto-Partyka, MK, Lydon, JP, Iruela-Arispe, ML, Generation of a mouse for conditional excision of progesterone receptor, *Genesis*, 44 (2006) 391-395.

[49] Mukherjee, A, Soyal, SM, Fernandez-Valdivia, R, DeMayo, FJ, Lydon, JP, Targeting reverse tetracycline-dependent transactivator to murine mammary epithelial cells that express the progesterone receptor, *Genesis*, 45 (2007) 639-646.

[50] Mukherjee, A, Soyal, SM, Li, J, Ying, Y, He, B, DeMayo, FJ, Lydon, JP, Targeting RANKL to a specific subset of murine mammary epithelial cells induces ordered branching morphogenesis and alveologenesis in the absence of progesterone receptor expression, *FASEB J*, 24 (2010) 4408-4419.

[51] Fata, JE, Kong, YY, Li, J, Sasaki, T, Irie-Sasaki, J, Moorehead, RA, Elliott, R, Scully, S, Voura, EB, Lacey, DL, Boyle, WJ, Khokha, R, Penninger, JM, The osteoclast differentiation factor osteoprotegerin-ligand is essential for mammary gland development, *Cell*, 103 (2000) 41-50.

[52] Cao, Y, Bonizzi, G, Seagroves, TN, Greten, FR, Johnson, R, Schmidt, EV, Karin, M, IKKalpha provides an essential link between RANK signaling and cyclin D1 expression during mammary gland development, *Cell*, 107 (2001) 763-775.

[53] Fantl, V, Stamp, G, Andrews, A, Rosewell, I, Dickson, C, Mice lacking cyclin D1 are small and show defects in eye and mammary gland development, *Genes Dev*, 9 (1995) 2364-2372.

[54] Srivastava, S, Matsuda, M, Hou, Z, Bailey, JP, Kitazawa, R, Herbst, MP, Horseman, ND, Receptor activator of NF-kappaB ligand induction via

Jak2 and Stat5a in mammary epithelial cells, *J Biol Chem*, 278 (2003) 46171-46178.

[55] Lee, HJ, Ormandy, CJ, Interplay between progesterone and prolactin in mammary development and implications for breast cancer, *Mol Cell Endocrinol*, 357 (2012) 101-107.

[56] Grimm, SL, Rosen, JM, The role of C/EBPbeta in mammary gland development and breast cancer, *J Mammary Gland Biol Neoplasia*, 8 (2003) 191-204.

[57] Seagroves, TN, Krnacik, S, Raught, B, Gay, J, Burgess-Beusse, B, Darlington, GJ, Rosen, JM, C/EBPbeta, but not C/EBPalpha, is essential for ductal morphogenesis, lobuloalveolar proliferation, and functional differentiation in the mouse mammary gland, *Genes Dev*, 12 (1998) 1917-1928.

[58] Robinson, GW, Johnson, PF, Hennighausen, L, Sterneck, E, The C/EBPbeta transcription factor regulates epithelial cell proliferation and differentiation in the mammary gland, *Genes Dev*, 12 (1998) 1907-1916.

[59] Gigliotti, AP, DeWille, JW, Lactation status influences expression of CCAAT/enhancer binding protein isoform mRNA in the mouse mammary gland, *J Cell Physiol*, 174 (1998) 232-239.

[60] Thangaraju, M, Rudelius, M, Bierie, B, Raffeld, M, Sharan, S, Hennighausen, L, Huang, AM, Sterneck, E, C/EBPdelta is a crucial regulator of pro-apoptotic gene expression during mammary gland involution, *Development*, 132 (2005) 4675-4685.

[61] Maier, E, Duschl, A, Horejs-Hoeck, J, STAT6-dependent and -independent mechanisms in Th2 polarization, *Eur J Immunol*, 42 (2012) 2827-2833.

[62] Khaled, WT, Read, EK, Nicholson, SE, Baxter, FO, Brennan, AJ, Came, PJ, Sprigg, N, McKenzie, AN, Watson, CJ, The IL-4/IL-13/Stat6 signalling pathway promotes luminal mammary epithelial cell development, *Development*, 134 (2007) 2739-2750.

[63] Kouros-Mehr, H, Slorach, EM, Sternlicht, MD, Werb, Z, GATA-3 maintains the differentiation of the luminal cell fate in the mammary gland, *Cell*, 127 (2006) 1041-1055.

[64] Asselin-Labat, ML, Sutherland, KD, Barker, H, Thomas, R, Shackleton, M, Forrest, NC, Hartley, L, Robb, L, Grosveld, FG, van der Wees, J, Lindeman, GJ, Visvader, JE, Gata-3 is an essential regulator of mammary-gland morphogenesis and luminal-cell differentiation, *Nat Cell Biol*, 9 (2007) 201-209.

[65] Hennighausen, L, Robinson, GW, Signaling pathways in mammary gland development, *Developmental Cell*, 1 (2001) 467-475.

[66] Horseman, ND, Zhao, W, Montecino-Rodriguez, E, Tanaka, M, Nakashima, K, Engle, SJ, Smith, F, Markoff, E, Dorshkind, K, Defective mammopoiesis, but normal hematopoiesis, in mice with a targeted disruption of the prolactin gene, *EMBO J*, 16 (1997) 6926-6935.

[67] Ormandy, CJ, Camus, A, Barra, J, Damotte, D, Lucas, B, Buteau, H, Edery, M, Brousse, N, Babinet, C, Binart, N, Kelly, PA, Null mutation of the prolactin receptor gene produces multiple reproductive defects in the mouse, *Genes Dev*, 11 (1997) 167-178.

[68] Ormandy, CJ, Binart, N, Kelly, PA, Mammary gland development in prolactin receptor knockout mice, *J Mammary Gland Biol Neoplasia*, 2 (1997) 355-364.

[69] Neubauer, H, Cumano, A, Muller, M, Wu, H, Huffstadt, U, Pfeffer, K, Jak2 deficiency defines an essential developmental checkpoint in definitive hematopoiesis, *Cell*, 93 (1998) 397-409.

[70] Parganas, E, Wang, D, Stravopodis, D, Topham, DJ, Marine, JC, Teglund, S, Vanin, EF, Bodner, S, Colamonici, OR, van Deursen, JM, Grosveld, G, Ihle, JN, Jak2 is essential for signaling through a variety of cytokine receptors, *Cell*, 93 (1998) 385-395.

[71] Wagner, KU, Krempler, A, Triplett, AA, Qi, Y, George, NM, Zhu, J, Rui, H, Impaired alveologenesis and maintenance of secretory mammary epithelial cells in Jak2 conditional knockout mice, *Mol Cell Biol*, 24 (2004) 5510-5520.

[72] Miyoshi, K, Cui, Y, Riedlinger, G, Robinson, P, Lehoczky, J, Zon, L, Oka, T, Dewar, K, Hennighausen, L, Structure of the mouse Stat 3/5 locus: evolution from Drosophila to zebrafish to mouse, *Genomics*, 71 (2001) 150-155.

[73] Liu, X, Robinson, GW, Gouilleux, F, Groner, B, Hennighausen, L, Cloning and expression of Stat5 and an additional homologue (Stat5b) involved in prolactin signal transduction in mouse mammary tissue, *Proc Natl Acad Sci U S A*, 92 (1995) 8831-8835.

[74] Liu, X, Robinson, GW, Wagner, KU, Garrett, L, Wynshaw-Boris, A, Hennighausen, L, Stat5a is mandatory for adult mammary gland development and lactogenesis, *Genes Dev*, 11 (1997) 179-186.

[75] Liu, X, Gallego, MI, Smith, GH, Robinson, GW, Hennighausen, L, Functional rescue of Stat5a-null mammary tissue through the activation of compensating signals including Stat5b, *Cell Growth Differ*, 9 (1998) 795-803.

[76] Udy, GB, Towers, RP, Snell, RG, Wilkins, RJ, Park, SH, Ram, PA, Waxman, DJ, Davey, HW, Requirement of STAT5b for sexual dimorphism of body growth rates and liver gene expression, *Proc Natl Acad Sci U S A*, 94 (1997) 7239-7244.

[77] Teglund, S, McKay, C, Schuetz, E, van Deursen, JM, Stravopodis, D, Wang, D, Brown, M, Bodner, S, Grosveld, G, Ihle, JN, Stat5a and Stat5b proteins have essential and nonessential, or redundant, roles in cytokine responses, *Cell*, 93 (1998) 841-850.

[78] Miyoshi, K, Shillingford, JM, Smith, GH, Grimm, SL, Wagner, KU, Oka, T, Rosen, JM, Robinson, GW, Hennighausen, L, Signal transducer and activator of transcription (Stat) 5 controls the proliferation and differentiation of mammary alveolar epithelium, *Journal of Cell Biology*, 155 (2001) 531-542.

[79] Liu, X, Robinson, GW, Hennighausen, L, Activation of Stat5a and Stat5b by tyrosine phosphorylation is tightly linked to mammary gland differentiation, *Mol Endocrinol*, 10 (1996) 1496-1506.

[80] Li, M, Liu, X, Robinson, G, Bar-Peled, U, Wagner, KU, Young, WS, Hennighausen, L, Furth, PA, Mammary-derived signals activate programmed cell death during the first stage of mammary gland involution, *Proc Natl Acad Sci U S A*, 94 (1997) 3425-3430.

[81] Kritikou, EA, Sharkey, A, Abell, K, Came, PJ, Anderson, E, Clarkson, RW, Watson, CJ, A dual, non-redundant, role for LIF as a regulator of development and STAT3-mediated cell death in mammary gland, *Development*, 130 (2003) 3459-3468.

[82] Schere-Levy, C, Buggiano, V, Quaglino, A, Gattelli, A, Cirio, MC, Piazzon, I, Vanzulli, S, Kordon, EC, Leukemia inhibitory factor induces apoptosis of the mammary epithelial cells and participates in mouse mammary gland involution, *Exp Cell Res*, 282 (2003) 35-47.

[83] Matsuda, M, Imaoka, T, Vomachka, AJ, Gudelsky, GA, Hou, ZY, Mistry, M, Bailey, JP, Nieport, KM, Walther, DJ, Bader, M, Horseman, ND, Serotonin regulates mammary gland development via an autocrine-paracrine loop, *Developmental Cell*, 6 (2004) 193-203.

[84] Nguyen, AV, Pollard, JW, Transforming growth factor beta3 induces cell death during the first stage of mammary gland involution, *Development*, 127 (2000) 3107-3118.

[85] Takeda, K, Noguchi, K, Shi, W, Tanaka, T, Matsumoto, M, Yoshida, N, Kishimoto, T, Akira, S, Targeted disruption of the mouse Stat3 gene leads to early embryonic lethality, *Proc Natl Acad Sci U S A*, 94 (1997) 3801-3804.

[86] Humphreys, RC, Bierie, B, Zhao, L, Raz, R, Levy, D, Hennighausen, L, Deletion of Stat3 blocks mammary gland involution and extends functional competence of the secretory epithelium in the absence of lactogenic stimuli, *Endocrinology*, 143 (2002) 3641-3650.

[87] Chapman, RS, Lourenco, PC, Tonner, E, Flint, DJ, Selbert, S, Takeda, K, Akira, S, Clarke, AR, Watson, CJ, Suppression of epithelial apoptosis and delayed mammary gland involution in mice with a conditional knockout of Stat3, *Genes Dev*, 13 (1999) 2604-2616.

[88] Kreuzaler, PA, Staniszewska, AD, Li, W, Omidvar, N, Kedjouar, B, Turkson, J, Poli, V, Flavell, RA, Clarkson, RW, Watson, CJ, Stat3 controls lysosomal-mediated cell death in vivo, *Nat Cell Biol*, 13 (2011) 303-309.

[89] Watson, CJ, Kreuzaler, PA, Remodeling mechanisms of the mammary gland during involution, *Int J Dev Biol*, 55 (2011) 757-762.

[90] Meraz, MA, White, JM, Sheehan, KC, Bach, EA, Rodig, SJ, Dighe, AS, Kaplan, DH, Riley, JK, Greenlund, AC, Campbell, D, Carver-Moore, K, DuBois, RN, Clark, R, Aguet, M, Schreiber, RD, Targeted disruption of the Stat1 gene in mice reveals unexpected physiologic specificity in the JAK-STAT signaling pathway, *Cell*, 84 (1996) 431-442.

[91] Veis, DJ, Sorenson, CM, Shutter, JR, Korsmeyer, SJ, Bcl-2-deficient mice demonstrate fulminant lymphoid apoptosis, polycystic kidneys, and hypopigmented hair, *Cell*, 75 (1993) 229-240.

[92] Jäger R, Herzer U, Schenkel J, Weiher H, Overexpression of Bcl-2 inhibits alveolar cell apoptosis during involution and accelerates c-myc-induced tumorigenesis of the mammary gland in transgenic mice, *Oncogene*, 15 (1997) 1787-1795.

[93] Gonzalez-Garcia, M, Perez-Ballestero, R, Ding, L, Duan, L, Boise, LH, Thompson, CB, Nunez, G, bcl-XL is the major bcl-x mRNA form expressed during murine development and its product localizes to mitochondria, *Development*, 120 (1994) 3033-3042.

[94] Krajewski, S, Krajewska, M, Shabaik, A, Wang, HG, Irie, S, Fong, L, Reed, JC, Immunohistochemical analysis of in vivo patterns of Bcl-X expression, *Cancer Res*, 54 (1994) 5501-5507.

[95] Motoyama, N, Wang, F, Roth, KA, Sawa, H, Nakayama, K, Negishi, I, Senju, S, Zhang, Q, Fujii, S, et al., Massive cell death of immature hematopoietic cells and neurons in Bcl-x-deficient mice, *Science*, 267 (1995) 1506-1510.

[96] Walton, KD, Wagner, KU, Rucker, EB, 3rd, Shillingford, JM, Miyoshi, K, Hennighausen, L, Conditional deletion of the bcl-x gene from mouse

mammary epithelium results in accelerated apoptosis during involution but does not compromise cell function during lactation, *Mech Dev*, 109 (2001) 281-293.

[97] Schorr, K, Li, M, Krajewski, S, Reed, JC, Furth, PA, Bcl-2 gene family and related proteins in mammary gland involution and breast cancer, *J Mammary Gland Biol Neoplasia*, 4 (1999) 153-164.

[98] Knudson, CM, Tung, KS, Tourtellotte, WG, Brown, GA, Korsmeyer, SJ, Bax-deficient mice with lymphoid hyperplasia and male germ cell death, *Science*, 270 (1995) 96-99.

[99] Heermeier, K, Benedict, M, Li, M, Furth, P, Nunez, G, Hennighausen, L, Bax and Bcl-xs are induced at the onset of apoptosis in involuting mammary epithelial cells, *Mech Dev*, 56 (1996) 197-207.

[100] Rucker, EB, 3rd, Hale, AN, Durtschi, DC, Sakamoto, K, Wagner, KU, Forced involution of the functionally differentiated mammary gland by overexpression of the pro-apoptotic protein bax, *Genesis*, 49 (2011) 24-35.

[101] Schorr, K, Li, M, Bar-Peled, U, Lewis, A, Heredia, A, Lewis, B, Knudson, CM, Korsmeyer, SJ, Jager, R, Weiher, H, Furth, PA, Gain of Bcl-2 is more potent than bax loss in regulating mammary epithelial cell survival in vivo, *Cancer Res*, 59 (1999) 2541-2545.

In: Mammary Glands
Editor: Edmund B. Rucker
ISBN: 978-1-62948-853-0

Chapter II

Mammary Gland Micro-Environment: From Stem Cells to Functional Mammary Glands

Hai-Jun Huang**, *Xia Peng, Li Zhou, Shun Lu, Min Xiang, Yun-Guo Qian, Qi-Shuang Gao and Si-Wen Jiang

Department of Animal Biotechnology and Cell Engineering,
Wuhan Institute of Animal and Veterinary Science,
Wuhan Academy of Agricultural Science Technology,
Wuhan, People's Republic of China

Abstract

Embryonic stem (ES) cells have been investigated in many animal models of severe injury and degenerative diseases. However, few studies have examined the ability of ES cells to improve the functional outcome following mammary gland injury. This study investigates the feasibility of implanting mouse ES cells labeled with enhanced green fluorescence protein in the developing mammary glands in order to acquire lineage-

* Corresponding author: Tel.: 0086-27- 88113301, Fax. : 0086-27- 88113300. Email address: paper2006@sina.cn (H.-J. Huang), jiangsiwen@mail.hzau.edu.cn (S.-W. Jiang).

committed cells in mammary (e.g., mammary gland epithelial cell or luminal cell). Cells implanted in high numbers (5×10^6 cells per mammary gland) survived in the majority of the mice and nearly 38.4% of the surviving cells were $CK18^+$ at 15 weeks following transplantation. These results provide a potential technical avenue for advanced stem cell-based therapies of breast diseases and mammary gland regeneration after partial breast ablation.

Keywords: Embryonic stem cells; Transplantation; Mammary Gland; Microenvironment; Survival; Differentiation

Introduction

Mammalian embryonic stem (ES) cells are pluripotent cells derived from the inner cell mass (ICM) of preimplantation embryos (Evans and Kaufman, 1981). They demonstrate the ability to differentiate and integrate into tissues and organs after transplantation according to environmental cues (Altschuler et al., 2008; Becerra et al., 2007; Bjorklund et al., 2002; Kim et al., 2005; Kudo et al., 2007; Motohashi et al., 2006; Regala et al., 2005; Robinson et al., 2005; Srivastava et al., 2006).

In addition, a previous study reported mammary glands formed from injected mammary epithelial cells that were engineered to express the *Escherichia coli* β-galactosidase gene as a reporter. These injected glands contained ductal and lobular cells which expressed the reporter when examined *in situ* more than 12 months later (Smith et al., 1991). These results indicated that stable recombinant gene expression can be achieved *in vivo* in reconstructed mammary glands without altering the growth properties of normal mammary epithelium. Rijnkels and collaborators confirmed this consequence (Rijnkels et al, 2001). Recently, several groups have reported that a single stem cell can generate a complete mammary gland (Alvi et al., 2003; Kordon et al., 1998; Shackleton et al., 2006; Welm et al., 2002). However, few studies have examined the ability of ES cells to improve the functional outcome following mammary gland injury or similar organ injury.

This study focuses on the feasibility of implanting mouse ES cells labelled with enhanced green fluorescence protein (eGFP) in the developing mammary glands in order to investigate the survival and functional integration of these cells in mammary glands. This could provide a potential technical avenue for advanced stem cell-based therapies of breast diseases and mammary gland regeneration after partial breast ablation.

Materials and Methods

Preparation of Mouse Embryonic Fibroblast Feeder Cells

Mouse embryonic fibroblast (MEF) feeder cells were produced using the Kun Ming mouse (purchased from Institute of Wuhan Biological Products, Wuhan, China) from isolated fetal fibroblasts at day 13 to 15 postcoitum as previously described (Nagy et al., 2003). Cells were mitotically inactivated by mitomycin C treatment (0.01 mg/ml; 37°C for three hours; Serva) when they had approached confluency. Fibroblasts were directly plated at a final density of 5×10^5 cells per ml onto 35 mm tissue culture dishes (Corning, NY) and cultured at 37℃ in a 5% CO_2-humidified atmosphere.

Culture of ES Cells

Murine ES D3 cell line were obtained from the Institute of Biochemistry and Cell Biology, Shanghai Institutes for Biological Sciences, Chinese Academy of Sciences. These cells were between passage number 25 and 30, and those cells displaying a normal karyotype were used (Zhou et al., 2007). ES D3 cells were maintained at 37°C in humidified air with 5% CO_2 in ES cell medium. This medium was comprised of Dulbecco's Modified Eagle's medium (DMEM; Sigma, St. Louis, MO) supplemented with 20% fetal bovine serum (FBS; Gibco), 2 mM L-glutamine (Gibco), 0.1mM β-mercaptoethanol (Sigma), 0.1 mM insulin (Serva, Heidelberg, Germany), 1mM sodium pyruvate (Sigma), 100 U/ml penicillin (Gibco) and 100 μg/ml streptomycin (Gibco). Tissue culture dishes (Corning, NY) were prepared prior to seeding by plating a confluent layer of MEFs. Once the ES colonies had grown to the optimum size before the onset of visible differentiation, the cells were harvested by digestion with a 0.25% trypsin-0.02 mM EDTA solution, then split 1:3 and seeded on to dishes freshly prepared with MEF feeder layers.

Generation and Culture of Enhanced Green Fluorescent Protein (eGFP) Expressing Cells

For cell transfection, ES-D3 cells were cultured in the above ES cell medium supplemented with 1,000 U/ml LIF (Chemicon, USA) without feeder layers. When they approached 80% confluency, the cells were transfected by Lipofection 2000 mediated gene transfer (Invitrogen) with an enhanced green fluorescence protein (eGFP)-N1 expression construct. pEGFP-N1 is a vector constructed with an eGFP driven by a CMV promoter (BD Biosciences Clontech). Stably transfected clones were selected using G418 (Promega) at 1000 μg/ml for 5 weeks and surviving cells were subsequently maintained in 500 μg/ml G418. The expression of eGFP in the selected clones was verified by fluorescence microscopy. Before transplantation, ES cells were collected, washed in phosphate-buffered saline (PBS, pH 7.3) and allowed to stand for 5 min at 1000rpm to allow cell clumps to settle. The remaining single cell suspension was diluted to a concentration of either 1×10^5 or 1×10^7 cells/100 μL.

Host Animals

Pregnant stage	2 weeks following implantation			15 weeks following implantation		
	Low	High	Vehicle	Low	High	Vehicle
Non-pregnancy	0/3	0/3	0/3	0/3	0/3	0/3
Early-pregnancy	0/3	0/3	0/3	0/3	0/3	0/3
Mid-Pregnancy	0/3	3/3	0/3	0/3	3/3	0/3
Late-pregnancy	0/3	3/3	0/3	0/3	2/3	0/3

Figure 1. The survival of EGFP expressing mouse ES cells implanted into the mammary glands of mice. Two or 15 weeks after EGFP expressing mouse ES-D3 cells implanted into the developing mammary glands, left inguinal #4 glands, were frozen in liquid nitrogen and embedded in Tissue-Tek OCT compound (Miles). Serial cryostat-sections of 6um were obtained and observed under a fluorescent microscope. "Low cells" were 1×10^5 ES-derived cells per mammary gland; "high cells" were 1×10^7 ES-derived cells per mammary gland.

A total of 72 host Kun Ming mice (female, 8-weeks old, weight approximately 20±2 g) were used in the study (Figure 1). These mice were maintained on a standard 12-h light: 12-h dark cycle with food and water available *ad libitum*. The animals were divided into four experimental groups:

1) Mice on day 1 of pregnancy (Early-Pregnancy) were injected with low dose cell-implants (1×10^5, n = 6) or high dose cell-implants (1×10^7, n = 6) or received sham surgery by injection of vehicle (medium, n=6).
2) Mice on day 9 of pregnancy (Mid-Pregnancy) were injected with low dose cell-implants (1×10^5, n = 6) or high dose cell-implants (1×10^7, n = 6) or received sham surgery by injection of vehicle (medium, n=6).
3) Mice on day 16 of pregnancy (Late Pregnancy) were injected with low dose cell-implants (1×10^5, n = 6) or high dose cell-implants (1×10^7, n = 6) or received sham surgery by injection of vehicle (medium, n=6).
4) Mice during non-pregnancy were injected with low dose cell-implants (1×10^5, n = 6) or high dose cell-implants (1×10^7, n = 6) or received sham surgery by injection of vehicle (medium, n=6).

Surgical Procedure

Mice were treated orally with Cyclosporine A (CSA, 20 mg/kg/day) (Neoral, Novartis, Australia), commencing the day before surgery for 14 days, then a dose of 10 mg/kg/day until sacrifice. For transplantation, recipient mice were anesthetized with an intra-peritoneal injection of 0.10 ml/10 g body weight of 4% (w/v) chloral hydrate, and the inguinal #4 glands fat pads were surgically exposed and cleared of all epithelial elements as described by DeOme (DeOme., 1959) with little modification. Each animal received a 0.1ml injection of either vehicle (e.g., medium) alone or suspension of 1×10^5 or 1×10^7 eGFP-expressing ES-D3 cells into the pair of "cleared" mammary fat pads (left and right both are 0.05ml). The wound was sutured with 5～6 stitches, but not wrapped. Mice were kept in separate cages under controlled conditions for light and temperature and given food and water *ad libitum*.

Fluorescent Microscopy and Immunohistochemistry

Half of the mice from each treatment group were sacrificed at 2 weeks following the operation, and the remainders were killed at 15 weeks following the transplantation. The following collections and assays were preformed immediately after sacrifice. For the survival and differentiation potency analyses, the inguinal #4 glands, including implants and surrounding tissue, were dissected and were split into two groups.

1) Left inguinal #4 glands were fixed overnight in 4% (w/v) paraformaldehyde in 0.1 M PBS (pH 7.3), washed with distilled water and placed into 30% (w/v) sucrose in PBS overnight. Afterwards, they were paraffin embedded, 6-μm serial sections were prepared for immunohistochemical detection of cytokeratin 18 (Boster, China) on one set of sections as previously described (Weiss et al., 2003). Briefly, tissue sections were rinsed in PBS, blocked in 10% goat serum (Invitrogen) for 1 h at room temperature and incubated with a mouse monoclonal antibody against cytokeratin 18 (1:150) at $4^{o}C$ overnight. After rinsing in PBS, samples were incubated for 2 h at room temperature with a goat anti-mouse secondary antibody (1:200; Jackson, West Grove, PA) conjugated to rhodamine. The specificity of the antibody was verified with negative controls.

2) Right inguinal #4 glands were digested into single cell suspension, and counted for CK18 staining. Briefly, mammary glands were minced into 1 mm^3 section, followed by a rinse in PBS, and then incubated with collagenase for 45 min at 37oC. After the cells were in a single-cell suspension, a cytospin centrifuge was used to prepare slides. Then they were fixed overnight in 4% (w/v) paraformaldehyde in 0.1 M PBS (pH 7.3), washed three times with distilled water, and stained with CK18 following the procedure described in the previous assay. In addition, slides used for cell counting were labelled with 10μg/ml (in PBS) bisbenzimide (Hoechst 33342, Sigma). All images were acquired on a fluorescence microscope (Leica Microsystems; Bannockburn, IL) using a Leica TCS SP2 laser confocal microscope (Leica) and were analyzed using Leica confocal software version 2.0 (Leica). Adobe Photoshop CS (Adobe, San Jose, CA) was used to prepare figures. The presence of a Hoechst-labelled nucleus in an eGFP-expressing cell enabled us to distinguish between adjacent donor cells and to obtain the total number of donor cells found in a single-cell suspension of each mammary gland sample. The number of cells expressing CK18 was counted and compared to the total number of donor cells found in each mammary sample. The ratio of CK18-positive cells was measured in ten random fields.

Results

Low Dose Cell Implants

When low dose cells were transplanted into mammary glands, no surviving cells were detected in host mice sacrificed 2 or 15 weeks following implantation, and no eGFP-expressing cells were observed in any of the vehicle-injected mice mammary glands (Figure 1).

High Dose Cell Implants

In mice transplanted with high dose eGFP expressing ES cells, implanted cells were easily detected by eGFP fluorescence at 2 and 15 weeks following transplantation (Figure 2A, B). At 2 weeks, surviving ES cells were observed in 100% of the animals (3 of 3) in the mid-Pregnancy and Late Pregnancy groups. At 15 weeks, fluorescent cells were found in 100% of the animals (3 of 3) in the mid-Pregnancy group and in 67% of the animals (2 of 3) in the Late Pregnancy group (Figure 1).

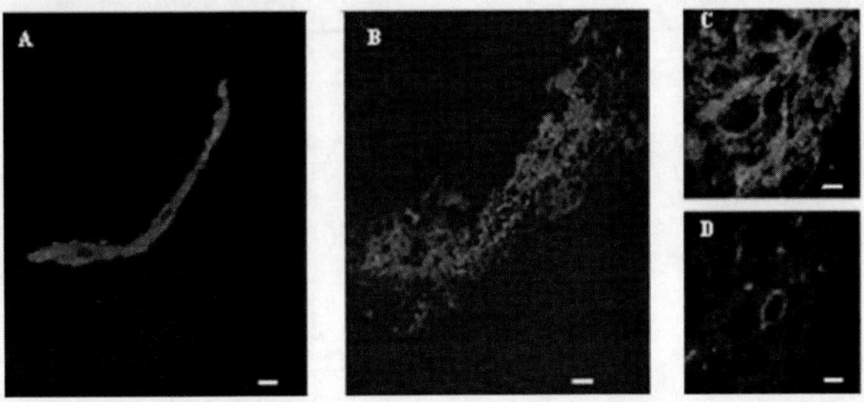

Figure 2. The survival and differentiation into $CK18^+$ cells of mES-D3 cells in developing mouse mammary glands 2 weeks (A) or 15 weeks (B) after transplantation. Left inguinal #4 glands were fixed overnight and serial sections of 6-µm thickness were performed for immunohistochemical detection of cytokeratin 18. Higher magnification of the boxed area of EGFP-positive cells in B (C, green) and CK18-positive cells (D, red) were seen in the cell grafts. All panels are sagittal sections. Scale bar, 1000µm (A and B); 50 µm (C and D).

At 2 weeks post-injection, the stem cells always aggregated within, or close to, the injection site (Figure 2A). The implanted cells were observed to have migrated to various sites throughout the mammary glands at 15 weeks after implantation (Figure 2B).

Cell counting revealed a relatively low survival rate (1.4 to 2.3%) of the transplanted cells (Figure 3). However, around 4.6% and 4.4% of the surviving cells were observed to be labelled with CK18 antibody at two weeks following transplantation in the mid-Pregnancy and Late Pregnancy groups, respectively (Figure 3). However, at 15 weeks postoperatively, nearly 38.4% of the surviving cells were found to be $CK18^+$ within the mammary parenchyma (Figure 3; Figure 2 C, D) while other groups showed very few $CK18^+$ cells. These results showed that these eGFP expressing ES-D3 cells differentiated into glandular epidermal related cells 15 weeks following transplantation.

Stage of pregnancy	Total cell number		CK18-positive cell number		Differentiation ratio (%)	
	2 weeks	15 weeks	2 weeks	15 weeks	2 weeks	15 weeks
Non-pregnancy (n=3)	2659	2937	0	0	0	0
Early-pregnancy (n=3)	3105	2594	0	0	0	0
Mid-Pregnancy (n=3)	2831	2752	130	531	4.6	19.3
Late-pregnancy (n=3)	3017	2483	133	954	4.4	38.4**

Figure 3. The ratio of mES-D3 cells in developing mammary glands differentiated into $CK18^+$ cells 2 weeks or 15 weeks after transplantation. Two or 15 weeks after transplantation, right inguinal #4 glands from 3 mice per group, were digested into single cell suspension, The $CK18^+$ cells were indicated by the percentage of mES cells differentiated into CK18-expressing cells. Note the significantly largest percentage of CK18-positive cells in Mid-Pregnancy group and Late-pregnancy group. A chi-square test was used for statistical tests. **$p<0.01$ vs. other groups.

Discussion

The mammary gland provides an excellent system to study questions pertaining to organogenesis and cell differentiation. The development of the gland is to a great extent governed by hormonal stimuli (Forsyth, 1986; Topper and Freeman, 1980). Before maturity, the epithelial tree develops slowly as it extends into the mammary fat pad during adolescence. Further development and differentiation of the gland takes place during pregnancy and lactation. Recently, several groups have reported that a single stem cell can generate a complete mammary gland (Kordon et al., 1998; Shackleton et al., 2006). More interestingly, Smith and his colleagues reported mammary glands formed from the injected mammary epithelial cells expressing the *Escherichia coli* β-galactosidase as a reporter gene. These glands contained ductal and lobular cells which expressed the β-galactosidase reporter when examined *in situ* more than 12 months later (Smith et al., 1991). This result indicated that stable recombinant gene expression can be achieved *in vivo* in the mammary gland without altering the growth properties of the normal mammary epithelia. Rijnkels and collaborators confirmed this finding (Rijnkels et al, 2001). Booth (Booth et al., 2008a, 2008b) and Boulanger (Boulanger et al., 2007, 2009) highlighted the ability of the mammary micro-environment to modify the intrinsic nature of cells transplanted from another adult tissue, therefore it is reasonable to expect that ES cells would respond and differentiate appropriately in this environment. Therefore, we hypothesized that the developing mammary gland tissues offer a niche in which injected eGFP-expressing ES cells can migrate and differentiate into the mammary gland-specific lineage-committed cells.

In this experiment, the eGFP gene that had been transfected into the injected ES cells, was not present in the cells of the KM mice used in this study. However, it was detected in the histological sections taken from injected glands as well as mammary gland cell suspensions, indicating that these cells had been derived from the ES cells. More importantly, we still detected the expression of eGFP and CK18 in mice mammary glands at 15 weeks after transplantation. These results indicated that mES-D3 cells can survive for a long time in the developing mammary glands and differentiate into epithelium type which can express a foreign gene (e.g., eGFP) long-term.

In addition, the low cell survival rate contrasted with reports from a previous study (Bjorklund et al., 2002), where implantation of similar numbers of mouse ES cells into the rat striatum resulted in well-integrated grafts in 56% of implanted animals. ES cells were found to have differentiated into stable, terminally differentiated, non-dividing phenotypes 9 weeks following implantation. The markedly lower survival of our low cell number implants in the present study could be due to a number of factors. First, the inherent variability due to the technical considerations of injecting 100 μl of a dilute cell suspension may have contributed to a poor graft survival efficiency in some of the animals, as discussed by others previously (Bjorklund et al., 2002). Second, in contrast to the brain, the mammary gland is comprised of a different biochemical environment which may have influenced the fate of cells following implantation. Third, the strain differences between the host animal and donor cells may have influenced graft survival. But interestingly, around 38.4% of the surviving cells were labelled with the glandular epidermis CK18 marker (Yang et al., 2001; Shackleton et al., 2006; Huang et al., 2010). Clearly, for future applications, more effort is needed to enhance the survival of implanted cells before this becomes an advanced stem cell-based therapy for breast diseases and mammary regeneration after partial breast ablation.

References

Altschuler, R.A., O'Shea, K.S., and Miller, J.M. 2008. Stem cell transplantation for auditory nerve replacement. *Hearing Research* 242: 110-116.

Alvi, A.J., Clayton, H., Joshi, C., Enver, T., Ashworth, A., Vivanco, M.M., Dale, T.C., and Smalley, M.J. 2003. Functional and molecular characterisation of mammary side population cells. *Breast Cancer Res.* 5: R1-R8.

Becerra, G.D., Tatko, L.M., Pak, E.S., Murashov, A.K., and Hoane, M.R. 2007. Transplantation of GABAergic neurons but not astrocytes induces recovery of sensorimotor function in the traumatically injured brain. *Behav. Brain. Res.* 179: 118-125.

Bjorklund, L.M., Sánchez-Pernaute, R., Chung, S., Andersson, T., Chen, L.Y.C., and McNaught, K.S.P. 2002. Embryonic stem cells develop into functional dopaminergic neurons after transplantation in a Parkinson rat model. *Proc. Natl. Acad. Sci. USA*. 99: 2344-2349.

Booth, B.W., Boulanger, C.A., and Smith, G.H. 2008a. Stem cells and the mammary microenvironment. *Breast. Dis*. 29:57-67.

Booth, B.W., Mack, D.L., Androutsellis-Theotokis, A., McKay, R.D., Boulanger, C.A., and Smith, G.H. 2008b. The mammary microenvironment alters the differentiation repertoire of neural stem cells. *Proc. Natl. Acad. Sci. USA*. 105:14891-14896.

Boulanger, C.A., Mack, D.L., Booth, B.W., and Smith, G.H. 2007. Interaction with the mammary microenvironment redirects spermatogenic cell fate in vivo. *Proc. Natl. Acad. Sci. USA*. 104: 3871-3876.

Boulanger, C.A., and Smith, G.H. 2009. Reprogramming cell fates in the mammary microenvironment. *Cell Cycle* 8:1127-1132.

Evans, M.J., and Kaufman, M.H. 1981. Establishment in culture of pluripotential cells from mouse embryos. *Nature* 292: 154-156.

Forsyth, I.A. 1986. Variation among species in the endocrine control of mammary growth and function: the roles of prolactin, growth hormone and placental lactogen. *J. Dairy. Sci.*69: 886-903.

Huang, H.J., Gao Q.S., Qian,.Y.G., Tao B.F., Xiang M., Peng J., Jiang S.W. 2010. Recombinant porcine beta-defensin 1 (PBD-1) expressed in the milk by transplanting transgenic mES-like derived cells into mouse mammary gland. *Cell Bio. Int.* 34: 1033-1040.

Kim, D., and Dressler, G.R. 2005. Nephrogenic Factors Promote Differentiation of Mouse Embryonic Stem Cells into Renal Epithelia. *J. Am. Soc. Nephrol.* 16: 3527-3534.

Kordon, E.C., and Smith, G.H. 1998. An entire functional mammary gland may comprise the progeny from a single cell. *Development* 125: 1921-1930.

Kudo, K., Abe, Y., Hu, D.L., Kijima, H., and Nakane, A. 2007. Colonization and differentiation of transplanted embryonic stem cells in the irradiated intestine of mice. Tohoku. *J. Exp. Med.* 212: 143-150.

DeOme, K. B., Faulkin, L. J., Bern, H. A., and Blair P. B. 1959. Development of mammary tumors from hyperplastic alveolar nodules transplanted into gland free mammary fat pads of female C3H mice. *Cancer. Res.* 19: 512-520.

Motohashi, T., Aoki, H., Yoshimura, N., and Kunisada T. 2006. Induction of melanocytes from embryonic stem cells and their therapeutic potential. *Pigment. Cell. Res.* 19: 284-289.

Nagy, A., Gertsenstein, M., Vintersten, K., and Behringer, R.R. 2003. *Manipulating the mouse embryo: a laboratory manual.* In Nagy, A., Gertsenstein, M. (ed.), Cold Spring Harbor Laboratory Press, New York, pp 453-506.

Regala, C., Duan, M., Zou, J., Salminen, and Olivius M., P. 2005. Xenografted fetal dorsal root ganglion, embryonic stem cell and adult neural stem cell survival following implantation into the adult vestibulocochlear nerve. *Exp. Neurol.* 193: 326-333.

Rijnkels, M., and Rosen J.M. 2001. Adenovirus-Cre-mediated recombination in mammary epithelial early progenitor cells. *J. Cell. Sci.* 114: 3147-3153.

Robinson, A.J., Meedeniya, A.C., and Hemsley K.M. 2005. Survival and engraftment of mouse embryonic stem cell-derived implants in the guinea pig brain. *Neurosci. Res.* 53: 161-168.

Shackleton, M., Vaillant, F., Simpson, K.J., Stingl, J., Smyth, G.K., Asselin-Labat, M.L., Wu, L., Lindeman, G.J., and Visvader J.E. 2006. Generation of a functional mammary gland from a single stem cell. *Nature*. 439: 84-88.

Smith, G.H., Gallahan, D., Zwiebel, J.A., Freeman, S.M., Bassin, R.H., and Callahan, R. 1991. Long-Term In Vivo Expression of Genes Introduced by Retrovirus-Mediated Transfer into Mammary Epithelial Cells. *J. Virol*. 65: 6365-6370.

Srivastava, A.S., Shenouda, S., Mishra, R., and Carrier E. 2006. Transplanted Embryonic Stem Cells Successfully Survive, Proliferate, and Migrate to Damaged Regions of the Mouse Brain. *Stem. Cells*. 24: 1689-1694.

Topper, Y.J., and Freeman C.S. 1980. Multiple hormone interactions in the developmental biology of the mammary gland. *Physiol. Rev*. 60: 1049-1056.

Weiss, M.L., Mitchell, K.E., Hix, J.E., Medicetty, S., El-Zarkouny, S.Z., Greiger, and Troyer D., D.L. 2003. Transplantation of porcine umbilical cord matrix cells into the rat brain. *Exp. Neurol.* 182: 288-299.

Welm, B.E., Tepera, S.B., Venezia, T., Graubert, T.A., Rosen, J.M., and Goodell, M.A. 2002. Sca-l (pos) cells in the mouse mammary gland represent an enriched progenitor cell population. *Dev. Biol*. 245: 42-56.

Yang, W., Hayward, S.W., Cao, M., Thayer, K.A., and Cunha, G.R. 2001. Cell differentiation lineage in the prostate. *Differentiation*. 68: 270-279.

Zhou, Q.J., Huang, Y.D., Xiang, L.X., Shao, J.Z., Zhou, G.S., Yao, H., Dai, L.C., and Lu Y.L. 2007. In vitro differentiation of embryonic stem cells into hepatocytes induced by fibroblast growth factors and bone morphological protein-4. *Int. J. Biochem. Cell. Biol*. 39: 1714-1721.

In: Mammary Glands
Editor: Edmund B. Rucker
ISBN: 978-1-62948-853-0

Chapter III

Environmental Chemicals and Mammary Gland Development

Erin Pias Hines[1] and Jennifer L. Rayner[2]*
[1]Office of Research and Development, National Center for Environmental Assessment, U.S. Environmental Protection Agency, RTP, NC, US
[2]Defense and Environmental Solutions, SRC, Inc. Arlington, VA, US

Abstract

The mammary gland is a dynamic tissue that undergoes multiple developmental changes over the course of the lifetime of a female. These developmental changes occur during *in utero* development, through the neonatal and peripubertal period, during puberty, and through pregnancy and lactation. As numerous changes occur in the mammary gland during these developmental periods, the mammary gland is sensitive to perturbations. Exposure to environmental chemicals during these sensitive periods has the potential to change the trajectory of breast development including affecting normal breast maturation, puberty, future lactational ability, and risk for breast cancer. Laboratory animal models are often employed to study mammary gland development across these sensitive windows. This chapter focuses on animal models that explore how mammary gland development is affected by environmental

* Correspondence: Erin P. Hines, Ph.D., U.S. EPA, ORD, NCEA, EMAG, B243-01, Research Triangle Park, NC 27711. Tel: (919) 541-4204. Email: hines.erin@epa.gov.

chemical exposure. The environmental chemicals reviewed in this chapter include: atrazine, bisphenol A (BPA), 1,1,1-trichloro-2,2-bis(p-chlorophenyl)ethane (DDT), polybrominated diphenylethers (PBDEs), perfluorooctanoic acid (PFOA), and 2,3,7,8-tetrachlorodibenzodioxin (TCDD). These chemicals have been shown to alter mammary gland development during life stages and this document looks to address the importance of age of exposure for developmental outcome.

Introduction

The mammary gland is a dynamic tissue that changes during multiple periods over a lifetime, developing both before and after birth. Laboratory animal models explore the potential for the trajectory and developmental progression of the mammary gland to be altered by exposure to environmental chemicals. These exposures could permanently alter the ability of a woman to breast feed her child or alter her risk for breast cancer. Normal mammary gland development involves endocrine pathways as well as exocrine, paracrine and growth hormone related contributions, which are all potentially sensitive to perturbations by environmental chemicals.

Increased mammary gland carcinogenesis has been reported in some rodent models in which environmental chemical exposure early in life altered mammary gland maturation, resulting in an excess presence of immature undifferentiated terminal end buds. Mammary gland development before puberty is characterized by epithelial invasion of the stroma. The terminal end buds are the highly proliferative structures at the tip or leading edge of the invading ducts as they grow into the stroma toward the lymph node. These undifferentiated terminal end buds are more susceptible to a future carcinogen than are terminal, differentiated tissues because they are rapidly dividing structures composed of many cell layers still undergoing development (Daniel and Silberstein 1987). The potential of exogenous environmental chemicals to disturb mammary gland development has been studied extensively in laboratory animals and the focus of this chapter is to summarize the effects of environmental chemicals including: atrazine, bisphenol A (BPA), 1,1,1-trichloro-2,2-bis(p-chlorophenyl)ethane (DDT), polybrominated diphenylethers (PBDEs), perfluorooctanoic acid (PFOA), and 2,3,7,8-tetrachlorodibenzodioxin (TCDD) on mammary gland development. These environmental chemicals have been reported by the National Health and

Nutrition Examination Survey (NHANES) as being detected in human participants of the program.

DDT

DDT is a synthetic insecticide with a legacy of widespread use as a mosquito repellant for reduction of typhoid and malaria. DDT is persistent in the environment with a long half-life and is still found in measurable amounts in current U.S. populations (NHANES), even though its use in the US has been banned since 1972 (EPA-20T-1002). DDT and its metabolites dichlorodiphenyldichloroethylene (DDE) and dichlorodiphenyldichloroethane (DDD) are endocrine disruptors showing estrogenic and anti-androgenic properties (Johnson et al. 2012). DDT and its metabolites are organochlorine compounds known to be lipophilic and partition to breast milk.

HER2/Neu mice, which do not metabolize DDT to DDE and DDD as humans do, were implanted with pellets that released p-DDD and p-DDE and were monitored for tumor multiplicity and tumor latency. While neither metabolite affected tumor multiplicity, both DDD and DDE decreased mammary tumor latency (Johnson et al. 2012). In another study, *in vitro* DDT exposure increased the estrogen-responsive mammary tumor cell proliferation (Robinson et al. 1985) in a dose-dependent fashion. Pubertal female Sprague Dawley rats exposed to op-DDT (50 μg/g subcutaneous, days 23, 25, 27, and 29 postpartum) had enhanced mammary gland differentiation and increased mammary gland epithelial cell proliferation; DDT caused an increase in synthesis or S-phase cells in terminal end buds and terminal ducts but not in lobules as measured with PCNA (Brown and Lamartiniere. 1995). Thus, in separate studies, DDT or its metabolites affected mammary gland tumors at various stages including tumor latency, shifts in mammary gland cell stages within the cell cycle, and mammary gland epithelial cell proliferation and differentiation.

There are few epidemiologic studies showing positive associations between DDT exposure and breast cancer. This may be because most of these studies assess DDT/DDE levels at the time of cancer diagnosis. A longitudinal or prospective study with DDT measurements taken peripubertally when breast formation and the sensitive terminal end buds of the mammary gland are present would be a better time to assess risk for future breast cancer development. One study employed such study design and found a positive association in girls exposed to higher concentrations of DDT (DDE) versus those with lower exposures, and risk increased as age of exposure decreased (Cohn et al. 2007). These girls were exposed during periods of uncontrolled, high application of DDT in the US. These results showed that girls exposed at an age younger than 14 were at increased risk for breast cancer than were girls greater than age 14, pointing to a sensitive window of exposure in breast development for future risk of cancer. Based upon the findings from this study, windows of exposure outside of the time at which cancer is assessed can inform future breast cancer risk.

PBDE

PBDEs are organobromine compounds that are used in applications as flame retardants and can be found in electronics, furniture, automobiles, polyurethane foams, and indoor dust among other sources. PBDEs are a class of chemicals that are persistent and ubiquitous and have been measured in breast milk.

Laboratory animal work has shown early life PBDE-exposure significantly stunted peri-pubertal mammary gland development of female offspring. Exposure of pregnant Long-Evans rats to the commercial flame retardant mixture DE-71 (oral gavage of 1.7, 10.2, or 30.6 mg/kg bw/day from gestational day (GD) 6 to weaning) produced female offspring at post-natal day (PND) 21 with stunted puberty-related mammary gland development characterized by less longitudinal epithelial cell growth (Kodavanti et al. 2010). The mammary glands of the DE-71 exposed female pups (10.2 and 30.6 mg/kg bw/day) exhibited a significant lack of outgrowth, with less lateral branching and limited development of terminal end buds. DE-71 has a relatively long half-life and detectable concentrations of the mixture DE-71 were reported in pup gastrointestinal contents (PND 4), dam milk (PND 10), and dam mammary glands (PND 22). DE-71 exposure produced severe hypothyroxinemia in dams and pups and delayed puberty in male pups (preputial separation), which may contribute mechanistically to the impaired mammary gland development noted in female offspring.

Few epidemiologic studies have asked whether exposure to PBDEs alters the risk for breast cancer. One case-control study with a small samples size (n=78 cases; 56 controls) asked if breast adipose levels of PBDEs were associated risk of breast cancer in women who were undergoing surgical biopsies in California (Hurley et al. 2011). In this study, no association of increased risk of breast cancer was reported in association with breast adipose concentrations of PBDEs measured near the time of diagnosis. Limitations to this study include sample size, the use of Californians who have among the highest levels of PBDEs ever reported due to strict California fire safety rule, and use of a PBDE sample measured at the time of diagnosis.

PFOA

PFOA is a synthetic eight-carbon surfactant found in numerous consumer applications including grease-proof, stain-proof products. PFOA does not readily degrade, is ubiquitous in the environment and persistent in humans with a half-life of years.

PFOA exposure during multiple developmental windows has been shown to affect rodent mammary gland development. Stunted mammary gland development of pups and dams (PND 10 and PND 20) has been demonstrated after gestational (GD 1-17, GD 8-17, GD 12-17) and lactational exposure of outbred CD-1 mice to PFOA (intrauterine/gestational and/or lactational dam/female pup PFOA exposure via 3 or 5 mg/kg bw/day oral gavage of dams) (White et al. 2007). Additionally, pup body weight was significantly decreased in this study from birth until PND 22 with PFOA exposure (dam lactational exposure 3 or 5 mg/kg bw/day oral gavage). Subsequent cross foster studies have shown that lactational PFOA exposure alone (3 or 5 mg/kg bw/day oral gavage of CD-1 dam during gestation) was sufficient to impair female offspring mammary gland development at PND 10 and PND 20 (White et al. 2009). Studies by the same lab at lower doses demonstrated that full gestational exposure of CD-1 dams to PFOA (GD 1-17, 0.3-3.0 mg/kg bw/day) resulted in extended presence of the terminal end bud structures in the mammary gland epithelium (Macon et al. 2011). Late gestational exposure of CD-1 mice also resulted in impaired mammary gland development, i.e., impaired epithelialization with poorer branching and differentiation in the mammary gland at doses as low as 0.01 mg/kg bw/day PFOA (oral gavage of dam from GD 10-17) (Macon et al. 2011). Thus, PFOA exposure *in utero* and lactationally has been shown to impair postnatal mammary gland development at multiple doses in CD-1 mice. Studies by a separate lab showed no mammary gland effects at PND 20 in female Sv/129 mouse pups (dams exposed to 3 mg/kg bw/day PFOA during GD 1-17) (Albrecht et al. 2013).

Like other known endocrine disrupting compounds, effects of PFOA on the mammary gland differ based upon timing of exposure. In another mouse strain, the C57BL/6 mouse, exposure across the peri-pubertal window (PND 21-50) either delayed (10 mg/kg bw/day) or accelerated (5 mg/kg bw/day) mammary gland development (Yang et al. 2009). In the inbred Balb/C mice, accelerated peri-pubertal mammary gland development was seen at both doses (5 and 10 mg/kg bw/day PFOA during PND 21-50) (Yang et al. 2009). Thus, strain sensitivity exists for mammary gland development at the peri-pubertal window, and possibly at other developmental windows. Mechanistic understanding of the effect of PFOA on steroid hormones was elucidated in studies with peri-pubertal PFOA exposure (5mg/kg bw/day PFOA) to C57BL/6 mice (Zhao et al. 2012) wherein PFOA mediated changes in progestin expression. Zhao et al. (2010) also studied mammary gland development with PFOA exposure but have since found that their wild-type control and knockout animals differentially metabolize PFOA (Zhao et al. 2012). Thus, peri-pubertal PFOA exposure differentially affected mammary gland development based on mouse strain and PFOA dose.

In the epidemiologic literature, a positive, albeit not statistically significant association between PFOA exposure and breast cancer was reported in a case-control study of Inuit women (Bonefeld-Jorgensen et al. 2011).

Atrazine

Atrazine, 2-chloro-4-ethylamino-6-isopropylamino-*s*-triazine, is a synthetic organochlorine herbicide used on food crops in the United States that is relatively persistent in the environment (Giddings et al. 2005) and has been detected in ground and surface waters (Balu et al. 1998). Atrazine and three of its metabolites, 2-chloro-4-amino-6-(isopropylamino)-s-triazine (DEA), 2-chloro-4-amino-6-(ethylamino)-s-triazine (DIA), and 2-chloro-4,6-diamino-s-chlorotriazine (DACT) are endocrine disruptors that disrupt the hypothalamic-pituitary-gonadal axis (USEPA, 2006). Atrazine does partition to milk although it is not a lipophilic compound (Stoker and Cooper 2007).

Long-Evans rats were dosed during pregnancy with atrazine (100 mg/kg bw/day) during a time period when mammary buds were increasing in size and the mammary tree was forming in the developing fetuses (GD 15-19). The female offspring of these rats exhibited persistent delayed mammary gland development up to adulthood (Rayner et al. 2004, 2005; Enoch et al. 2007; Moon et al. 2007). Low doses of atrazine and its metabolites administered to pregnant Long-Evans rats during the same time period resulted in female offspring with delayed mammary gland development as long at postnatal day 60 (Enoch et al. 2007). The delayed development observed in gestationally exposed pups included decreased branching and delayed migration through the mammary fat pad prior to puberty and the presence of terminal end buds beyond puberty.

Studies assessing cancer in rodents found that adult female Sprague-Dawley rats fed atrazine in their diets developed mammary tumors earlier, with an increase in incidence, than control animals (Wetzel et al. 1994). The same tumor response was not observed when female Fisher 344 or ovariectomized Sprague-Dawley rats were treated the same way (Eldridge et al. 1999b; Wetzel et al. 1994).

There are epidemiologic studies showing both positive and negative associations between atrazine and breast cancer. Three studies, including two on rural Kentucky populations and one on a Leicestershire United Kingdom population, found positive associations between atrazine (levels in ground or surface water or pesticide application) and breast cancer rates (Kettles et al. 1997; Muir et al. 2004). Three studies, including one on rural cases in Wisconsin, the population of Kentucky, and the population in Lincolnshire, United Kingdom, found no association between atrazine and breast cancer rates (Hopenhayn-Rich et al. 2002, Muir et al. 2004, McElroy et al. 2007).

TCDD

TCDD is an organochlorine that is highly persistent and causes varied effects in mammalian species including immune, reproductive, teratogenic, and carcinogenic effects (Birnbaum and Fenton 2003). TCDD is a product of incineration and industrial application, and was a contaminant of the Vietnam War defoliant Agent Orange. TCDD is an endocrine disruptor and has been measured in serum and breast milk in several countries (LaKind et al. 2011). TCDD is a lipophilic compound with a half-life in humans of 7-8 years (Kerger et al. 2006). TCDD is known to bind to the aromatic hydrocarbon receptor to induce its mode of action (Safe 1995).

Several studies have examined the effects of TCDD on mammary gland development. C57BL/6J mice dosed with TCDD during pregnancy on GD 0,

7, and 14 had delayed pregnancy-related mammary gland differentiation evidenced by decreased branching, smaller and fewer lobulo-alveolar clusters, and less ductal branching (Vorderstrasse et al. 2004; Collins et al. 2009). The offspring of these mice died within 24 hours of birth due to impaired lactational ability of the dams (Vorderstrasse et al. 2004). In addition to impaired dam pregnancy-related mammary gland development, TCDD stunted mammary gland development in Long-Evans, Holtzmann, and Sprague-Dawley rat offspring exposed on GD 15 (oral gavage of 1 μg TCDD/kg bw) (Brown et al. 1998; Fenton et al. 2002; Lewis et al. 2001; Jenkins et al. 2007). Because of TCDD's persistence or long half-life, exposure likely continued beyond the initial dosing. Jenkins et al. (2007) cross-fostered offspring to unexposed dams to prevent lactational exposure to TCDD. In these studies, delayed mammary gland development was observed as early as postnatal day 4 and remained stunted well into the adult stage of life (PND 50). At PND 50 there were significant increases in the non-differentiated terminal end bud structures. Decreased levels of β-casein have been reported with TCDD exposure, demonstrating a functional effect on mammary gland and epithelial function both *in vivo* and *in vitro* (Collins et al. 2009). In summary, gestational TCDD exposure impaired mammary gland development of the dam and stunted lactational capacity to the extent that offspring died by 24 hours after birth.

The role of TCDD in cancer was explored after gestational exposure to TCDD increased chemically-induced mammary tumors in offspring. The Sprague-Dawley rats exposed *in utero* on GD 15 to TCDD (oral gavage of dam with 1 μg TCDD/kg bw) were treated with DMBA (30 mg/kg bw/day) on PND 50 to induce tumors (Brown et al., 1998; Jenkins et al. 2007). Offspring were cross-fostered at birth to prevent lactational exposure. Tumors were detected earlier and the incidence was increased in offspring exposed to TCDD (Brown et al. 1998).

Epidemiologic studies of populations exposed to high levels of dioxin showed an elevated risk (increased hazard ratio based on serum TCDD concentrations) for breast cancer in women from the dioxin-contaminated area of Seveso, Italy (Warner et al. 2002, Warner et al. 2011). In a study of occupational exposure to dioxins in Hamburg, Germany, female pesticide plant workers with known dioxin exposure had increased breast cancer mortality when compared to women from the same city without occupational exposure (Manuwald et al. 2012). An elevated incidence of breast cancer was reported in the population near a dioxin generating point-source in Chapaevsk,

Russia, where elevated levels of dioxins have been measured in the air, soil, drinking water, and cow's milk.

BPA

BPA is a diphenolic compound used in the manufacture of epoxy resins and polycarbonate plastics. BPA can be found in plastics, linings to metal cans, indoor dust, thermal paper receipts and dental sealants (Calafat et al. 2005). BPA is ubiquitous in the environment and in humans and has a relatively short half-life (Calafat et al. 2005). BPA has been shown to be estrogenic and is thought to be an endocrine disrupting compound. Some laboratory animal studies with BPA have shown non-monotonic dose-responsive curves.

At blood concentrations of BPA relevant to human exposure, studies in rhesus monkeys showed that *in utero* exposure to BPA altered the development of the mammary gland (400 µg BPA/kg bw/day administered to dams from GD100-term, with unconjugated BPA concentration of 0.68 ± 0.312 ng/mL of maternal serum) (Tharp et al. 2012). Newborn female monkey mammary glands were more developed and there was a significant increase in the number of terminal end buds per ductal unit. The most relevant route of administration of BPA is the oral route, as that is the means by which humans are exposed to BPA. Other routes of administration including via subcutaneous osmotic pumps or injection may miss first pass metabolism and have different clearance kinetics and bioavailability (Lamartiniere et al. 2011). BPA exposure to CD-1 mice during pregnancy (subcutaneous osmotic pump delivering 25 and 250 µg/kg BPA bw/day) altered the development and tissue organization of female rodent offspring (Markey et al. 2001). BPA was shown to modulate fetal mammary gland development through the transciptome of the stroma (GD 8-GD 18 250 ng BPA/kg bw via osmotic pump) (Wadia et al. 2013). Mammary glands of BPA-exposed female offspring had significant differences in the rate of ductal migration into the stroma at 1 month of age, and significant increases in the percentage of terminal end buds, alveolar buds, terminal ducts, and ducts at 6 months of age (Markey et al. 2001). Perinatal BPA exposure to dams (25 or 250 ng BPA/kg bw/day via subcutaneous osmotic pump from GD 9 to postpartum day 4) caused significant changes to the peri-pubertal (4 months of age) female CD-1 mouse mammary gland including an increased number of TEBs, decreased apoptosis in the TEBs, increased percentage of cells expressing the progesterone receptor (PR), and increased lateral branching (Munoz-de-Toro 2005). In a separate study, *in utero* BPA exposure (25 pg/kg bw/day GD8-23 via osmotic pump in dam) caused changes in the adult female offspring (PND 110, PND 180) mammary gland including increased number of hyperplastic ducts and increased stromal nuclear density (Durando et al. 2007). In humans, increased ductal density is a risk factor for the development of breast cancer (McCormack and dos Santos Silva 2006).

The role of BPA in cancer of the mammary gland has been assessed using multiple models. Early life exposure to BPA alters the mammary gland developmental trajectory, affecting the time during which mitotically competent terminal end buds are present in the mammary gland, and potentially increasing the carcinogenic susceptibility of the mammary gland. The following studies use animal models with early life BPA exposure and follow carcinogenicity and related endpoints in adult animals. Female rodents that spontaneously develop mammary tumors, MMTV-erbB2 mice, received oral exposure to BPA (2.5, 25, 250, or 2,500 μg BPA/L in drinking water from 56-252 days of age, with respective estimated daily intake of 0.5, 5, 50 or 500 μg/kg BPA bw/day) (Jenkins et al. 2011). This chronic oral BPA exposure induced significant decreases in mammary gland tumor latency, increased tumor multiplicity, tumor burden, and incidence of metastasis only at the lowest dose of BPA tested in the MMTV-erbB2 mice. In another model of mammary cancer, lactational exposure to BPA increased tumor multiplicity and reduced tumor latency in a dose-dependent fashion in female Sprague Dawley CD rat offspring with dimethylbenzanthracene (DMBA)-induced mammary cancer (Jenkins et al. 2009). Nursing dams were orally exposed to 0, 25, or 250 μg BPA/kg bw/day from 2-20 days postpartum and offspring were exposed to 30mg DMBA/kg bw at PND 50 (Jenkins et al. 2009); milk BPA concentrations were not determined. *In utero* BPA exposure (GD 10-21, Sprague Dawley CD rats, dam oral gavage of 25 or 250 μg BPA/kg bw) shifted the timing of mammary gland carcinogenic sensitivity to DMBA (Betancourt et al. 2011). Fetal BPA exposure (Wistar-Furth rat dam exposure to 2.5, 25, 250 and 1000 μg BPA/kg bw/day via osmotic pump GD8-post-partum day 1) induced a significant increase in mammary gland ductal hyperplasia and carcinoma *in situ* at PND 50 in female offspring above the background vehicle-control incidence in the absence of any additional treatment aimed at increasing tumor development (Murray et al. 2007). Following *in utero* BPA exposure (25 pg/kg bw/day GD 8-23 via osmotic pump in dam), a sub-carcinogenic dose of N-nitroso-N-methyl urea (25 mg/kg

NMU at PND 50) caused rodents to develop increased percentages of neoplastic and preneoplastic lesions in the mammary gland (Durando et al. 2007).

In another study, cancer risk was followed after gestational exposure of the mammary-tumor prone FVB/N strain mouse dams to 25 or 250 μg/kg bw BPA/day during pregnancy and subsequent DMBA carcinogen (1 mg/100 μl) challenge at PND 35 and PND 42 (Weber Lozada et al. 2011). BPA increased DMBA tumor susceptibility in a dose-dependent manner (Weber Lozada et al. 2011).

Conclusion

This chapter examines the effects on mammary gland development of a few of the environmental chemicals that humans are exposed to and that have been detected in their bodies. It also highlights critical periods of mammary gland development during which exposure to these chemicals results in adverse changes in growth and development that may be evident long after the exposure is over.

Chemicals including PBDE, PFOA, TCDD, BPA, and atrazine delayed mammary gland development when administered during critical periods of development. Other chemicals including DDT and BPA (lower dose) accelerated mammary gland development. Exposures during critical periods of development either with or without exposure to a carcinogenic compound were also found to cause an increase in tumor incidence in the animal models utilized. Environmental chemicals are often ubiquitous and humans are exposed to them daily. This chapter covers only a few of the chemicals to which we are exposed, but shows that they may have an impact on our lives that may have long-lasting consequences.

Acknowledgment

This article was peer-reviewed by Madison Macon and Geneice Lehmann, respectively of NIEHS and the US EPA, RTP, NC.

Disclaimer

This document has been reviewed in accordance with U.S. Environmental Protection Agency policy and approved for publication. Mention of trade names or commercial products does not constitute endorsement or recommendation for use. The views expressed in this article are those of the authors and do not necessarily reflect the views or policies of the U.S. Environmental Protection Agency.

References

Albrecht PP, Torsell NE, Krishnan P, Ehresman DJ, Frame SR, Chang SC, Butenhoff JL, Kennedy GL, Gonzalez FJ, Peters JM. A species difference in the peroxisome proliferator-activated receptor α-dependent response to the developmental effects of perfluorooctanoic acid. *Toxicol Sci.* 2013 Feb; 131(2):568-82.

Balu K, Holden PW, Johnson LC, Cheung MW. Summary of Ciba Crop Protection groundwater monitoring study for atrazine and its degradation products in the United States. In: *Pesticide Transformation Products: Fate and Significance in the Environment* (Somasundaram L, Coats JR, eds.), ACS Symposium Series. Washington, DC: American Chemical Society, 1998 pp. 227–238.

Betancourt AM, Eltoum IA, Desmond RA, Russo J, Lamartiniere CA. In utero exposure to bisphenol A shifts the window of susceptibility for mammary carcinogenesis in the rat. *Environ Health Perspect.* 2010 Nov; 118(11):1614-9.

Brown NM and Lamartiniere CM. Xenoestrogens Alter Mammary Gland Differentiation and Cell Proliferation in the Rat. *Eviron Health Perspect.* 1995 Jul-Aug: 103 (7-8), 1995.

Brown NM, Manzolillo PA, Zhang JX, Wang J, Lamartiniere CA. Prenatal TCDD and predisposition to mammary cancer in the rat. *Carcinogenesis.* 1998 Sep; 19(9):1623-1629.

Birnbaum LS and Fenton SE. Cancer and developmental exposure to endocrine disruptors. *Environ Health Perspect.* 2003 Apr 2003; 111(4):389-394.

Bonefeld-Jorgensen EC, Long M, Bossi R, Ayotte P, Asmund G, Krüger T, Ghisari M, Mulvad G, Kern P, Nzulumiki P, Dewailly E. Perfluorinated compounds are related to breast cancer risk in Greenlandic Inuit: a case control study. *Environ Health.* 2011 Oct 6; 10:88.

Cohn BA, Wolff MS, Cirillo PM, Sholtz RI. DDT and breast cancer in young women: new data on the significance of age at exposure. *Environ Health Perspect.* 2007 Oct; 115(10):1406–14.

Collins LL, Lew BJ, Lawrence BP. TCDD exposure disrupts mammary epithelial cell differentiation and function. *Reprod Toxicol.* 2009 Jul; 28(1):11-7.

Daniel CW and Silberstein GB. Postnatal development of the rodent mammary gland. In: Neville MC, Daniel CW (eds.). The Mammary Gland: Development, Regulation, and Function. Plenum Press, New York. 1987 pp. 3-36.

Durando M, Kass L, Piva J, Sonnenschein C, Soto AM, Luque EH, Muñoz-de-Toro M. Prenatal bisphenol A exposure induces preneoplastic lesions in the mammary gland in Wistar rats. *Environ Health Perspect.* 2007 Jan; 115(1):80-6.

Eldridge JC, Wetzel LT, Stevens JT, Simpkins JW. The mammary tumor response in triazine-treated female rats: a threshold-mediated interaction with strain and species-specific reproductive senescence. *Steroids.* 1999 Sep; 64(9): 672-678.

Enoch RR, Stanko JP, Greiner SN, Youngblood GL, Rayner JL, Fenton SE. Mammary gland development as a sensitive end point after acute prenatal exposure to an atrazine metabolite mixture in female Long-Evans rats. *Environ Health Perspect.* 2007 Apr; 115(4): 541-547.

EPA-20T-1002, Suspended, cancelled and restricted use pesticides; U. S. Environmental Protection Agency, Office of Pesticide Programs, U. S. Government Printing Office: Washington, DC, 1990.

Fenton SE, Hamm JT, Birnbaum LS, Youngblood GL. Persistent abnormalities in the rat mammary gland following gestational and lactational exposure to 2,3,7,8-tetrachlorodibenzo-p-dioxin (TCDD). *Toxicol Sci.* May 2002; 67(1):63-74.

Giddings JM, Anderson TA, Hall LW, Jr, Hosman AJ, Kendall RJ, Richards RP, et al. In Atrazine in North American Surface Waters: A Probabilistic Aquatic Ecological Risk Assessment. SETAC Press; Pensacola, FL.: 2005. pp. 108–112.

Hopenhayn-Rich, Stump ML, Browning SR. Regional assessment of atrazine exposure and incidence of breast and ovarian cancers in Kentucky. *Arch Environ Contam Toxicol.* 2002 Jan; 42(1): 127-136.

Hurley S, Reynolds P, Goldberg D, Nelson DO, Jeffrey SS, Petreas M. Adipose levels of polybrominated diphenyl ethers and risk of breast cancer. *Breast Cancer Res Treat.* 2011 Sep; 129(2):505-11.

Jenkins S, Rowell C, Wang J, Lamartiniere CA. Prenatal TCDD exposure predisposes for mammary cancer in rats. *Reprod Toxicol.* 2007 Apr-May; 23(3):391-6.

Jenkins S, Wang J, Eltoum I, Desmond R, Lamartiniere CA. Chronic oral exposure to bisphenol A results in a nonmonotonic dose response in mammary carcinogenesis and metastasis in MMTV-erbB2 mice. *Environ Health Perspect.* 2011 Nov; 119(11):1604-9.

Jenkins S, Raghuraman N, Eltoum I, Carpenter M, Russo J, Lamartiniere CA. Oral exposure to bisphenol a increases dimethylbenzanthracene-induced mammary cancer in rats. *Environ Health Perspect.* 2009 Jun; 117(6):910-5.

Johnson NA, Ho A, Cline JM, Hughes CL, Foster WG, Davis VL. Accelerated mammary tumor onset in a HER2/Neu mouse model exposed to DDT metabolites locally delivered to the mammary gland. *Environ Health Perspect.* 2012 Aug; 120(8):1170–1176.

Kerger BD, Leung HW, Scott P, Paustenbach DJ, Needham LL, Patterson DG Jr, Gerthoux PM, Mocarelli P. Age- and concentration-dependent elimination half-life of 2,3,7,8-tetrachlorodibenzo-p-dioxin in Seveso children. *Environ Health Perspect.* 2006 Oct; 114(10):1596-602.

Kettles MA, Browning SR, Prince TS, Horstman SW (1997) Triazine herbicide exposure and breast cancer incidence: an ecologic study of Kentucky counties. *Environ Health Perspect* 105: 1222-1227.

Kodavanti PR, Coburn CG, Moser VC, MacPhail RC, Fenton SE, Stoker TE, Rayner JL, Kannan K, Birnbaum LS. Developmental exposure to a commercial PBDE mixture, DE-71: neurobehavioral, hormonal, and reproductive effects. *Toxicol Sci.* 2010 Jul; 116(1):297-312.

LaKind JS, Berlin, Jr. CM, Fenton SE. Environmental Chemicals in Breast Milk. In: Nriagu, J.O. (ed.) *Encyclopedia of Environmental Health*, 2011 volume 2, pp. 347-356. Burlington: Elsevier.

Lamartiniere CA, Jenkins S, Betancourt AM, Wang J, Russo J. Exposure to the Endocrine Disruptor Bisphenol A Alters Susceptibility for Mammary Cancer. *Horm Mol Biol Clin Investig.* 2011 Mar 1; 5(2):45-52.

Lewis BC, Hudgins S, Lewis A, et al. In utero and lactational treatment with 2,3,7,8-tetrachlorodibenzo-p-dioxin impairs mammary gland differentiation but does not block the response to exogenous estrogen in the postpubertal female rat. *Toxicol Sci.* 2001 Jul; 62(1):46-53.

Macon MB, Villanueva LR, Tatum-Gibbs K, Zehr RD, Strynar MJ, Stanko JP, White SS, Helfant L, Fenton SE. Prenatal perfluorooctanoic acid exposure in CD-1 mice: low-dose developmental effects and internal dosimetry. *Toxicol Sci.* 2011 Jul; 122(1): 135-145.

Manuwald U, Velasco Garrido M, Berger J, Manz A, Baur X. Mortality study of chemical workers exposed to dioxins: follow-up 23 years after chemical plant closure. *Occup Environ Med.* 2012 Sep; 69(9):636-642.

Markey, C.M., Luque, E.H., Munoz de Toro, M., Sonnenschein, C., Soto, A.M. *In utero* exposure to bisphenol A alters the development and tissue organization of the mouse mammary gland. *Biol. Reprod.* 2001 Oct; 65(4): 1215-1223.

McCormack VA, dos Santos Silva I. Breast density and parenchymal patterns as markers of breast cancer risk: a meta-analysis. *Cancer Epidem Biomar.* 2006 Jun; 15(6):1159–1169.

McElroy JA, Gangnon RE, PA Newcomb, Kanarek MS, HA Anderson, JV Brook, A Trentham-Dietz, Remington PL. Risk of breast cancer for women living in rural areas from adult exposure to atrazine from well water in Wisconsin. *J Exposure Sci Environ Epidemiol.* 2007 Mar: 17(2): 207-214.

Moon HJ, Han SY, Shin J-H, Kang IH, Kim TS, Hong JH, Kim S-H, Fenton SE. Gestational exposure to nonylphenol causes precious mammary gland development in female rat offspring. *J Reprod Devel.* 2007 Apr: 53(2): 333-344.

Muir K, Rattanamongkolgul S, Smallman-Raynor M, Thomas M, Downer S, Jenkinson C (2004) Breast cancer incidence and its possible spatial association with pesticide application in two counties of England. *Public Health.* 2004 Oct: 118(7): 512-520.

Murray TJ, Maffini MV, Ucci AA, Sonnenschein C, and Soto AM. Induction of mammary gland ductal hyperplasias and carcinoma in situ following fetal bisphenol A exposure. *Reprod Toxicol.* 2007 Apr-May; 23(3): 383-390.

Rayner JL, Wood C, Fenton SE (2004) Exposure parameters necessary for delayed puberty and mammary gland development in Long-Evans rats exposed in utero to atrazine. *Toxicol Appl Pharmacol.* 2004 Feb; 195(1): 23-34.

Rayner JL, Enoch RR, Fenton SE (2005) Adverse effects of prenatal exposure to atrazine during a critical period of mammary gland growth. *Toxicol Sci.* 2005 Sep; 87(1): 255-266.

Safe SH. Modulation of gene expression and endocrine response pathways by 2,3,7,8-tetrachlorodibenzo-p-dioxin and related compounds. *Pharmacol Ther*. 1995; 67(2):247-281. Review.

Stoker TE and Cooper RL. Distribution of 14C-atrazine following an acute lactational exposure in Wistar rats. *Reprod Toxicol* 2007 Jun; 23(4): 607-610.

Tharp AP, Maffini MV, Hunt PA, VandeVoort CA, Sonnenschein C, Soto AM. Bisphenol A alters the development of the rhesus monkey mammary gland. *Proc Natl Acad Sci U S A*. 2012 May; 109(21):8190-8195.

USEPA (United States Environmental Protection Agency). Triazine Cumulative Risk Assessment March 28, 2006. Available: *http://www.epa.gov/oppsrrd1/REDs/triazine_ cumulative_risk.pdf.*

Vorderstrasse BA, Fenton SE, Bohn AA, Cundiff JA, Lawrence BP. A novel effect of dioxin: exposure during pregnancy severely impairs mammary gland differentiation. *Toxicol Sci.* 2004 Apr; 78(2):248-257.

Wadia PR, Cabaton NJ, Borrero MD, Rubin BS, Sonnenschein C, Shioda T, Soto AM. Low-Dose BPA Exposure Alters the Mesenchymal and Epithelial Transcriptomes of the Mouse Fetal Mammary Gland, *PLoS ONE*. 2013 May; 8(5): e63902.

Warner M, Eskenazi B, Mocarelli P, Gerthoux PM, Samuels S, Needham L, Patterson D, Brambilla P. Serum dioxin concentrations and breast cancer risk in the Seveso Women's Health Study. *Environ Health Perspect*. 2002 Jul; 110(7):625-8.

Warner M, Mocarelli P, Samuels S, Needham L, Brambilla P, Eskenazi B. Dioxin exposure and cancer risk in the Seveso Women's Health Study. *Environ Health Perspect*. 2011 Dec; 119(12):1700-5.

Weber Lozada K, Keri RA. Bisphenol A increases mammary cancer risk in two distinct mouse models of breast cancer. *Biol Reprod*. 2011 Sep; 85(3):490-7.

Wetzel LT, Luempert LC III, Breckenridge CB, Tisdel MO, Stevens JT, Thakur AK, Extrom PJ, Eldridge JC. Chronic effects of atrazine on estrus and mammary tumor formation in female Sprague–Dawley and Fischer 344 rats. *J Toxicol Environ Health* 1994 Oct;43(2):182–196.

White SS, Calafat AM, Kuklenykik Z, Villanueva L, Zehr RD, Helfant L, Strynar MJ, Lindstrom AB, Thibodeauz JR, Wood C, Fenton SE. Gestational PFOA exposure of mice is associated with altered mammary gland development in dams and female offspring. *Toxicol Sci.* 2007 Mar; 96(1): 133-144.

White SS, Kato K, Jia LT, Basden BJ, Calafat AM, Hines EP, Stanko JP, Wolf CJ, Abbott BD, Fenton SE. Effects of perfluorooctanoic acid on mouse mammary gland development and differentiation resulting from cross-foster and restricted gestational exposures. *Reprod Toxicol.* 2009 Jun; 27(3-4): 289-298.

Yang C, Tan YS, Harkema JR, Haslam SZ. Differential effects of peripubertal exposure to perfluorooctanoic acid on mammary gland development in C57Bl/6 and Balb/c mouse strains. *Reprod Toxicol* 2009 Jun; 27 (3-4):299-306.

Zhao Y, Tan YS, Haslam SZ, Yang C. Perfluorooctanoic acid effects on steroid hormones and growth factor levels mediate stimulation of peripubertal mammary gland development in C57Bl/6 mice. *Toxicol Sci* 2010 May; 115(1): 214-224.

Zhao Y, Tan YS, Strynar MJ, Perez G, Haslam SZ, Yang C. Perfluorooctanoic acid effects on ovaries mediate its inhibition of peripubertal mammary gland development in Balb/c and C57Bl/6 mice. *Reprod Toxicol*. 2012 Jul; 33(4):563-76.

In: Mammary Glands
Editor: Edmund B. Rucker
ISBN: 978-1-62948-853-0

Chapter IV

Epigenetic Contributions to Mammary Gland Development and Breast Cancer Risk

Kurt B. Hodges[1,2], Dana Bazzoun[3], Kimberly M. McDole[1], Rabih Talhouk[3] and Sophie A. Lelièvre*[1]

[1]Department of Basic Medical Sciences and Center for Cancer Research, Purdue University, West Lafayette, IN, US
[2]Department of Pathology and Laboratory Medicine, Indiana University School of Medicine
[3]Biology Department, American University of Beirut, Beirut, Lebanon

Abstract

Understanding the biology of the mammary gland is essential for deciphering the molecular mechanisms behind breast cancer, a leading cause of death in women worldwide. There has been a dramatic shift from a genetic to a mixed genetic/epigenetic perception of breast cancer.

* Corresponding author: Sophie A. Lelièvre, 625 Harrison Street, Dept. Basic Medical Sciences, Lynn Hall, West Lafayette, IN 7907-2026, US. Phone: (765) 496-7793. Fax: (765) 494-0781, lelievre@purdue.edu.

Indeed, the expression of genes involved in mammary gland development is not only regulated by DNA sequence modifications, but it is also under the control of molecular alterations of the chromatin structure which defines an epigenetic pattern of the development process. Epigenomics' contribution to the normal development of the breast and its role, in addition to that of genomics, in explaining the existence of various breast cancer subtypes is increasingly being recognized. It is inevitable to comprehend the epigenetic landscape that dictates normal mammary gland development to better understand, predict and treat breast cancer. Our goal in this chapter is to provide an overview of how epigenetic factors like DNA methylation and histone modifications contribute to normal mammary gland development and how alterations in the epigenetic pattern modulate breast cancer risk. In particular, we aim to address the epigenetic attributes of mammary stem cells that underlie the formation of the mammary gland and their deregulations that may lead to tumor initiation and progression. We also highlight tissue architecture - defined as the mechanical and biochemical interactions between cells and their environment- that supports the proper structure and function of the mammary gland and its implication in breast cancer risk. Finally, we discuss the relationship between nutrition and epigenetics that is critical during normal breast development and the influence of dietary factors on the risk of breast cancer development.

Introduction

The lifetime risk for women to develop breast cancer is increasing worldwide [1]. Based on current incidence rates it is estimated that one out of every eight women born today will be diagnosed with breast cancer at some time during her life. It has become clear that genetic mutations alone account for only a small percentage of risk leading to breast cancer. Mounting evidence supports a central role of tissue architecture in the regulation of normal and cancerous tissue behaviors via epigenetic control of gene transcription (i.e., the control of DNA accessibility to the transcriptional machinery), especially in stem and progenitor cells that drive mammary gland development. Further evidence comes from environmental factors, notably diet, that impact breast cancer risk by deregulating the epigenetic mechanisms controlling cell fate [2]. In this chapter, we define stages of normal mammary gland development and architecture based on the epigenetic regulation of stem cell fate and outline links with breast cancer development. We scrutinize the organization of the double-layered mammary epithelial architecture that is essential for breast homeostasis under microenvironmental influence. Finally, we discuss epigenetic mechanisms underlying the nutritional impact on breast cancer risk in light of stem cell and tissue architectural features.

A. Mammary Gland Development, Tissue Architecture and Breast Cancer Risk

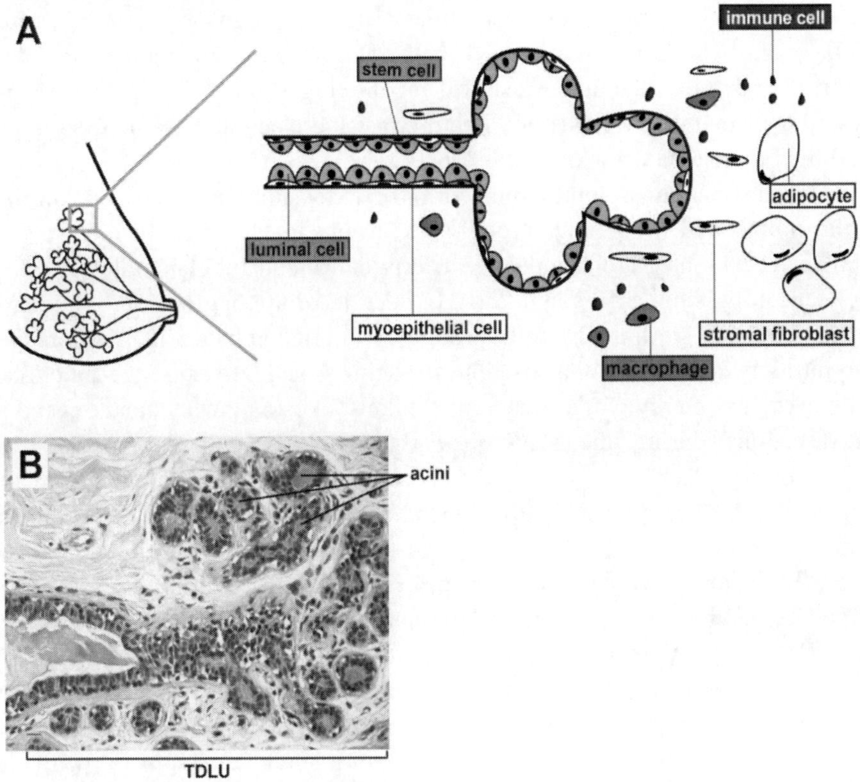

Figure 1. Organization of the mammary gland. A. The schematic shows the branched ductal network terminating into lobules. B. Simplified representation of the different cell types in the TDLU. The drawing displays fewer acini than those normally associated with a TDLU. Luminal and myoepithelial cells line the TDLUs, and stem cells have been reported to be mainly found in the terminal duct connected to acini. Some of the luminal cells in the acini make contact with the BM that delineates the epithelium. Cells usually found in the stroma are also represented. C. H&E stained tissue section of a TDLU from normal breast tissue. (Picture slightly modified from Grafton et al Integr Biol, 2011). Size bar, 30 μm.

The organization of the mammary epithelium and microenvironmental cues impinging on the breast tissue are major regulators of normal mammary gland development and function [3]. In response to hormones the breast undergoes dramatic remodeling with duct growth as well as formation of glandular structures during puberty, pregnancy and lactation, and dissolution of glandular structures during involution following lactation. Phases of development are driven by pools of mammary stem cells that self-renew and differentiate as needed. The dynamic organization of the breast during normal growth as well as recurrent development during pregnancy and menstrual cycles makes this organ particularly vulnerable to environmental factors that might disrupt normal homeostasis by modulating stem cells. Understanding how normal mammary tissue architecture is established and maintained might shed light on mechanisms of breast cancer risk.

The adult mammary epithelium forms an extensive ductal network starting at the nipple and branching through the stroma to end distally into several lobules. The lobules are composed of terminal ductal lobular units (TDLUs) each encompassing a terminal (distal) duct leading to glandular structures called acini that are lined by milk producing luminal cells. A TDLU branches into intralobular ductules that end into the acini. The TDLUs are the functional units of the mammary gland; they radiate like spokes on a wheel and expand in all directions during the growth of the mammary gland, especially in pregnancy and lactation (Figure 1). These structures are separated from the surrounding stroma by a specialized extracellular matrix (ECM), the basement membrane (BM). The stroma is a type of fibrous connective tissue composed of the ECM and a variety of cell types including fibroblasts, macrophages, adipocytes, endothelial cells and inflammatory cells that secrete soluble factors and ECM components, hence contributing to the homeostasis of the mammary gland. The mammary epithelium is composed of two cell types, the luminal cells and myoepithelial cells. They organize into bilayered structures coordinated by cell adhesion molecules during fetal development, with the myoepithelial cells located basally against the luminal cells [4]. The major architectural feature of the mammary epithelium is the basoapical polarity axis with cell-cell tight junctions at the apical pole facing the lumen and cell-BM junctions (hemidesmosomes) resulting from the interaction between laminin-332 and $\alpha6/\beta4$ integrins at the basal pole (Figure 2) [5, 6]. Cytoskeletal proteins have an important architectural function and bridge signals between ECM and nucleus. They are also a means to characterize the two cell layers [7, 8]. The luminal cells express cytokeratins (CK) 8, 18, and 19. They form a continuous layer lining the ducts, are cuboidal-shaped and contain smooth oval nuclei oriented perpendicularly to the lumen.

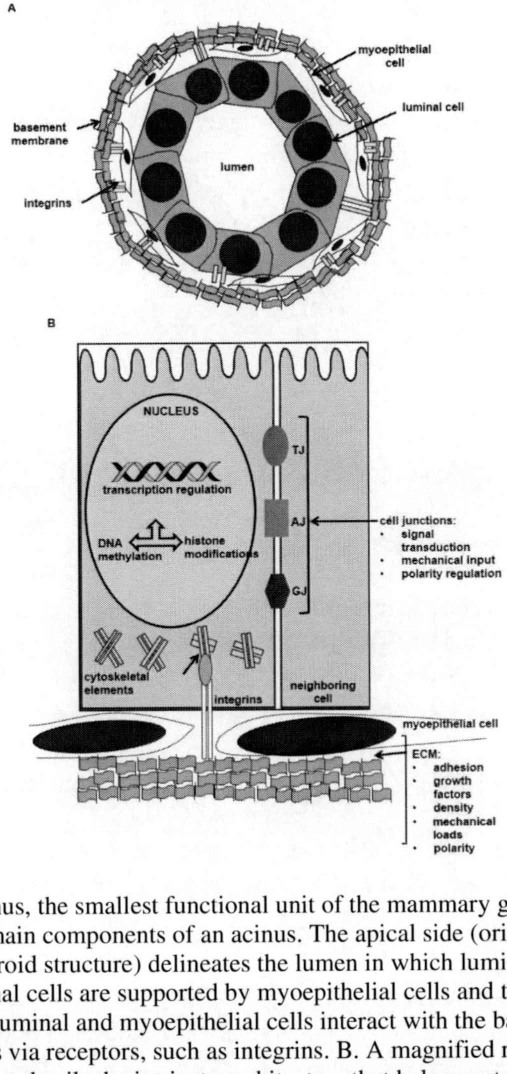

Figure 2. The acinus, the smallest functional unit of the mammary gland. A. Drawing representing the main components of an acinus. The apical side (oriented towards the center of the spheroid structure) delineates the lumen in which luminal cells secrete. Basally, the luminal cells are supported by myoepithelial cells and the basement membrane. Both luminal and myoepithelial cells interact with the basement membrane (BM) components via receptors, such as integrins. B. A magnified region of luminal-luminal cell contact details the intricate architecture that helps control gene expression in luminal epithelial cells, with specific subcellular localization of cell-cell junctions (tight junctions [TJs], adherens junctions [AJs] and gap junctions [GJs]), which depending on their structure, provide cellular adhesion, cell-cell communication and regulate polarity and mediate mechanical input into the interior of the cell. The BM plays an integral role in modulating signaling networks that convey information to the cell nucleus to modulate epigenetic marks (e.g., DNA methylation, histone modifications) through integrins and cytoskeletal elements.

The myoepithelial cells are spindle-shaped and express basal CK5 and 14, α-smooth muscle actin and myosin. They are responsible for the contractile capability of the epithelium. These cells form a continuous layer oriented parallel to the long axis of the duct; whereas they are discontinuous in the lobules where they form a basket-like network around the acini, allowing luminal cell-BM contacts that are crucial for normal development [7, 9]. Histochemical staining suggests that mammary stem cells have an intermediate suprabasal location in the epithelium [10-12]. Common progenitor cells expressing cytoskeletal proteins characteristic of both luminal and myoepithelial cells (e.g., $CK19^+$ and $CK14^+$) have been proposed to give rise to these two cell lineages (Figure 3) [13].

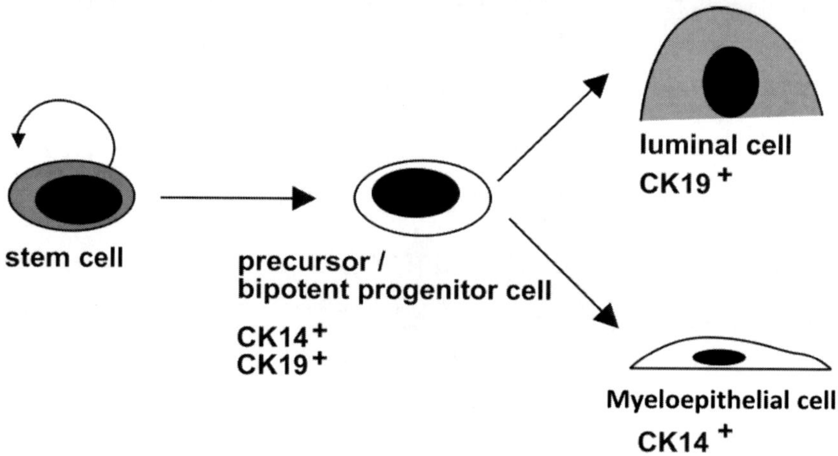

Figure 3. Hypothetical model of CK14+/CK19+ precursor/bipotent cells as a source of luminal and myoepithelial cell lineages during cycles of proliferation and differentiation in the mammary gland. These cell types can be identified by a variety of cell markers including, in particular, cytoskeletal proteins.

Once the rudimentary ductal structures are formed during fetal development, the breast tissue remains relatively quiescent until puberty when, in response to ovarian hormones and local growth factors, a dramatic expansion of the mammary stem cell compartment occurs. Epithelial cell proliferation and migration is accompanied with marked ductal elongation and lobulogenesis [14]. This stage requires production and organization of BM components including collagen IV and laminins-111 and -332 by the myoepithelial cells, hence providing the signaling necessary to establish and maintain the function of the new epithelial structures [15]. For example, expression of the milk protein β-casein has been shown to be controlled by laminins-111 and β1-integrin signaling [16]. Moreover, alterations in BM components reproduced in three-dimensional (3D) cultures of mammary luminal epithelial cells prevent acinar differentiation [17, 18]. In addition to BM components, myoepithelial cells secrete growth factors and matrix metalloproteinases (MMPs) like MMP2 and MMP3 that are essential for tissue remodeling during normal development [19].

Following puberty the mammary epithelium undergoes sequential waves of proliferation and apoptosis associated with tissue remodeling with each menses period [20]. A major structural and functional change is associated with pregnancy as the mammary epithelium undergoes further branching morphogenesis and differentiation under the control of NOTCH and ~~Gata-~~ GATA3 signaling pathways. This stage promotes the formation of additional lobules and milk producing luminal cells [21, 22]. The stroma is also modified during pregnancy as illustrated by the loss of lipid content in adipocytes and by angiogenesis [23, 24]. After cessation of lactation, the mammary epithelium incurs massive cell death via apoptosis resulting in a remodeled tissue that morphologically resembles the pre-pregnancy state, with the exception that more glandular tissue remains compared to before pregnancy [25]. Interestingly, reproductive history has been associated with the modulation of breast cancer risk [26]. A large international case control study reported that women who had their first childbirth under 20 years of age showed a 50% reduction in breast cancer cases compared to nulliparous women, suggesting a protective effect of early parity [27]. The protection mechanisms are not fully understood, but it has been suggested that pregnancy-induced changes in tissue architecture and the degree of differentiation of the mammary epithelium may impart a safeguard mechanism in the susceptibility of the breast to cancer [28, 29].

Although cancer arises from the epithelium, the mammary stroma plays a considerable role in breast cancer risk [30]. This microenvironment modulates tissue specific differentiation, growth and even polarity of the normal mammary epithelium [31]. The cellular components of the mammary stroma, notably adipocytes and fibroblasts have been implicated in cancer initiation and progression [32]. Moreover, ECM components and stromal gene expression profiles have been informative to identify specific breast cancer subtypes, including the aggressive basal-like breast cancer, and may predict clinical outcomes [33, 34]. Some of these findings corroborate epidemiologic evidence that high mammographic breast tissue density and postmenopausal obesity/adiposity are breast cancer risk factors [35-39].

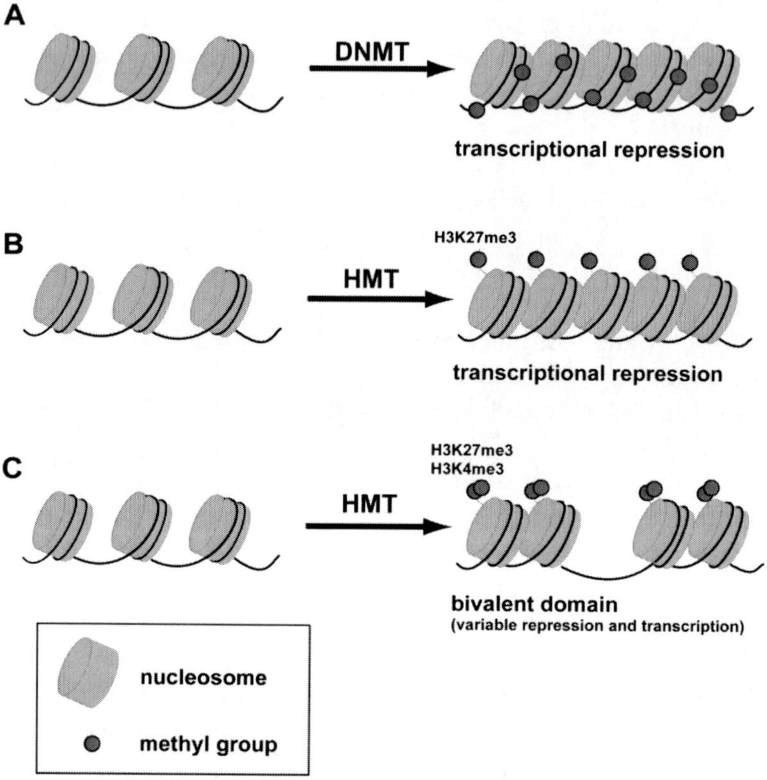

Figure 4. Schematic of nucleosomes distributed along the DNA and of some of the epigenetic modifications that control chromatin structure and gene transcription. A. DNA methylation via DNA methyl transferases (DNMTs) often leads to compaction of chromatin and transcriptional silencing of target genes during development and differentiation. B. Histone modifications involve methylation via histone methyl-transferases (HMT), which can also trigger a decrease in transcription depending on the type of lysine that is methylated (e.g., H3K27 vs. H3K4). This type of modification leading to chromatin remodeling occurs for instance during stem/progenitor cell differentiation. C. H3K27me3, a repressive mark, can coexist with H3K4me3, commonly found in actively transcribed chromatin, to form bivalent domains that keep developmentally important genes in "ready state" for transcriptional repression or activation.

Furthermore, epidemiologic data link chronic inflammation (such as chronic mastitis), a condition that involves strong stromal reaction, to increased breast cancer risk, whereas nonsteroidal anti-inflammatory drugs may decrease breast cancer risk [40, 41]. Overall microenvironmental conditions and epithelial structure exert considerable control over the risk of tumor onset. As we will further discuss in chapter II, loss of tissue polarity is an early event associated with increased breast cancer risk [42, 43]. Yet, how different breast cancer types can be specifically determined by such changes remains an important source of research efforts.

Breast cancer is a heterogeneous disease with tremendous variations with regard to molecular and clinical features. The current concept is that both genetic and epigenetic transforming events occur in different types of stem and progenitor cells, resulting in deregulated self-renewal and differentiation pathways, including Wnt/β-catenin, Notch and hedgehog signaling [44]. In general, breast cancer is classified according to receptor status (e.g., ER+ and ER-) and molecular subtypes reflected by gene expression patterns [45]. There are at least five molecular subtypes: luminal A (ER+ and/or PR+, HER2-), luminal B (ER+ and/or PR+, HER2+), triple negative (TN) basal-like (ER-, PR-, HER2-), HER2 type (ER-, PR-, HER2+), and claudin-low [46-48]. While the distinct cell types at the origin of the different molecular subtypes of breast cancer are still debated, it is postulated that these cancers may be initiated in different stem/progenitor cells and possess distinct DNA methylation patterns [49, 50]. For example, luminal A subtype is associated with hypermethylation of the SOX1 gene [51]. It is the most frequent subtype, accounting for more than 75% of all breast cancers, and has the most favorable clinical outcome partly because it can be treated with targeted anti-estrogen therapy. In contrast, aggressive TN basal-like breast cancers, the incidence of which has been increasing in young women worldwide, are difficult to treat because they typically lack expression of hormone receptors and HER2. These tumors are frequently associated with an altered function of *BRCA* genes via mutations or epigenetic silencing following promoter methylation [52, 53]. One of the highest levels of risk for breast cancer is associated with germ-line mutations in the *BRCA1* gene, predisposing women to a lifetime risk of breast cancer up to 85% [54]. In addition to its role as a tumor suppressor and in DNA repair, *BRCA1* is also involved in epithelial architectural integrity. Indeed *BRCA1* haploinsufficiency has been associated with impaired cytoskeletal organization and loss of epithelial polarity in 3D cell culture [43]. Loss of the bilayered epithelial architecture and thus, polarity with piling-up of cells is among the earliest changes that pathologists can observe in breast tissues associated with increased breast cancer risk. Other signs of alterations are abnormalities in nuclear morphology, such as loss of proper orientation of the nucleus and modifications in the chromatin pattern. Changes in chromatin structure (an epigenetic visualization) also occur during the course of normal mammary epithelial growth and differentiation as they reflect modifications in gene transcription. Emerging evidence that mammary stem cells are the targets of factors, like diet and ionizing radiation, that alter epigenetic mechanisms and increase breast cancer risk requires a better understanding of epigenetic principles and mechanisms underlying normal mammary gland development and of the etiology of breast cancer [2, 55].

B. Epigenetic Mechanisms and Control of Cell Phenotype

The concept of epigenetics is evolving and several definitions have been proposed [56, 57]. Strictly speaking, epigenetics is the study of changes at the gene level that lead to modifications in transcription without necessitating alterations in the DNA sequence. Epigenetic modifications can be transmitted through cell division. Factors with epigenetic impact include proteins binding to chromatin and long noncoding RNAs that exert an effect on chromatin organization and thus, impact the accessibility of factors involved in gene transcription [58-62]. Epigenetic modifications correspond to chemical alterations involving DNA methylation and histone modifications. Although there is emerging evidence that long noncoding RNAs are important regulators of gene transcription [63], there are currently limited data regarding their role in breast cancer and they will not be discussed here.

The large set of possible epigenetic modifications provides a mechanism for cellular diversity and transcriptional plasticity by directing which genes will be transcribed and when [64]. Certain modifications like DNA methylation are stable, which in some pathologies contributes to the propagation of characteristics of diseased cells across generations [65]. Environmental factors can sustainably influence the epigenome via DNA methylation, affecting tissue phenotype many years later or even in offspring. DNA methylation plays a central role in the mammary gland. It occurs during lineage commitment and leads to progressive silencing of genes that encode homeobox and polycomb group (PcG) proteins in addition to other genes that regulate stem cell functions [66, 67]. DNA methylation is regulated by a family of DNA methyltransferases (DNMTs) and involves enzymatic addition of a single carbon methyl group on the C5 position of cytosine bases. Cytosines can be grouped within CpG islands that exist in the promoter or first exon of 60-70% of known genes [68]. DNA methylation inhibits transcriptional initiation by interfering with the binding of certain transcription factors and attracting methyl binding proteins (MBPs) that interact with other proteins and/or complexes that control chromatin [69]. Precise DNA methylation patterns are generated by the cooperative activity of *de novo* DNA methyltransferases DNMT3a and DNMT3b,. These enzymes are expressed throughout the cell cycle and establish DNA methylation patterns early in development [70]. The original DNA methylation pattern is sustained largely by maintenance enzyme DNMT1 [71]. As will be illustrated in section III of this chapter, DNMTs are regulated by dietary factors, establishing a link between nutrition, epigenetic regulation and breast cancer risk [68]. DNA methylation also impacts gene expression via an interaction with chromatin modifying enzymes that influences the types of histone modifications in gene promoters.

The nucleosomes, which are the basic building blocks of chromatin, contain about 147 base pairs of DNA wrapped around histone proteins with a globular C-terminal domain and an unstructured N-terminal tail [72]. The N-terminal tail can undergo a variety of modifications including acetylation, methylation, phosphorylation and ubiquitylation on specific residues, resulting in regional or tissue-specific modifications of the chromatin structure and gene transcription [73]. Methylation of lysines and/or arginines can also be of different forms such as mono-, di- or trimethylation for lysines and mono- or dimethylation for arginines [61, 62]. More than 20 histone modifications work in concert with DNA methylation to regulate key cellular processes such as transcription, replication and DNA repair [74]. Histone modifications can have both repressive and activating functions depending upon the type of modifications, the residues modified, and the form of modification [75]. Trimethylation of the lysine 9 and lysine 27 residues of histone H3 (i.e., H3K9me3 and H3K27me3 respectively) are well understood [76]. For example methylated H3K9 serves as a binding site for the chromodomain-containing heterochromatin protein 1 (HP1) and induces transcriptional repression of the target genes. H3K27me3 is mediated by the enzyme EZH2 of PcG repressive complexes and plays an important role in cellular differentiation. It also recruits DNA methyltransferases and adds an additional layer of epigenetic control of gene transcription [77]. In contrast, H3K4me3 and H3K9 acetylation (H3K9ac) are associated with active genes. These and other modifications form a histone code that marks chromatin regions for transcription activation or repression. The pattern of histone modifications determines the structure and activity of different chromatin regions; it is controlled by a balance of enzymes such as histone acetyltransferase (HAT) that transfers an acetyl group from acetyl CoA and histone deacetylase (HDAC) that removes the acetyl group [78].

Variations in global levels of histone acetylation and methylation have been shown to correlate with breast cancer subtypes and clinical outcome [79]. In addition, the bivalent epigenome of stem cells with simultaneous presence of transcription repressive (H3K27me3) and permissive (H3K4me3) marks on a number of genes might make these cells particularly sensitive to environmental influence (Figure 4). Yet the link between epigenetic modifications, specific cell types and modifications in the architecture of the mammary gland that modulate breast cancer risk is difficult to unravel, hence impairing the development of successful breast cancer risk reduction strategies. The major gap in identifying cellular targets for epigenetic modifications that lead to increased breast cancer risk requires additional efforts to elucidate the epigenetic mechanisms involved in breast cancer onset. In the next three sections of this chapter we investigate the strength of the link between epigenetics and tissue architecture as it directs breast homeostasis and review the knowledge of diet-epigenetic interactions during normal development that impinge on the mammary gland.

Part I. Epigenetics and Mammary Stem Cells

Women seem more at risk from environmental exposure of the breast at certain points in their lifelong developmental time-line, with a peak of impact on breast cancer incidence from exposure to risk factors before puberty [2]. It is reasonable to postulate that specific exposures may modify the epigenome of stem cells responsible for organogenesis and differentiation in a way that allows them to survive, but results in altered tissue architecture, setting the stage for breast cancer initiation. The existence of long-lived modifications in the mammary gland was dramatically demonstrated in the study of survivors of the 1945 atomic bombings of Hiroshima and Nagasaki. Women exposed to ionizing radiation before age 20 had the highest rates of breast cancer [80]. A variety of conventional environmental exposures including chest radiographs, mammograms and other diagnostic tests also increases breast cancer risk. This is particularly evident in women with *BRCA1* or *BRCA2* breast susceptibility gene mutations exposed to these radiation-generating tests prior to age 30 [81]. These findings suggest that the environmental impact on the mammary epithelium and/or the stroma during "windows of susceptibility" alter the risk of developing breast cancer. Indeed, the breast might be more sensitive to damage before and during puberty as well as during pregnancy when there is rapid expansion and activation of mammary stem cells.

The mammary gland does not completely mature until pregnancy, therefore there remains a pool of self-renewing stem cells during extended periods of time [11, 12]. In fact, the breast undergoes regeneration over decades under hormonal control. Thus, it appears that the breast might be vulnerable to epigenetic insults that could accumulate over time. A better understanding of how epigenetic factors regulate stem cell fate and contribute to normal mammary gland development and breast cancer risk is warranted. Moreover, mammary stem cells ought to be well-characterized so that major epigenetic mechanisms controlling their self-renewal and differentiation potential can be studied and altered epigenetic patterns leading to tumor initiation and progression can be identified.

Identification and Characterization of Normal Mammary Stem Cells

Mammary stem cells were first identified and extensively studied in mouse models [82]. However, there are limited data on these cells in humans. Substantial efforts to identify markers of human mammary stem cells have relied on flow cytometry for cell surface markers including MUC1, EpCAM, CD49f, CD10, CD44 and CD24, followed by *in vitro* colony and 3D cell culture assays [83-85]. $CD44^{+}$ mammary epithelial cells are part of a hierarchy of cells with stem characteristics that differentiate into luminal and myoepithelial cells forming the ducts and lobules of the breast [86, 87]. Al-Hajj and colleagues prospectively identified mammary cells with stem properties by demonstrating the tumorigenic potential of $CD44^{high}/CD24^{low}$ lineage (-) cells compared to $CD44^{low}/CD24^{low}$ cells [88]. Subsequent studies have provided additional evidence supporting the idea that $CD44^{high}/CD24^{low}$ mammary epithelial cells have characteristics associated with stem cells [89]. Nevertheless, most of the stem cell information in the breast comes from cancer studies. Noteworthy is the frequency of tumor cells positive for stem cell-like and more differentiated cell markers that bears clinical significance; it varies according to the tumor subtype with basal-like tumors having the highest frequency of $CD44^{+}/CD24^{-}$ cells compared to other subtypes studied [90]. The site of normal mammary stem cells has been elusive. Yet, studies are revealing a niche at a narrow region of the TDLU that serves not only as the site for the proliferation of the mammary epithelium and duct branching during pregnancy, but also as the site of origin of most breast cancers [91].

Hormonal Influence on Stem Cells Associated with the Normal Mammary Gland

Estrogen and progesterone are key regulators of mammary gland development and their effects are mediated by estrogen receptors (ER) alpha (ERα) and beta (ERβ) and progesterone receptors (PR) A and B. Absence of ovarian function results in failure of mammary gland development [92]. Moreover, ERα knockout mice develop only rudimentary ducts, which further illustrates the obligate role of estrogen in mammary gland development [93]. Approximately 15-30% of luminal epithelial cells in premenopausal women express ERα and PR as detected by immunohistochemistry whereas these receptors are not present in the myoepithelial cells [94-96]. In contrast, ERβ expression is present in both luminal and myoepithelial cells as well as in some stromal cells including fibroblasts [97]. Conflicting reports surround the hormone receptor status of mammary stem cells [10]. The current idea is that although these cells lack ER receptors they might indirectly respond to the estrogen stimulation of luminal cells. Indeed, estrogen action on ER+ luminal cells induces expression of amphiregulin, a member of the epidermal growth factor receptor (EFGR) family [98, 99]. Amphiregulin is subsequently cleaved, possibly allowing an action on EGFR positive stromal cells which, in turn, directly or indirectly stimulate mammary stem cells [91].

The lifetime exposure of women to estrogen has been strongly linked to breast cancer risk [100]. In addition to physiologic exposure to estrogen, hormone replacement therapy in postmenopausal women is associated with invasive breast cancer and increased risk of ductal carcinoma *in situ* [101]. Thus, it is important to understand the impact of steroid hormones on mammary stem cells [102, 103]. Mammary stem cells have been shown to be highly responsive to steroid signaling in mice. For instance, pregnancy is marked by an elevated serum level of progesterone that works with prolactin to drive the expansion of the mammary stem cell pool by up to 14-fold [104]. It is possible that steroid hormone control of mammary stem cells may account for the transient increase in breast cancer risk in humans that has been associated with pregnancy [26]. Moreover, the breast undergoes repeated cycles of hormonally driven expansion of stem/progenitor cell populations during menses that may explain the increased breast cancer risk associated with a greater number of menstrual cycles linked to early onset of puberty and late onset menopause [105].

Epigenetic Regulation of Mammary Stem Cell Differentiation Potential

Mammary stem cells undergo changes in gene transcription patterns as they differentiate into progenitor subsets with defined lineage potentials. These transcriptional alterations are proposed to result from chromatin reorganization during differentiation that establish and maintain lineage-specific transcriptional networks. For example, gene expression profiling studies have shown that genes important for maintaining pluripotency and self-renewal such *SUZ12* are hypomethylated in $CD44^+$ cells compared to the more differentiated $CD24^+$ mammary epithelial cells, suggesting that progressive epigenetic silencing marked by promoter DNA methylation is an important step in mammary epithelial differentiation [106]. Epigenetic control of the Notch signaling pathway also regulates mammary stem cell function and commitment to luminal cell lineage; deregulation of this pathway leads to breast cancer [107]. Although the molecular mechanisms are not fully understood, studies have shown that BRCA1 plays a critical role in mammary stem cell regulation including differentiation and lineage commitment of ER- mammary stem/progenitor cells into ER+ luminal cells, possibly through activation of the Notch signaling pathway [108, 109].

As mentioned earlier, ERα signaling plays a key role in the hormonal control of mammary stem/progenitor cell proliferation. The mechanisms involve dynamic interaction of epigenetic modifiers such as HATs and HDACs, that are influenced by coactivators and corepressors, respectively [110]. In mice, emerging evidence suggests that ERα signaling has the potential to contribute to epigenetic changes in mammary stem cells through paracrine signaling from RANKL [111]. Because epigenetic alterations are reversible, there may be opportunities in the future to develop novel therapeutic strategies to reverse ERα-driven epigenetic changes.

In humans, there is evidence that some of the epigenetic mechanisms that govern embryonic stem cell differentiation are active in adult stem cells of the breast. These mechanisms might play a role in determining stem cell fate including self-renewal or lineage commitment. In general, stem cells follow well-defined epigenetic programs that control the differentiation of their progeny [86]. These programs might involve progressive restriction of stem cell plasticity and acquisition of cell-type specific features via epigenetic regulation. Both DNA and histone modifications have been implicated in mammary stem cell self-renewal signaling pathways. Yet, the bivalent (H3K27me3/H3K4me3) histone marks are considered crucial for the plasticity of mammary stem cells that is necessary for normal mammary gland development and maintenance [112]. Genome wide chromatin immunoprecipitation studies have demonstrated that bivalent epigenetic domains allow transcription factors to be poised for rapid transcriptional activation upon differentiation [113]. Generation of the first comprehensive epigenomic profile of $CD44^+$ mammary stem cells and the more differentiated $CD24^+$ luminal progenitors revealed differences in the presence of bivalent domains in genes central to the development process [114], illustrating the plasticity of the epigenome in the mammary gland.

As illustrated so far, the importance of both epithelial tissue organization and stem cells in breast homeostasis is well established. These features are influenced by signaling between the cells and their microenvironment with a direct impact on the cell nucleus and ultimately the epigenome, hence modifying breast cancer risk. In the next section we explore tissue architecture defined by the mechanical and biochemical interactions between cells and their environment, and discuss the implications of alterations in such architecture for breast cancer onset.

Part II. Epigenetics and Mammary Epithelial Architecture

The establishment of correct mammary epithelial tissue organization, regardless of the developmental stage or incremental growth initiated from stem and progenitor cells, depends on proper cell-cell, cell-ECM, and ECM-nucleus interactions. It is governed via reciprocal exchange of mechanical and biochemical stimuli underlying changes in cell shape, nuclear structure and ultimately the epigenome.

Cell-ECM and ECM-Nucleus Interplay During Mammary Differentiation

The dynamic stages of mammary gland development highlighted in the introduction require flexibility in the tissue architecture intimately linked to cell-ECM and ECM-nucleus interactions [115]. The ECM plays an essential role in regulating normal tissue and tumor development in the mammary gland by supplying and controlling signals from the surrounding environment. The continuous interplay between ECM and nucleus influences nuclear architecture which, in turn, through epigenetic mechanisms, regulates gene expression and consequently differentiation and morphogenesis of the mammary epithelium [116].

Breast cancer risk has been correlated with mammographic density, a measure of the radiodense fibroglandular tissue that composes the ECM. The majority of studies on this matter reported two- to six-fold increased risk for the highest breast densities compared with the lowest risk categories [117]. Furthermore, several studies have revealed an association between increased mammographic density and cell proliferation within the stroma and the epithelium. Beside the cell compartment, increased breast density also encompasses enhanced fibrillar collagen deposition [118, 119]. The long established association between stromal fibrosis and breast density confirms the extensive role played by the ECM in this phenomenon [120-124]. Interestingly, breast tissue from persons with high breast density displays not only twice the collagen area compared to those with low breast density, but also a significantly larger cell nucleus area [119]. Mechanistically, it has been proposed that collagen composition in particular, and higher breast density in general, lead to a more rigid ECM which, in turn, induces high local mechanical loads altering focal adhesion and Rho GTPase signaling pathways associated with a transformed phenotype and higher breast cancer risk [125, 126]. Another possibility is that increased stromal collagen might affect mammary fibroblasts that stimulate mammary epithelial cells to secrete specific soluble growth factors, hence increasing the risk of developing breast cancer [127-130].

The investigation of nuclear modifications might bring important cues regarding the nature of the ECM impact on the modulation of breast cancer risk. During the course of mammary gland differentiation, the size and heterochromatin distribution of the cell nucleus vary as visualized by light microscopy. For instance in the rabbit mammary gland, during early gestation the nuclei have irregular shapes with folds and invaginations, nucleoli are either at the periphery or the interior of the nucleus, and DNA staining appears diffused throughout the nucleoplasm with concentration at the periphery. Later on, during lactation, the nucleoplasm becomes clearer as heterochromatin clusters appear throughout. These observations suggest that with certain differentiation stages, a global nuclear reorganization occurs during which the nuclear space becomes divided into fewer but larger subcompartments [131]. In addition, H4K20me3 foci appear more compact in lactating mammary epithelial cells compared to nonlactating cells. These foci are located more frequently at the nuclear periphery in lactating mammary cells, while they are distributed throughout the nucleus in virgin and pregnant mammary epithelial cells [132-134].

The interconnection between epigenetic mechanisms, nuclear organization and microenvironmental cues has been extensively examined in 3D cell culture models that resemble to a certain extent *in vivo* conditions. For non-neoplastic luminal epithelial cells, such conditions are achieved by providing BM component laminin 111 for instance, which stimulates endogenous BM organization. Under these conditions, cells form spherical polarized structures that mimic mammary acini, as opposed to the flat monolayer that they display in standard 2D culture conditions. For example, the non-neoplastic S1 cell population of the HMT-3522 progression series, derived from a benign breast fibrocystic lesion, is able to differentiate into basoapically polarized acinus-like structures upon deposition of endogenous BM components (e.g., laminin-332 and collagen IV) [135, 136].

During differentiation of human breast acini, high order chromatin is modified with a concentration of heterochromatin at the periphery of a central nucleolus and a ring of DNase sensitive chromatin at the outmost nuclear periphery [137]. In addition, splicing factor speckles become fewer and larger, further highlighting modifications in global nuclear compartmentalization. The nuclear protein, TIN2, which is usually part of the chromosome-end protection machinery, clusters into a single large perinucleolar domain that colocalizes with heterochromatin upon mammary acinar differentiation. Truncated TIN2 is incapable of forming these large domains, which results in impaired cell growth arrest, hence affecting an essential feature of the differentiation process [138]. Beyond global nuclear organization, cell-ECM interactions also control the expression of specific genes.

Convincing evidence linking ECM to the control of differentiation genes in mammary epithelial cells has been the identification of the bovine β-casein ECM response element, BCE-1, in the promoter region of certain genes [139]. In addition, culturing mammary epithelial cells in the presence of ECM appears necessary for the expression of the whey acidic protein mammary differentiation gene, probably through the down regulation of TGF-α, confirming the immense role that the ECM plays in directing the differentiation of the mammary epithelium [140].

Epigenetic mechanisms that control changes in chromatin organization and gene expression necessary to modulate the cell phenotype are an integral part of how ECM impacts the cell nucleus [116]. The shape of the cell that changes in response to the ECM has been shown to regulate the expression of chromatin proteins. When human mammary epithelial cells are cultured in 3D conditions, acetylated histone H4 levels decrease while HP1γ (a trimethyl H3K9-binding protein), H3K9 and MeCP2 levels increase in comparison to 2D culture conditions [18, 141].

A possible differential impact of ECM signaling depending on the genes is the compartmentalization of gene groups to regions of the nucleus with different accessibility to epigenetic modifiers [142]. The mechanisms that control genome compartmentalization and higher order chromatin organization in response to the ECM remain poorly understood. The structural nuclear protein, nuclear mitotic apparatus (NuMA), has been shown to contribute to the control of chromatin structure and organization in the mammary epithelium.

Impaired acinar differentiation and altered BM integrity occur upon induced redistribution of NuMA [17, 42, 137, 143]. These phenotypic changes are preceded by the reorganization of higher order chromatin, as shown by redistribution of euchromatin and heterochromatin markers [137]. Interestingly NuMA distribution is dependent on ECM signaling, notably through hemidesmosomes, which in turn, determines NuMA's influence on early chromatin modifications that are part of the DNA damage response [144].

Epithelial differentiation not only involves changes in the ECM and the nucleus but it is also illustrated by the asymmetrical distribution of cell junction and polarity-specific proteins within the cells to form the basoapical polarity axis. As illustrated below, these proteins appear to play a role in the epigenetic control of mammary differentiation and thus, breast cancer risk.

Cell-Cell Contact and Polarity Control of Epigenetic Mechanisms

Epithelial polarity contributes to the coordination of cell behavior within the monolayered luminal epithelium of the bilayered structure. The formation of junction complexes at cell–cell contacts contributes to the architecture of the epithelium during development and tissue remodeling by mediating the adhesion of cells to one another in an orderly manner. These cell junctions also mediate communication by allowing the passage of signals and metabolites between neighboring cells. They are classified into tight junctions (TJ), adherens junctions (AJ), and gap junctions (GJ) (Figure 2B). These junctions consist of transmembrane proteins with intracellular domains that enable the interaction with partner signaling molecules. In addition, the investigation of polarity in Drosophila has led to the characterization of a highly conserved set of proteins now classified into three functional groups: Crumbs, Scribble (Scrib) and Partition (Par). These polarity proteins and the cell junction proteins act in concert and affect each others' localization, leading to the formation of the normal differentiated epithelium. They also impinge on signal transduction pathways involved in normal and cancer cell functions [145].

The establishment of the mammary epithelial polarity axis is under ECM influence, necessitating at least the presence of laminin 111 and collagen IV [146]. In turn, apical polarity contributes to nuclear localization. Its disruption, like in the preinvasive neoplastic epithelium, leads to the relocalization of the cell nucleus away from the basal side [147]. Increasing evidence supports the idea that the loss of apical polarity is necessary for tumor development. Indeed, only acinar cells with disrupted polarity can be pushed into the cell cycle as shown in 3D cell culture, making apical polarity a candidate biomarker for breast cancer risk [42]. Silencing of *BRCA1* appears to impair the polarization of mammary epithelial cells through the alteration of intracellular cytoskeletal organization as reflected by larger and less circular acinar growth indicative of a preneoplastic phenotype compared to controls [43]. Overall, the essential contribution of polarity to mammary epithelial differentiation implies that variations in the expression and/or localization of components of the polarity complex may modulate breast cancer risk.

Cell junction molecules provide a structural continuum among cells and integrate signals from the cell surroundings to modulate cell function and often gene expression. They independently contribute to the maintenance of tissue morphology and homeostasis but still display overlapping localization and multiple interactions with each other. From the apical to the basal cellular poles of the normal epithelium are first the TJs, the belt-like structures that control the diffusion of molecules into the intercellular space by acting as selectively permeable barriers at the apical region of cells. They are major contributors to tissue polarity as they mark the boundaries between apical and basolateral membranes, hence preventing the movement of proteins and other macromolecules from one domain of the membrane to another. Basolaterally are AJs which are the first junctions established between two contacting cells during cell junction formation. Their presence has been suggested to be a requirement for the initiation and stabilization of other intercellular junctions, including TJs, desmosomal junctions and GJs. Also located at epithelial cell–

cell contacts are GJs [148]. They form clusters of intercellular channels with numerous functions including rapid transmission of action potentials, and diffusion of metabolites, nutrients, second messengers such as calcium ions, inositol-triphosphate (IP3) and cyclic nucleotides that ultimately affect gene transcription, proliferation, and apoptosis. Functional GJs have been found in the murine mammary gland [149]. Some of their components connexin (Cx) 26 and Cx43 are normally present in the human mammary gland [150]. Cxs, through their C-termini have acquired an important signaling role beyond classical GJ-dependent roles [151]). For example, Cx43, Cx30 and Cx26 were reported to form a complex with ZO-2 and β-catenin at the membrane of mammary epithelial murine cells in the differentiated state of these cells as shown by the production of β-casein, a milk precursor [149]. Several cell junction proteins have been documented to alter gene expression levels through epigenetic mechanisms. For example, core TJs proteins ZO-1 and ZO-2 were found to translocate to the cell nucleus upon disruption of tight junctions and have been linked to oncogenesis. ZO-1 displays its epigenetic regulatory effects via ZONAB, a y-box ZO-1 nucleic acid binding protein. When ZO-1 is down-regulated by RNA interference, ZONAB becomes free to enter the nucleus and induce the transcription of histone 4 and high mobility group I protein, which, in turn, can affect the epigenetic make-up of cancer related genes coding for c-jun, c-Myc, PCNA, and cyclin D1 [152]. Another report indicates that ZO-2 is involved in the repression of cell cycle genes such as cyclin D1 via the recruitment of HDAC1 at its gene promoter region in non-neoplastic epithelial kidney cells [153].

Polarity proteins also contribute to the epigenetic control of the expression of genes involved in differentiation and cell homeostasis. It has been reported that Par proteins activate the ras-MAPK pathway in oncogene-transformed fibroblasts, leading to enhanced phosphorylation of histones H1 and H3 that imposes a more relaxed structure of cancer promoting genes such as *c-MYC* and *c-FOS*, leading to their overexpression [154, 155]. In a non-neoplastic kidney cell line, MDCKII, Scrib was shown to modify LPP, a zyxin-related protein, which then translocated to the nucleus to activate genes encoding proteases implicated in breast cancer metastasis [156]. In addition, Dlg was reported to form a complex with tumor suppressor adenomatous polyposis coli enabling G0/G1 to S cell cycle transition blockage via an association with euchromatin and a change in the accessibility of polymerases to target genes in Drosophila [157]. Little information is available in the breast. However, our initial investigation of the expression of genes responding to changes in the integrity of apical polarity suggests that some of these genes code for enzymes involved in epigenetic mechanisms (Cárdenas-Mora et al., submitted), further supporting apical polarity as a critical feature for the control of breast cancer risk.

As illustrated so far, the importance of the organization of the mammary epithelium to prevent cancer onset is paramount. The contributions of the ECM and gene expression to normal mammary gland development happen within the context of a continuum that involves tissue specific organization from the cell membrane to the cell nucleus. It is essential to understand how environmental factors might influence the epigenome depending on the structural development and status of the mammary gland. Therefore, in the last section of this chapter, we turn our attention to the gene-diet interaction in normal development and how long-term phenotypic consequences can arise from dietary influence during specific stages of development.

Part III. Nutritional Impact on the Epigenetic Control of Mammary Development

Nutrition has a strong influence on the epigenetic mechanisms that regulate development. One of the most striking illustrations of this phenomenon is seen in the honeybee. Indeed, a difference only in the nutrient source fed to genetically identical immature larvae is capable of altering DNMT3 levels, which later will differentially specify the phenotypes determining reproductive capacity, body physical features, and social/work position of the adult bee for its entire lifetime [158]. This example highlights the fact that epigenetically-driven plasticity in response to nutrient supply during development is a highly-conserved phenomenon. There is now considerable evidence in animal and human studies for the *in utero* induction of a range of disease-susceptibility phenotypes determined by the lifelong epigenetic modification of genes impacted by maternal nutrition during embryogenesis [159].

Nutrition-Epigenome Interaction Affecting the Mammary Gland

In mammals, a range of critical developmental time-windows is particularly vulnerable to the nutritional impact on the epigenome. These time-windows include the periconceptional period, embryonic stage, mid- and late gestation, postnatal/postweaning period, and puberty [160]. Among these time-windows, the influence of environmental factors on the epigenome during embryogenesis is the most thoroughly studied. During this time, the mammalian genome undergoes two waves of global DNA demethylation completely erasing the instructions for gene expression contained in the specific pattern that these methyl-groups once provided [161]. Immediately after demethylation, *de novo* methylation establishes a new pattern, providing a mechanism for the opportunity to respond and adjust to the environment with every generation. By convention, the first wave of demethylation occurs in primordial germ cells during gametogenesis, whereas the second wave of demethylation happens shortly after zygote formation at the time of fertilization.

During gametogenesis, the developing embryo (F1) generates primordial germ cells that will differentiate into gamete precursors, giving rise to the next generation (F2). In males, the DNA methylation pattern of primordial germ cells is reestablished during embryonic development. In females, on the other hand, the primordial germ cells remain unmethylated until maturation in the F1 adult when successive cohorts are remethylated at puberty and during each estrous cycle. Thus, nutrient intake by the mother (F0) during gametogenesis in the F1 embryo can impact the epigenome of primordial germ cells, regardless of the sex of the embryo. Eventually, these epigenetic marks and their effect on gene expression will be transmitted through cell-divisions to the developing tissues, including breast, of the F2 individuals produced by the adult F1 offspring. Importantly, the primordial germ cells that reside in F1 females in a state of DNA hypomethylation remain perpetually vulnerable to the effects of dietary intake of nutrients modulating DNA methylation. For the primordial germ cells to become remethylated with the fidelity that will properly reset their developmental trajectory, mistakes must be prevented. The hypomethylated DNA must be maintained in some subsets of primordial germ cells for up to many decades. Second, the subsequent remethylation of DNA, in each new wave of differentiated gametes prior to ovulation at each monthly estrous cycle, relies on optimum dietary intake and homeostasis of one-carbon nutrient factors that supply the methyl-donors for this reaction. The epigenetic marks laid down in the primordial germ cells and differentiating gametes will be passed to the stem cells of all tissue types, including mammary stem cells. Unfortunately, studies that evaluate the effects of prenatal diet-epigenome interaction in humans as they relate to breast cancer risk specifically are lacking. Yet, there is a known relationship between folate, a one-carbon metabolism regulator, and breast cancer risk [2]. In rats, folate deficiency before tumor initiation is associated with a reduced risk of developing mammary tumors, suggesting that high dietary folate may increase the progression of cancer. On a more general scale, maternal mouse dietary intake of one-carbon nutrients has been shown to impact histone modifications in both the adult offspring and their progeny [162]. In humans, an effect on birth weight, diabetes, and cardiovascular disease has been observed in the F2 offspring of F1 individuals who were either maternally or paternally exposed to decreased food availability. Specifically, the individuals who were exposed sixty years earlier to famine *in utero,* during the Dutch Hunger Winter in 1944-45, had DNA hypomethylation of the Insulin Growth Factor (*IGF*) 2 gene compared with their unexposed, same-sex siblings [163].

The second wave of DNA demethylation occurs immediately after fertilization in the preimplantation embryo. In this new hypomethylated state, genes that were specific to differentiated, specialized haploid gametes are now turned off and genes that maintain the pluripotency of diploid embryonic stem cells are turned on instead, imparting the potential for development of a new individual [164]. Rapid demethylation of the paternal genome occurs first (except for imprinted genes, retrotransposons, heterochromatin around centromeres, and some repetitive elements). Then demethylation of the maternal genome follows with a relatively slower demethylation pattern. In this phase, DNMT1 is responsible for maintaining the methylation of imprinted genes [165]. Imprinted genes (e.g., *IGF1* & 2) are genes for which it is critical for correct development that only one parental allele is expressed while the complimentary allele remains methylated and silenced throughout life. If this methylation is not established properly during embryogenesis, there is an increased expression of the gene product. Notably, the *IGF1* gene overexpression is associated with increased risk of breast cancer [166]. Maternal nutrition has the potential to permanently affect DNA methylation in the developing embryo by redirecting methylation-specific events, which could eventually be reflected in the breast tissue if genes important for breast homeostasis were influenced, hence altering the risk for developing cancer. Persistent differential epigenetic effects were demonstrated in the ~9-year-old children of Gambian women exposed to seasonal variation in nutritional status. Especially, DNA methylation at metastable epialleles was elevated in blood samples from children conceived during the nutritionally challenged rainy season, providing the first evidence of a permanent systemic effect of the periconceptional environment on the human epigenome [167]. It would be important to identify any change in breast cancer risk in this population in follow-up studies. As mentioned earlier with the Dutch Winter Hunger study, follow-up of adults sixty years after prenatal exposure to famine revealed persistent hypomethylation of the growth-regulatory imprinted gene *IGF2* in association with increased risk of several chronic diseases, including obesity, a known factor for the modulation of breast cancer risk [163]. The *IGF2* gene is hypermethylated in 17 month-old offspring of mothers in The Netherlands who are supplemented with the current United States of America (USA) periconceptional folic acid recommendation of 400 mg daily. This epigenetic consequence is occurring even in a country without the nation-wide folic acid supplementation that is experienced in the USA [168]. These findings show how easily the epigenetic pattern of genomic DNA, notably of available genes at the time of exposure, can be influenced by dietary factors that impact on methylation pathways during susceptible developmental time-windows.

Occurring simultaneously with DNA methylation/remethylation in the embryo, there is also widespread rearrangement of histone modifications resulting from the interaction of stem cell regulating PcG and trithorax group (txG) proteins. The PcG and txG proteins control the activity (and/or are subunits) of histone methylating and demethylating enzymes and are interconnected with DNA methylation during subsequent reestablishment, or rewriting of the new epigenetic code in embryonic stem cells [169]. The bivalent chromatin gene-activating mark H3K4me3 (product of txG protein ASH1) and gene-silencing mark H3K27me3 (product of PcG protein EZH2) become redistributed within chromosomes to allow sequential expression of temporally-appropriate genes during embryogenesis while tissue-specific genes remain silenced until they are needed.

Certain histone-based epigenetic alterations of great importance for stem cells have been linked to increased susceptibility of developing breast cancer. EZH2 and H3K27me3 protein levels were increased, as revealed by immunohistochemistry, in biopsies of normal tissue from women who later (at least 12 years) developed breast cancer, compared to women who remained breast cancer-free. In this study it was impossible to know how long the breast epithelium of these women had been harboring this epigenetic imbalance; it could feasibly have been established as far back as during embryogenesis or gametogenesis. Also, nutrient intake during puberty and early life offer another layer of influence that could affect mammary tissue differently depending on the epigenetic landscape that has already been established *in utero*. Interestingly, in this same study, EZH2 was also increased in normal breast tissue, notably in luminal progenitors, of individuals carrying a germ-line *BRCA1* mutation linked to higher risk of developing breast cancer, compared to noncarriers [170]. Evidently, only a small fraction of women who develop breast cancer have a mutation in known breast cancer susceptibility genes and, not all women who carry a genetic mutation conferring increased risk will necessarily develop breast cancer. Therefore, we need studies that will address how diet *in utero* and early life imparts an epigenetic background that imposes breast cancer risk or protects against the disease in women with and those without genetic mutations.

Epigenetic modifications are likely to continue to occur with morphogenesis of the breast during puberty and pregnancy. For example, in the murine mammary gland, promoter hypomethylation of pregnancy induced noncoding RNA (Pinc), the expression of which is persistently upregulated during lactation, is established even before pregnancy in the virgin mammary gland between three and six weeks (onset of puberty) of age [60]. As reported above, epigenetic changes that occur in immature mammary epithelial cells as they proliferate and differentiate into acini have been studied in cultured human mammary epithelial HMT3522-S1 cells and revealed increased levels of proteins (MeCP2, HP1γ) binding to epigenetic marks associated with gene silencing [18]. In this same study, preventing DNA methylation led to the absence of formation of apical polarity, suggesting that this architectural feature of breast cancer risk may depend on the earlier establishment of an epigenetic pattern in the immature mammary epithelial cells. We need human tissue-based studies that characterize the developmental progression of changes in DNA and histone methylation in the breast from birth, through adolescence and puberty, until pregnancy and lactation. Most of these studies will only be possible in tissue culture. In particular, as many nutrients linked to the modulation of breast cancer risk have been reported to have an impact during prepubertal exposure, it will be important to develop *in vitro* models of human breast epithelium that reproduce the immature stage and differentiation to a mature stage [2].

Overall, studies reported in the literature support the hypothesis that aberrant epigenetic alterations in the breast epithelium that accompany cancer occur early during susceptible developmental time-windows when there is widespread reformatting of epigenetic patterns. Since diet induces epigenetic modifications which can persist with fidelity through many cell divisions and cell generations and can also permanently lie latent in quiescent and slowly-dividing stem cells, the implication is that the epigenetic effects superinmposed by foods on breast cancer risk will remain with an individual long after the food has been consumed, extending to offspring as well. Notwithstanding the fact that the majority of epigenetic programming is established early in life, some of these initial patterns might be modified or even reversed later on by pharmacological agents and through dietary factors. For instance, stress-induced hypomethylation and concomitant increased expression of the glucocorticoid receptor gene in neonatal rat hippocampus can be reversed in adulthood by supplementation of one-carbon nutrients, folic acid and methionine, used for DNA and histone methylation [171]. It seems possible that the ability for *de novo* DNA methylation/demethylation could persist in the mammary gland throughout adulthood as it does in the brain [172] owing to the similarity of these two tissues in their lifelong developmental plasticity. With the realization of the influence of nutrition on chronic disease, like obesity and diabetes, in later life of the adult offspring, it is now recognized that breast cancer risk might also be affected by maternal diet, especially the supply of one-carbon nutrients [173]. Errors due to aberrant DNA methylation that occur during embryogenesis, including gametogenesis, will be harbored in the embryonic stem cells, eventually being passed to progenitor cells of many different tissues as the embryo develops, including the breast. It is timely and essential to understand which nutrients affect the epigenome of the mammary gland and the underlying mechanisms. Moreover, understanding the potential for nutrients to reverse adverse environmental effects on epigenetic determinants of health vs. disease is one of the pillars of primary breast cancer prevention.

Epigenetic Influence of Nutrients on Breast Cancer Risk

Early-life developmental time-windows of vulnerability offer some explanation for the apparent lack of association between adult diet and breast cancer risk. Diet during adult life may indeed not be the best predictor of breast cancer risk; it is not a period of particular increased epigenetic vulnerability or epigenetic reprogramming. In a PubMed database review of all prospective studies that relate candidate nutrient factors to the incidence of breast cancer or to gene-diet interactions, no correlation could be drawn between risk of developing breast cancer and any particular dietary factor considered in the search, including adolescent diet, fat intake, consumption of fruit and vegetables, antioxidant vitamins A, C, E, and β-carotene, dairy products (including vitamin D), soy products and isoflavones, green tea, heterocyclic amines, and carbohydrates, glycemic index and glycemic load [174]. To date, only the avoidance of postmenopausal weight gain and limiting the consumption of alcohol in adulthood are considered by international public health organizations to be associated with reduced breast cancer risk [175]. Certain foods or nutrient factors may, nevertheless, have a protective effect against breast cancer by virtue of their ability to preserve or restore epigenetic modifications that are associated with development and maintenance of normal tissue architecture, namely apical polarity. In the next few paragraphs we highlight some of the nutrients that have been shown to influence the epigenome of the breast.

Folate is an essential micronutrient found naturally in beef liver, green vegetables, peas, nuts, and beans and that can be supplemented in food as the synthetic product, folic acid. It is critical to proper methylation of DNA and histones because it transfers methyl-moieties and regulates many of the enzymes used in one-carbon metabolism reactions in the cell. Folate regulates DNA methyltransferases which maintain methylation (DNMT1) and establish *de novo* methylation (DNMT3a and DNMT3b) [176]. Dietary folate deficiency causes global hypomethylation of DNA, which is a hallmark, and early event, of all cancers [177]. This type of hypomethylation leads to genomic instability and impaired DNA repair [178]. Folate deficiency paradoxically also causes early hypermethylation of promoters on specific genes [179]. With the advent of mandatory folic acid (the synthetic form of folate) fortification of wheat flour products in North America in 1998, aimed at reducing neural tube defects in light of the seriously deficient folate status of much of the population at that time, excessive folic acid in the diet has now become a concern [180]. Ominously, dietary supplementation of folic acid to pregnant rats, at a level selected to represent the likely average post-fortification total folate intake in North American populations taking multivitamins (including prenatal), caused hypomethylation of DNA and increased mammary tumors in the offspring. Similar effects were seen in mammary glands of rats in the same study that received folic acid supplement only during prepuberty; these rats had increased mammary tumors and decreased DNMT1 activity [181]. At present, there is no information concerning the effect of maternal folic acid supplementation on breast cancer risk in humans. However, a retrospective evaluation of cervical biopsies comparing samples obtained in the post- to those from the prefolic acid fortification period in Canada revealed an increase in a histone modification that, in this study, was associated with higher grades of cervical cancer, H3K9me2. Even in biopsies of normal tissue H3K9me2 was higher after the fortification was instituted than before [182]. This finding implies that supplementation of synthetic folic acid may influence epigenetic marks linked to cancer even ahead of time in cancer-free women. Similar studies are necessary to evaluate histone modifications as well as DNA methylation in breast tissue under various nutrient conditions and during different time-windows of increased vulnerability to epigenetic remodeling.

Soya is one of the most studied of food ingredients known to be associated with breast cancer prevention and to have epigenetic effects that are passed to the next generation. Although epidemiological studies are not clear-cut, in Asian countries with high soya intake, breast cancer incidence is reduced compared to populations where soya intake is lower, and intake during childhood especially is associated with reduced breast cancer risk in both pre- and postmenopausal women [183, 184]. In mice, transgenerational epigenetic effects of soya were confirmed when maternal dietary genistein (the active ingredient of soya) induced increased methylation of the Agouti gene in the offspring, producing a visible coat-color pattern. The methylation status of the Agouti gene is conveniently linked to other methylation-responsive genes in mice that are associated with lower cancer risk [185]. A key signaling pathway that regulates progenitor cells, Wnt/β-catenin, responds to soy and genistein, and it has been suggested that early life exposure may affect the epigenetic regulation of this pathway during differentiation of progenitor cells in the breast [2, 186]. Unequivocal evidence of epigenetic response by the breast tissue to soya intake in humans has been observed in the ductal lavage of breast cancer-free premenopausal women revealing DNA hypermethylation in the promoters of two genes associated with proliferation regulation in mammary epithelial cells, *RARβ2* coding for the retinoic acid receptor β2 and *CCND2* coding for cyclin D2 [187].

There have been many studies over the decades to find a causal link between breast cancer risk and dietary fats, but the conclusions have been mixed. The issue is that both the increased energy intake and the resultant adiposity that occur along with an increased fat intake are distinct entities and are impossible to separate experimentally in humans. To assess only the variable of increased dietary fat, the total energy of the control diet has to be increased to the same level as that in the high-fat diet. In rodent studies, where these variables can be controlled, a high-fat diet is consistently shown to promote increased incidence of chemically-induced mammary tumors [188]. It has been pointed out that the difference in dietary fat intake between low-fat and high-fat consuming individuals is relatively small in North America and may contribute to undetected differences between diets in humans that are linked to breast cancer risk in rodents, such as cancer-protection by ω3 fatty acids and cancer promotion by ω6 fatty acids [189]. Worldwide epidemiology studies are needed that span the global diversity of dietary fat intake in order to identify the link(s) to breast cancer risk. Interestingly, ω6 fatty acid arachidonic acid disrupts apical polarity in breast acini in 3D culture [190].

Another confounding factor is that dietary fats are a heterogeneous collection of many different classes of lipids, and individual lipids can have an assortment of functionally distinct stereoisomers. Besides serving as backbone building blocks for complex macromolecules and organelles in the cell, many fats also act as signaling molecules for several cell processes. There is a lack of research on the effect of dietary fat or of individual lipid species on the epigenome of the mammary epithelial cells per se; yet, an epigenetic relationship with breast cancer risk is suggested by the transgenerational effects of dietary fat and specific fats in rodents. Increased proliferation and density in normal mammary epithelium of rats occurs after exposure to a maternal high-fat diet [191]. DNA hypomethylation of the ER gene in normal mammary tissue is associated with increased mammary tumors in rats exposed to maternal high-fat diets [192]. Increased of mammary tumor incidence also occurs in rats that received high maternal levels of a specific single fatty acid, ω6 linoleic acid [193]. Studies like these, showing an impact of maternal diet on the offspring's cancer risk, support a link between breast cancer risk and epigenetic response to dietary fats. A decrease in breast cancer risk related to the type of dietary fat has been shown to depend on the timing of the exposure in rats, further suggesting an epigenetic influence. Prepubertal consumption of ω3 fatty acids and of ω7 fatty acid conjugated linoleic acid (CLA) by rats later reduces tumor incidence [193, 194]. Recently, we observed that the c-9, t-11 isomer of CLA affects acinar differentiation and formation of apical polarity as well as certain histone modifications differently depending on the timing of its supplementation to the cell culture medium of non-neoplastic mammary epithelial cells (i.e., immature vs. mature or differentiated epithelium) (Lelièvre laboratory, unpublished results). Cell culture studies that employ the 3D culture method recapitulating the epigenetic mechanism-driven differentiation of the human mammary epithelium that occurs in the body are a convenient method to help decipher the timing and epigenetic response to dietary fats that impact breast cancer risk [195].

Vitamin D, 1,25 $(OH)_2D$, is a lipid-based molecule which, besides its conventional role in calcium homeostasis, has been linked to breast cancer protection in epidemiologic as well as animal studies [196]. The possibility of vitamin D influence on the epigenome is drawn from the regulation of its actions through vitamin D receptor-mediated control of gene transcription [197]; mice lacking the vitamin D receptor have increased mammary gland proliferation and mammary tumors [198]. However, the epigenetic connection between vitamin D and breast cancer risk remains to be established.

Carotenoids, which include vitamin A, are another family of lipids that, like dietary fats, encompasses a variety of compounds and thus, would be expected to have differential effects on both the epigenome and breast cancer risk. The genes for two tumor suppressors against breast cancer, *RARβ2* in non-neoplastic MCF10A mammary cells and glutathione S-transferase P1 (*GSTP1*) in breast cancer cells, are demethylated by the carotenoid, lycopene, epigenetically promoting their expression [199]. This observation supports earlier work demonstrating that women who subsequently developed breast cancer had displayed a lower serum level of β-carotene and lycopene compared to women who remained breast cancer-free [200]. A first-time longitudinal study reporting repeated measurements over six years revealed both α-carotene and β-carotene associations with reduced incidence of breast cancer. On the other hand, in that same study, γ-tocopherol was associated with increased risk of breast cancer [201]. Like for vitamin D, research on the epigenetic effects of these molecules is warranted.

Overall the influence of diet on the epigenome, notably in early stages of development with strong involvement of stem cells, cannot be ignored when studying breast cancer risk. As a review of the literature highlights, some nutrients are particularly associated with risk for certain forms of breast cancer while other nutrients are protective, yet only in certain situations or life stages [2]. To clearly classify environmental impacts, cell culture models that mimic the mammary gland in terms of cell-type specific developmental interactions necessary for tissue architecture maintenance will be needed. Ultimately, a combination of models from real tissue and 3D culture will enable the identification of pathways and cell types involved in the risk of developing the different classes of breast cancer.

Conclusion

In this chapter, we have emphasized the importance of mammary stem cells, tissue architecture and the interplay between the nucleus and the ECM in the control of chromatin structure and gene transcription during normal mammary gland development. One of the research directions to further decipher the gene-environment relationship in the context of disease risk is the development of models of risk for laboratory investigation. The fact that different factors of breast cancer risk are related to tissue architecture (e.g., tissue polarity, cell density) warrants working in tissue context when investigating mechanisms that promote or prevent tumor onset. Studies in animal models have yielded unparalleled insights into the cellular and epigenetic aspects of normal mammary gland development and breast cancer; however, there are limitations in fully mimicking the human neoplastic disease with such models. Three-dimensional cell culture models that recapitulate phenotypically normal breast acini *in vivo* are very useful alternatives to animal models, and cultures of such acini have proven to be very useful for the understanding of the control of tissue architecture over cell behavior. Yet, it is important to remember that in the breast epithelium, acini are connected to the branching mammary duct system via the terminal ducts that are the site of the mammary stem cell niche and where most tumors form. Therefore, the next wave of 3D cell culture models to investigate breast cancer onset is on its way [195, 202]. It is based on microengineering and microfabrication technologies used to create "organs-on-a-chip" that better mimic the microstructure and biomechanical functionalities of tissues. Major challenges in building these new breast ductal models are to integrate mammary stem and progenitor cells in appropriate proportions as well as different components of the stroma. The relation between genes and the environment is most critical to modulate cancer risk, therefore new technologies that permit the study of the epigenome on per cell type basis, like those developed for microscopy [203], will provide the necessary tools to readily decipher the link between cell type, epigenetic impact and environmental influence.

Acknowledgments

We thank Dr. Pierre-Alexandre Vidi for help with the preparation of some of the figures and Tracy A. Bender for preparation of the manuscript. We acknowledge support from a Unesco-L'Oreal fellowship (to DB), the National Institutes of Health (CA171704 to SAL), the Purdue Discovery Park Oncological Sciences Center and Center for Cancer Research. SAL and RT are members of the International Breast Cancer & Nutrition (IBCN) collaboration.

References

[1] Ferlay J, Shin HR, Bray F, Forman D, Mathers C, Parkin DM. GLOBOCAN 2008 v2.0, Cancer Incidence and Mortality Worldwide: IARC CancerBase No. 10 [Internet]. Lyon, France: International Agency for Research on Cancer; 2010 [cited 2013 08/01]; Available from: *http://globocan.iarc.fr.*

[2] Teegarden D, Romieu I, Lelièvre SA. Redefining the impact of nutrition on breast cancer incidence: is epigenetics involved? *Nutrition research reviews.* 2012;25(1):68-95.

[3] Bissell MJ, Radisky DC, Rizki A, Weaver VM, Petersen OW. The organizing principle: microenvironmental influences in the normal and malignant breast. *Differentiation; research in biological diversity.* 2002;70(9-10):537-46.

[4] Runswick SK, O'Hare MJ, Jones L, Streuli CH, Garrod DR. Desmosomal adhesion regulates epithelial morphogenesis and cell positioning. *Nature cell biology.* 2001;3(9):823-30.

[5] Chanson L, Brownfield D, Garbe JC, Kuhn I, Stampfer MR, Bissell MJ, et al. Self-organization is a dynamic and lineage-intrinsic property of mammary epithelial cells. *Proceedings of the National Academy of Sciences of the United States of America.* 2011;108(8):3264-9.

[6] Taddei I, Faraldo MM, Teuliere J, Deugnier MA, Thiery JP, Glukhova MA. Integrins in mammary gland development and differentiation of mammary epithelium. *Journal of mammary gland biology and neoplasia.* 2003;8(4):383-94.

[7] Gudjonsson T, Adriance MC, Sternlicht MD, Petersen OW, Bissell MJ. Myoepithelial cells: their origin and function in breast morphogenesis and neoplasia. *Journal of mammary gland biology and neoplasia.* 2005;10(3):261-72.

[8] Sheetz MP. Cell control by membrane-cytoskeleton adhesion. *Nature reviews Molecular cell biology.* 2001;2(5):392-6.

[9] Fata JE, Werb Z, Bissell MJ. Regulation of mammary gland branching morphogenesis by the extracellular matrix and its remodeling enzymes. *Breast cancer research : BCR.* 2004;6(1):1-11.

[10] Clarke RB, Spence K, Anderson E, Howell A, Okano H, Potten CS. A putative human breast stem cell population is enriched for steroid receptor-positive cells. *Developmental biology.* 2005;277(2):443-56.

[11] Gudjonsson T, Villadsen R, Nielsen HL, Ronnov-Jessen L, Bissell MJ, Petersen OW. Isolation, immortalization, and characterization of a human breast epithelial cell line with stem cell properties. *Genes & development.* 2002;16(6):693-706.

[12] Villadsen R, Fridriksdottir AJ, Ronnov-Jessen L, Gudjonsson T, Rank F, LaBarge MA, et al. Evidence for a stem cell hierarchy in the adult human breast. *The Journal of cell biology.* 2007;177(1):87-101.

[13] Fridriksdottir AJ, Petersen OW, Ronnov-Jessen L. Mammary gland stem cells: current status and future challenges. *The International journal of developmental biology.* 2011;55(7-9):719-29.

[14] Topper YJ, Freeman CS. Multiple hormone interactions in the developmental biology of the mammary gland. *Physiological reviews.* 1980;60(4):1049-106.

[15] Gusterson BA, Warburton MJ, Mitchell D, Ellison M, Neville AM, Rudland PS. Distribution of myoepithelial cells and basement membrane proteins in the normal breast and in benign and malignant breast diseases. *Cancer research.* 1982;42(11):4763-70.

[16] Streuli CH, Bailey N, Bissell MJ. Control of mammary epithelial differentiation: basement membrane induces tissue-specific gene expression in the absence of cell-cell interaction and morphological polarity. *The Journal of cell biology.* 1991;115(5):1383-95.

[17] Lelièvre SA, Weaver VM, Nickerson JA, Larabell CA, Bhaumik A, Petersen OW, et al. Tissue phenotype depends on reciprocal interactions between the extracellular matrix and the structural organization of the nucleus. *Proceedings of the National Academy of Sciences of the United States of America.* 1998;95(25):14711-6.

[18] Plachot C, Lelièvre SA. DNA methylation control of tissue polarity and cellular differentiation in the mammary epithelium. *Experimental cell research.* 2004;298(1):122-32.

[19] Lu P, Weaver VM, Werb Z. The extracellular matrix: a dynamic niche in cancer progression. *The Journal of cell biology.* 2012;196(4):395-406.

[20] Navarrete MA, Maier CM, Falzoni R, Quadros LG, Lima GR, Baracat EC, et al. Assessment of the proliferative, apoptotic and cellular renovation indices of the human mammary epithelium during the follicular and luteal phases of the menstrual cycle. *Breast cancer research : BCR.* 2005;7(3):R306-13.

[21] Asselin-Labat ML, Sutherland KD, Barker H, Thomas R, Shackleton M, Forrest NC, et al. Gata-3 is an essential regulator of mammary-gland

morphogenesis and luminal-cell differentiation. *Nature cell biology*. 2007;9(2):201-9.

[22] Buono KD, Robinson GW, Martin C, Shi S, Stanley P, Tanigaki K, et al. The canonical Notch/RBP-J signaling pathway controls the balance of cell lineages in mammary epithelium during pregnancy. *Developmental biology*. 2006;293(2):565-80.

[23] Neville MC, Medina D, Monks J, Hovey RC. The mammary fat pad. *Journal of mammary gland biology and neoplasia*. 1998;3(2):109-16.

[24] Djonov V, Andres AC, Ziemiecki A. Vascular remodelling during the normal and malignant life cycle of the mammary gland. *Microscopy research and technique*. 2001;52(2):182-9.

[25] Russo J, Russo IH. Development of the human breast. *Maturitas*. 2004;49(1):2-15.

[26] Kobayashi S, Sugiura H, Ando Y, Shiraki N, Yanagi T, Yamashita H, et al. *Reproductive history and breast cancer risk. Breast cancer*. 2012;19(4):302-8.

[27] MacMahon B, Cole P, Lin TM, Lowe CR, Mirra AP, Ravnihar B, et al. Age at first birth and breast cancer risk. *Bulletin of the World Health Organization*. 1970;43(2):209-21.

[28] Russo J, Lynch H, Russo IH. Mammary gland architecture as a determining factor in the susceptibility of the human breast to cancer. *The breast journal*. 2001;7(5):278-91.

[29] Russo J, Moral R, Balogh GA, Mailo D, Russo IH. The protective role of pregnancy in breast cancer. *Breast cancer research : BCR*. 2005;7(3):131-42.

[30] Bissell MJ, Kenny PA, Radisky DC. Microenvironmental regulators of tissue structure and function also regulate tumor induction and progression: the role of extracellular matrix and its degrading enzymes. *Cold Spring Harbor symposia on quantitative biology*. 2005;70:343-56.

[31] Xu R, Boudreau A, Bissell MJ. Tissue architecture and function: dynamic reciprocity via extra- and intra-cellular matrices. *Cancer metastasis reviews*. 2009;28(1-2):167-76.

[32] Mao Y, Keller ET, Garfield DH, Shen K, Wang J. Stromal cells in tumor microenvironment and breast cancer. *Cancer metastasis reviews*. 2013;32(1-2):303-15.

[33] Bergamaschi A, Tagliabue E, Sorlie T, Naume B, Triulzi T, Orlandi R, et al. Extracellular matrix signature identifies breast cancer subgroups with different clinical outcome. *The Journal of pathology*. 2008;214(3):357-67.

[34] Finak G, Bertos N, Pepin F, Sadekova S, Souleimanova M, Zhao H, et al. Stromal gene expression predicts clinical outcome in breast cancer. *Nature medicine*. 2008;14(5):518-27.

[35] Assi V, Warwick J, Cuzick J, Duffy SW. Clinical and epidemiological issues in mammographic density. *Nature reviews Clinical oncology*. 2012;9(1):33-40.

[36] Boyd NF, Martin LJ, Yaffe MJ, Minkin S. Mammographic density and breast cancer risk: current understanding and future prospects. *Breast cancer research : BCR*. 2011;13(6):223.

[37] Ghosh K, Brandt KR, Reynolds C, Scott CG, Pankratz VS, Riehle DL, et al. Tissue composition of mammographically dense and non-dense breast tissue. *Breast cancer research and treatment*. 2012;131(1):267-75.

[38] Martin LJ, Boyd NF. Mammographic density. Potential mechanisms of breast cancer risk associated with mammographic density: hypotheses based on epidemiological evidence. *Breast cancer research : BCR*. 2008;10(1):201.

[39] Yang XR, Chang-Claude J, Goode EL, Couch FJ, Nevanlinna H, Milne RL, et al. Associations of breast cancer risk factors with tumor subtypes: a pooled analysis from the Breast Cancer Association Consortium studies. *Journal of the National Cancer Institute*. 2011;103(3):250-63.

[40] Lambe M, Johansson AL, Altman D, Eloranta S. Mastitis and the risk of breast cancer. *Epidemiology*. 2009;20(5):747-51.

[41] Takkouche B, Regueira-Mendez C, Etminan M. Breast cancer and use of nonsteroidal anti-inflammatory drugs: a meta-analysis. *Journal of the National Cancer Institute*. 2008;100(20):1439-47.

[42] Chandramouly G, Abad PC, Knowles DW, Lelièvre SA. The control of tissue architecture over nuclear organization is crucial for epithelial cell fate. *Journal of cell science*. 2007;120(Pt 9):1596-606.

[43] Maxwell CA, Benitez J, Gomez-Baldo L, Osorio A, Bonifaci N, Fernandez-Ramires R, et al. Interplay between BRCA1 and RHAMM regulates epithelial apicobasal polarization and may influence risk of breast cancer. *PLoS biology*. 2011;9(11):e1001199.

[44] Roarty K, Rosen JM. Wnt and mammary stem cells: hormones cannot fly wingless. *Current opinion in pharmacology*. 2010;10(6):643-9.

[45] Peppercorn J, Perou CM, Carey LA. Molecular subtypes in breast cancer evaluation and management: divide and conquer. *Cancer investigation*. 2008;26(1):1-10.

[46] Sotiriou C, Neo SY, McShane LM, Korn EL, Long PM, Jazaeri A, et al. Breast cancer classification and prognosis based on gene expression profiles from a population-based study. *Proceedings of the National Academy of Sciences of the United States of America.* 2003;100(18):10393-8.

[47] Perou CM, Borresen-Dale AL. Systems biology and genomics of breast cancer. *Cold Spring Harbor perspectives in biology*. 2011;3(2).

[48] Sorlie T, Perou CM, Tibshirani R, Aas T, Geisler S, Johnsen H, et al. Gene expression patterns of breast carcinomas distinguish tumor subclasses with clinical implications. *Proceedings of the National Academy of Sciences of the United States of America.* 2001;98(19):10869-74.

[49] Holm K, Hegardt C, Staaf J, Vallon-Christersson J, Jonsson G, Olsson H, et al. Molecular subtypes of breast cancer are associated with characteristic DNA methylation patterns. *Breast cancer research : BCR.* 2010;12(3):R36.

[50] Polyak K. Breast cancer: origins and evolution. *The Journal of clinical investigation*. 2007;117(11):3155-63.

[51] Bediaga NG, Acha-Sagredo A, Guerra I, Viguri A, Albaina C, Ruiz Diaz I, et al. DNA methylation epigenotypes in breast cancer molecular subtypes. *Breast cancer research : BCR.* 2010;12(5):R77.

[52] Millikan RC, Newman B, Tse CK, Moorman PG, Conway K, Dressler LG, et al. Epidemiology of basal-like breast cancer. *Breast cancer research and treatment.* 2008;109(1):123-39.

[53] Molyneux G, Smalley MJ. The cell of origin of BRCA1 mutation-associated breast cancer: a cautionary tale of gene expression profiling. *Journal of mammary gland biology and neoplasia.* 2011;16(1):51-5.

[54] Narod SA, Foulkes WD. BRCA1 and BRCA2: 1994 and beyond. *Nature reviews Cancer*. 2004;4(9):665-76.

[55] Prise KM, Saran A. Concise review: stem cell effects in radiation risk. *Stem cells*. 2011;29(9):1315-21.

[56] Dupont C, Armant DR, Brenner CA. Epigenetics: definition, mechanisms and clinical perspective. *Seminars in reproductive medicine*. 2009;27(5):351-7.

[57] Waddington CH. The epigenotype. *Endeavour*. 1942;1:18-20.

[58] Berger SL. The complex language of chromatin regulation during transcription. *Nature*. 2007;447(7143):407-12.

[59] Lelièvre SA. Tissue polarity-dependent control of mammary epithelial homeostasis and cancer development: an epigenetic perspective. *Journal of mammary gland biology and neoplasia.* 2010;15(1):49-63.

[60] Rijnkels M, Kabotyanski E, Montazer-Torbati MB, Hue Beauvais C, Vassetzky Y, Rosen JM, et al. The epigenetic landscape of mammary gland development and functional differentiation. *Journal of mammary gland biology and neoplasia.* 2010;15(1):85-100.

[61] Wang GG, Allis CD, Chi P. Chromatin remodeling and cancer, Part II: ATP-dependent chromatin remodeling. *Trends in molecular medicine.* 2007;13(9):373-80.

[62] Wang GG, Allis CD, Chi P. Chromatin remodeling and cancer, Part I: Covalent histone modifications. *Trends in molecular medicine.* 2007;13(9):363-72.

[63] Guttman M, Rinn JL. Modular regulatory principles of large non-coding RNAs. *Nature.* 2012;482(7385):339-46.

[64] Bloushtain-Qimron N, Yao J, Shipitsin M, Maruyama R, Polyak K. Epigenetic patterns of embryonic and adult stem cells. *Cell cycle.* 2009;8(6):809-17.

[65] Daxinger L, Whitelaw E. Transgenerational epigenetic inheritance: more questions than answers. *Genome research.* 2010;20(12):1623-8.

[66] Jones PA, Liang G. Rethinking how DNA methylation patterns are maintained. *Nature reviews Genetics.* 2009;10(11):805-11.

[67] Reddington JP, Pennings S, Meehan RR. Non-canonical functions of the DNA methylome in gene regulation. *The Biochemical journal.* 2013;451(1):13-23.

[68] Auclair G, Weber M. Mechanisms of DNA methylation and demethylation in mammals. *Biochimie.* 2012;94(11):2202-11.

[69] Bird A. DNA methylation patterns and epigenetic memory. *Genes & development.* 2002;16(1):6-21.

[70] Kinney SR, Pradhan S. Regulation of expression and activity of DNA (cytosine-5) methyltransferases in mammalian cells. *Progress in molecular biology and translational science.* 2011;101:311-33.

[71] Song J, Teplova M, Ishibe-Murakami S, Patel DJ. Structure-based mechanistic insights into DNMT1-mediated maintenance DNA methylation. *Science.* 2012;335(6069):709-12.

[72] Luger K, Mader AW, Richmond RK, Sargent DF, Richmond TJ. Crystal structure of the nucleosome core particle at 2.8 A resolution. *Nature.* 1997;389(6648):251-60.

[73] Turner BM. The adjustable nucleosome: an epigenetic signaling module. *Trends in genetics : TIG*. 2012;28(9):436-44.

[74] Kouzarides T. Chromatin modifications and their function. *Cell*. 2007;128(4):693-705.

[75] Sharma S, Kelly TK, Jones PA. Epigenetics in cancer. *Carcinogenesis*. 2010;31(1):27-36.

[76] Bartova E, Krejci J, Harnicarova A, Galiova G, Kozubek S. Histone modifications and nuclear architecture: a review. *The journal of histochemistry and cytochemistry : official journal of the Histochemistry Society*. 2008;56(8):711-21.

[77] Vire E, Brenner C, Deplus R, Blanchon L, Fraga M, Didelot C, et al. The Polycomb group protein EZH2 directly controls DNA methylation. *Nature*. 2006;439(7078):871-4.

[78] Jenuwein T, Allis CD. Translating the histone code. *Science*. 2001;293(5532):1074-80.

[79] Elsheikh SE, Green AR, Rakha EA, Powe DG, Ahmed RA, Collins HM, et al. Global histone modifications in breast cancer correlate with tumor phenotypes, prognostic factors, and patient outcome. *Cancer research*. 2009;69(9):3802-9.

[80] Tokunaga M, Norman JE, Jr., Asano M, Tokuoka S, Ezaki H, Nishimori I, et al. Malignant breast tumors among atomic bomb survivors, Hiroshima and Nagasaki, 1950-74. *Journal of the National Cancer Institute*. 1979;62(6):1347-59.

[81] Haffty BG, Lee C. Exposure to diagnostic levels of radiation prior to age 30 increases the risk of breast cancer in BRCA1/2 carriers. *Evidence-based medicine*. 2013;18(4):e40.

[82] Espada J, Esteller M. Mouse models in epigenetics: insights in development and disease. *Briefings in functional genomics*. 2013;12(3):279-87.

[83] Shackleton M, Vaillant F, Simpson KJ, Stingl J, Smyth GK, Asselin-Labat ML, et al. Generation of a functional mammary gland from a single stem cell. *Nature*. 2006;439(7072):84-8.

[84] Shipitsin M, Campbell LL, Argani P, Weremowicz S, Bloushtain-Qimron N, Yao J, et al. Molecular definition of breast tumor heterogeneity. *Cancer cell*. 2007;11(3):259-73.

[85] Stingl J, Eirew P, Ricketson I, Shackleton M, Vaillant F, Choi D, et al. Purification and unique properties of mammary epithelial stem cells. *Nature*. 2006;439(7079):993-7.

[86] Huang TH, Esteller M. Chromatin remodeling in mammary gland differentiation and breast tumorigenesis. *Cold Spring Harbor perspectives in biology.* 2010;2(9):a004515.
[87] Visvader JE. Keeping abreast of the mammary epithelial hierarchy and breast tumorigenesis. *Genes & development.* 2009;23(22):2563-77.
[88] Al-Hajj M, Wicha MS, Benito-Hernandez A, Morrison SJ, Clarke MF. Prospective identification of tumorigenic breast cancer cells. *Proceedings of the National Academy of Sciences of the United States of America.* 2003;100(7):3983-8.
[89] Mani SA, Guo W, Liao MJ, Eaton EN, Ayyanan A, Zhou AY, et al. The epithelial-mesenchymal transition generates cells with properties of stem cells. *Cell.* 2008;133(4):704-15.
[90] Park SY, Lee HE, Li H, Shipitsin M, Gelman R, Polyak K. Heterogeneity for stem cell-related markers according to tumor subtype and histologic stage in breast cancer. *Clinical cancer research : an official journal of the American Association for Cancer Research.* 2010;16(3):876-87.
[91] Joshi PA, Di Grappa MA, Khokha R. Active allies: hormones, stem cells and the niche in adult mammopoiesis. *Trends in endocrinology and metabolism: TEM.* 2012;23(6):299-309.
[92] Laron Z, Pauli R, Pertzelan A. Clinical evidence on the role of estrogens in the development of the breasts. *Proc R Soc Edinburgh B1.* 1989;95:13-22.
[93] Bocchinfuso WP, Korach KS. Mammary gland development and tumorigenesis in estrogen receptor knockout mice. *Journal of mammary gland biology and neoplasia.* 1997;2(4):323-34.
[94] Jacquemier JD, Hassoun J, Torrente M, Martin PM. Distribution of estrogen and progesterone receptors in healthy tissue adjacent to breast lesions at various stages--immunohistochemical study of 107 cases. *Breast cancer research and treatment.* 1990;15(2):109-17.
[95] Petersen OW, Hoyer PE, van Deurs B. Frequency and distribution of estrogen receptor-positive cells in normal, nonlactating human breast tissue. *Cancer research.* 1987;47(21):5748-51.
[96] Speirs V, Skliris GP, Burdall SE, Carder PJ. Distinct expression patterns of ER alpha and ER beta in normal human mammary gland. *Journal of clinical pathology.* 2002;55(5):371-4.
[97] Russo J, Ao X, Grill C, Russo IH. Pattern of distribution of cells positive for estrogen receptor alpha and progesterone receptor in relation to

proliferating cells in the mammary gland. *Breast cancer research and treatment*. 1999;53(3):217-27.

[98] Ciarloni L, Mallepell S, Brisken C. Amphiregulin is an essential mediator of estrogen receptor alpha function in mammary gland development. *Proceedings of the National Academy of Sciences of the United States of America*. 2007;104(13):5455-60.

[99] McBryan J, Howlin J, Napoletano S, Martin F. Amphiregulin: role in mammary gland development and breast cancer. *Journal of mammary gland biology and neoplasia*. 2008;13(2):159-69.

[100] Key TJ, Pike MC. The role of oestrogens and progestagens in the epidemiology and prevention of breast cancer. *European journal of cancer & clinical oncology*. 1988;24(1):29-43.

[101] Luo J, Cochrane BB, Wactawski-Wende J, Hunt JR, Ockene JK, Margolis KL. Effects of menopausal hormone therapy on ductal carcinoma in situ of the breast. *Breast cancer research and treatment*. 2013;137(3):915-25.

[102] Anderson E. The role of oestrogen and progesterone receptors in human mammary development and tumorigenesis. *Breast cancer research : BCR*. 2002;4(5):197-201.

[103] Stingl J. Estrogen and progesterone in normal mammary gland development and in cancer. *Hormones & cancer*. 2011;2(2):85-90.

[104] Joshi PA, Jackson HW, Beristain AG, Di Grappa MA, Mote PA, Clarke CL, et al. Progesterone induces adult mammary stem cell expansion. *Nature*. 2010;465(7299):803-7.

[105] Kelsey JL, Gammon MD, John EM. Reproductive factors and breast cancer. *Epidemiologic reviews*. 1993;15(1):36-47.

[106] Bloushtain-Qimron N, Yao J, Snyder EL, Shipitsin M, Campbell LL, Mani SA, et al. Cell type-specific DNA methylation patterns in the human breast. *Proceedings of the National Academy of Sciences of the United States of America*. 2008;105(37):14076-81.

[107] Reedijk M. Notch signaling and breast cancer. *Advances in experimental medicine and biology*. 2012;727:241-57.

[108] Foulkes WD. BRCA1 functions as a breast stem cell regulator. *Journal of medical genetics*. 2004;41(1):1-5.

[109] Liu S, Ginestier C, Charafe-Jauffret E, Foco H, Kleer CG, Merajver SD, et al. BRCA1 regulates human mammary stem/progenitor cell fate. *Proceedings of the National Academy of Sciences of the United States of America*. 2008;105(5):1680-5.

[110] Mann M, Cortez V, Vadlamudi RK. Epigenetics of Estrogen Receptor Signaling: Role in Hormonal Cancer Progression and Therapy. *Cancers.* 2011;3(3):1691-707.

[111] Asselin-Labat ML, Vaillant F, Sheridan JM, Pal B, Wu D, Simpson ER, et al. Control of mammary stem cell function by steroid hormone signalling. *Nature.* 2010;465(7299):798-802.

[112] Bernstein BE, Mikkelsen TS, Xie X, Kamal M, Huebert DJ, Cuff J, et al. A bivalent chromatin structure marks key developmental genes in embryonic stem cells. *Cell.* 2006;125(2):315-26.

[113] Schubeler D, MacAlpine DM, Scalzo D, Wirbelauer C, Kooperberg C, van Leeuwen F, et al. The histone modification pattern of active genes revealed through genome-wide chromatin analysis of a higher eukaryote. *Genes & development.* 2004;18(11):1263-71.

[114] Maruyama R, Choudhury S, Kowalczyk A, Bessarabova M, Beresford-Smith B, Conway T, et al. Epigenetic regulation of cell type-specific expression patterns in the human mammary epithelium. *PLoS genetics.* 2011;7(4):e1001369.

[115] Ferguson JE, Schor AM, Howell A, Ferguson MW. Changes in the extracellular matrix of the normal human breast during the menstrual cycle. *Cell and tissue research.* 1992;268(1):167-77.

[116] Lelièvre SA. Contributions of extracellular matrix signaling and tissue architecture to nuclear mechanisms and spatial organization of gene expression control. *Biochimica et biophysica acta.* 2009;1790(9):925-35.

[117] McCormack VA, dos Santos Silva I. Breast density and parenchymal patterns as markers of breast cancer risk: a meta-analysis. *Cancer epidemiology, biomarkers & prevention : a publication of the American Association for Cancer Research, cosponsored by the American Society of Preventive Oncology.* 2006;15(6):1159-69.

[118] Alowami S, Troup S, Al-Haddad S, Kirkpatrick I, Watson PH. Mammographic density is related to stroma and stromal proteoglycan expression. *Breast cancer research : BCR.* 2003;5(5):R129-35.

[119] Li T, Sun L, Miller N, Nicklee T, Woo J, Hulse-Smith L, et al. The association of measured breast tissue characteristics with mammographic density and other risk factors for breast cancer. *Cancer epidemiology, biomarkers & prevention : a publication of the American Association for Cancer Research, cosponsored by the American Society of Preventive Oncology. 2005;*14(2):343-9.

[120] Bartow SA, Mettler FA, Black WC. Correlations between radiographic patterns and morphology of the female breast. *Rad Patterns Morph.* 1997;13:263-75.

[121] Bland KI, Kuhns JG, Buchanan JB, Dwyer PA, Heuser LF, O'Connor CA, et al. A clinicopathologic correlation of mammographic parenchymal patterns and associated risk factors for human mammary carcinoma. *Annals of surgery*. 1982;195(5):582-94.

[122] Bright RA, Morrison AS, Brisson J, Burstein NA, Sadowsky NS, Kopans DB, et al. Relationship between mammographic and histologic features of breast tissue in women with benign biopsies. *Cancer*. 1988;61(2):266-71.

[123] Urbanski S, Jensen HM, Cooke G, McFarlane D, Shannon P, Kruikov V, et al. The association of histological and radiological indicators of breast cancer risk. *British journal of cancer*. 1988;58(4):474-9.

[124] Wellings SR, Wolfe JN. Correlative studies of the histological and radiographic appearance of the breast parenchyma. *Radiology*. 1978;129(2):299-306.

[125] Paszek MJ, Zahir N, Johnson KR, Lakins JN, Rozenberg GI, Gefen A, et al. Tensional homeostasis and the malignant phenotype. *Cancer cell*. 2005;8(3):241-54.

[126] Wozniak MA, Desai R, Solski PA, Der CJ, Keely PJ. ROCK-generated contractility regulates breast epithelial cell differentiation in response to the physical properties of a three-dimensional collagen matrix. *The Journal of cell biology*. 2003;163(3):583-95.

[127] Allinen M, Beroukhim R, Cai L, Brennan C, Lahti-Domenici J, Huang H, et al. Molecular characterization of the tumor microenvironment in breast cancer. *Cancer cell*. 2004;6(1):17-32.

[128] Bavik C, Coleman I, Dean JP, Knudsen B, Plymate S, Nelson PS. The gene expression program of prostate fibroblast senescence modulates neoplastic epithelial cell proliferation through paracrine mechanisms. *Cancer research*. 2006;66(2):794-802.

[129] Chung LW, Baseman A, Assikis V, Zhau HE. Molecular insights into prostate cancer progression: the missing link of tumor microenvironment. *The Journal of urology*. 2005;173(1):10-20.

[130] Orimo A, Gupta PB, Sgroi DC, Arenzana-Seisdedos F, Delaunay T, Naeem R, et al. Stromal fibroblasts present in invasive human breast carcinomas promote tumor growth and angiogenesis through elevated SDF-1/CXCL12 secretion. *Cell*. 2005;121(3):335-48.

[131] Kress C, Ballester M, Devinoy E, Rijnkels M. Epigenetic modifications in 3D: nuclear organization of the differentiating mammary epithelial cell. *Journal of mammary gland biology and neoplasia.* 2010;15(1):73-83.

[132] Martens JH, O'Sullivan RJ, Braunschweig U, Opravil S, Radolf M, Steinlein P, et al. The profile of repeat-associated histone lysine methylation states in the mouse epigenome. *The EMBO journal.* 2005;24(4):800-12.

[133] Biron VL, McManus KJ, Hu N, Hendzel MJ, Underhill DA. Distinct dynamics and distribution of histone methyl-lysine derivatives in mouse development. *Developmental biology.* 2004;276(2):337-51.

[134] Arney KL, Fisher AG. Epigenetic aspects of differentiation. *Journal of cell science.* 2004;117(Pt 19):4355-63.

[135] Briand P, Petersen OW, Van Deurs B. A new diploid nontumorigenic human breast epithelial cell line isolated and propagated in chemically defined medium. *In vitro cellular & developmental biology : journal of the Tissue Culture Association.* 1987;23(3):181-8.

[136] Petersen OW, Ronnov-Jessen L, Howlett AR, Bissell MJ. Interaction with basement membrane serves to rapidly distinguish growth and differentiation pattern of normal and malignant human breast epithelial cells. *Proceedings of the National Academy of Sciences of the United States of America.* 1992;89(19):9064-8.

[137] Abad PC, Lewis J, Mian IS, Knowles DW, Sturgis J, Badve S, et al. NuMA influences higher order chromatin organization in human mammary epithelium. *Molecular biology of the cell.* 2007;18(2):348-61.

[138] Kaminker P, Plachot C, Kim SH, Chung P, Crippen D, Petersen OW, et al. Higher-order nuclear organization in growth arrest of human mammary epithelial cells: a novel role for telomere-associated protein TIN2. *Journal of cell science.* 2005;118(Pt 6):1321-30.

[139] Xu R, Spencer VA, Bissell MJ. Extracellular matrix-regulated gene expression requires cooperation of SWI/SNF and transcription factors. *The Journal of biological chemistry.* 2007;282(20):14992-9.

[140] Butcher DT, Alliston T, Weaver VM. A tense situation: forcing tumour progression. *Nature reviews Cancer.* 2009;9(2):108-22.

[141] Le Beyec J, Xu R, Lee SY, Nelson CM, Rizki A, Alcaraz J, et al. Cell shape regulates global histone acetylation in human mammary epithelial cells. *Experimental cell research.* 2007;313(14):3066-75.

[142] Brown KE, Baxter J, Graf D, Merkenschlager M, Fisher AG. Dynamic repositioning of genes in the nucleus of lymphocytes preparing for cell division. *Molecular cell.* 1999;3(2):207-17.

[143] Knowles DW, Sudar D, Bator-Kelly C, Bissell MJ, Lelièvre SA. Automated local bright feature image analysis of nuclear protein distribution identifies changes in tissue phenotype. *Proceedings of the National Academy of Sciences of the United States of America.* 2006;103(12):4445-50.

[144] Vidi PA, Chandramouly G, Gray M, Wang L, Liu E, Kim JJ, et al. Interconnected contribution of tissue morphogenesis and the nuclear protein NuMA to the DNA damage response. *Journal of cell science.* 2012;125(Pt 2):350-61.

[145] Bazzoun D, Lelièvre S, Talhouk R. Polarity proteins as regulators of cell junction complexes: implications for breast cancer. *Pharmacology & therapeutics.* 2013;138(3):418-27.

[146] Plachot C, Chaboub LS, Adissu HA, Wang L, Urazaev A, Sturgis J, et al. Factors necessary to produce basoapical polarity in human glandular epithelium formed in conventional and high-throughput three-dimensional culture: example of the breast epithelium. *BMC biology.* 2009;7:77.

[147] Konska G, Guillot J, De Latour M, Fonck Y. Expression of Tn antigen and N-acetyllactosamine residues in malignant and benign human breast tumors detected by lectins and monoclonal antibody 83D4. *International journal of oncology.* 1998;12(2):361-7.

[148] Guttman JA, Finlay BB. Tight junctions as targets of infectious agents. *Biochimica et biophysica acta.* 2009;1788(4):832-41.

[149] Talhouk RS, Mroue R, Mokalled M, Abi-Mosleh L, Nehme R, Ismail A, et al. Heterocellular interaction enhances recruitment of alpha and beta-catenins and ZO-2 into functional gap-junction complexes and induces gap junction-dependant differentiation of mammary epithelial cells. *Experimental cell research.* 2008;314(18):3275-91.

[150] Talhouk RS, Elble RC, Bassam R, Daher M, Sfeir A, Mosleh LA, et al. Developmental expression patterns and regulation of connexins in the mouse mammary gland: expression of connexin30 in lactogenesis. *Cell and tissue research.* 2005;319(1):49-59.

[151] Herve JC, Bourmeyster N, Sarrouilhe D. Diversity in protein-protein interactions of connexins: emerging roles. *Biochimica et biophysica acta.* 2004;1662(1-2):22-41.

[152] Sourisseau T, Georgiadis A, Tsapara A, Ali RR, Pestell R, Matter K, et al. Regulation of PCNA and cyclin D1 expression and epithelial morphogenesis by the ZO-1-regulated transcription factor ZONAB/DbpA. *Molecular and cellular biology*. 2006;26(6):2387-98.
[153] Huerta M, Munoz R, Tapia R, Soto-Reyes E, Ramirez L, Recillas-Targa F, et al. Cyclin D1 is transcriptionally down-regulated by ZO-2 via an E box and the transcription factor c-Myc. *Molecular biology of the cell.* 2007;18(12):4826-36.
[154] Dunn KL, Davie JR. Stimulation of the Ras-MAPK pathway leads to independent phosphorylation of histone H3 on serine 10 and 28. *Oncogene*. 2005;24(21):3492-502.
[155] Dunn KL, Espino PS, Drobic B, He S, Davie JR. The Ras-MAPK signal transduction pathway, cancer and chromatin remodeling. *Biochemistry and cell biology = Biochimie et biologie cellulaire*. 2005;83(1):1-14.
[156] Petit MM, Meulemans SM, Alen P, Ayoubi TA, Jansen E, Van de Ven WJ. The tumor suppressor Scrib interacts with the zyxin-related protein LPP, which shuttles between cell adhesion sites and the nucleus. *BMC cell biology*. 2005;6(1):1.
[157] Ishidate T, Matsumine A, Toyoshima K, Akiyama T. The APC-hDLG complex negatively regulates cell cycle progression from the G0/G1 to S phase. *Oncogene*. 2000;19(3):365-72.
[158] Kucharski R, Maleszka J, Foret S, Maleszka R. Nutritional control of reproductive status in honeybees via DNA methylation. *Science*. 2008;319(5871):1827-30.
[159] Burdge GC, Hanson MA, Slater-Jefferies JL, Lillycrop KA. Epigenetic regulation of transcription: a mechanism for inducing variations in phenotype (fetal programming) by differences in nutrition during early life? *The British journal of nutrition*. 2007;97(6):1036-46.
[160] Sinclair KD, Lea RG, Rees WD, Young LE. The developmental origins of health and disease: current theories and epigenetic mechanisms. *Society of Reproduction and Fertility supplement*. 2007;64:425-43.
[161] Reik W. Stability and flexibility of epigenetic gene regulation in mammalian development. *Nature*. 2007;447(7143):425-32.
[162] Cropley JE, Suter CM, Beckman KB, Martin DI. Germ-line epigenetic modification of the murine A vy allele by nutritional supplementation. *Proceedings of the National Academy of Sciences of the United States of America*. 2006;103(46):17308-12.
[163] Heijmans BT, Tobi EW, Stein AD, Putter H, Blauw GJ, Susser ES, et al. Persistent epigenetic differences associated with prenatal exposure to

famine in humans. *Proceedings of the National Academy of Sciences of the United States of America.* 2008;105(44):17046-9.

[164] Hemberger M, Dean W, Reik W. Epigenetic dynamics of stem cells and cell lineage commitment: digging Waddington's canal. Nature reviews *Molecular cell biology.* 2009;10(8):526-37.

[165] Nafee TM, Farrell WE, Carroll WD, Fryer AA, Ismail KM. Epigenetic control of fetal gene expression. *BJOG : an international journal of obstetrics and gynaecology.* 2008;115(2):158-68.

[166] Endogenous Hormones Breast Cancer Collaborative Group, Key TJ, Appleby PN, Reeves GK, Roddam AW. Insulin-like growth factor 1 (IGF1), IGF binding protein 3 (IGFBP3), and breast cancer risk: pooled individual data analysis of 17 prospective studies. *The lancet oncology.* 2010;11(6):530-42.

[167] Waterland RA, Kellermayer R, Laritsky E, Rayco-Solon P, Harris RA, Travisano M, et al. Season of conception in rural gambia affects DNA methylation at putative human metastable epialleles. *PLoS genetics.* 2010;6(12):e1001252.

[168] Steegers-Theunissen RP, Obermann-Borst SA, Kremer D, Lindemans J, Siebel C, Steegers EA, et al. Periconceptional maternal folic acid use of 400 microg per day is related to increased methylation of the IGF2 gene in the very young child. *PloS one*. 2009;4(11):e7845.

[169] Richly H, Aloia L, Di Croce L. Roles of the Polycomb group proteins in stem cells and cancer. *Cell death & disease.* 2011;2:e204.

[170] Ding L, Erdmann C, Chinnaiyan AM, Merajver SD, Kleer CG. Identification of EZH2 as a molecular marker for a precancerous state in morphologically normal breast tissues. *Cancer research.* 2006;66(8):4095-9.

[171] Weaver IC, Champagne FA, Brown SE, Dymov S, Sharma S, Meaney MJ, et al. Reversal of maternal programming of stress responses in adult offspring through methyl supplementation: altering epigenetic marking later in life. *The Journal of neuroscience : the official journal of the Society for Neuroscience.* 2005;25(47):11045-54.

[172] Guo JU, Su Y, Zhong C, Ming GL, Song H. Hydroxylation of 5-methylcytosine by TET1 promotes active DNA demethylation in the adult brain. Cell. 2011;145(3):423-34.

[173] Jirtle RL, Skinner MK. Environmental epigenomics and disease susceptibility. *Nature reviews Genetics.* 2007;8(4):253-62.

[174] Michels KB, Mohllajee AP, Roset-Bahmanyar E, Beehler GP, Moysich KB. Diet and breast cancer: a review of the prospective observational studies. *Cancer*. 2007;109(12 Suppl):2712-49.

[175] Boyle P, Levin B, International Agency for Research on Cancer., World Health Organization. *World cancer report 2008. Lyon, Geneva:* International Agency for Research on Cancer; Distributed by WHO Press; 2008. 510 p.

[176] Kim KC, Friso S, Choi SW. DNA methylation, an epigenetic mechanism connecting folate to healthy embryonic development and aging. *The Journal of nutritional biochemistry*. 2009;20(12):917-26.

[177] Wild L, Flanagan JM. Genome-wide hypomethylation in cancer may be a passive consequence of transformation. *Biochimica et biophysica acta.* 2010;1806(1):50-7.

[178] Wilson AS, Power BE, Molloy PL. DNA hypomethylation and human diseases. *Biochimica et biophysica acta.* 2007;1775(1):138-62.

[179] Crott JW, Liu Z, Keyes MK, Choi SW, Jang H, Moyer MP, et al. Moderate folate depletion modulates the expression of selected genes involved in cell cycle, intracellular signaling and folate uptake in human colonic epithelial cell lines. *The Journal of nutritional biochemistry.* 2008;19(5):328-35.

[180] Eichholzer M, Tonz O, Zimmermann R. Folic acid: a public-health challenge. *Lancet*. 2006;367(9519):1352-61.

[181] Ly A, Lee H, Chen J, Sie KK, Renlund R, Medline A, et al. Effect of maternal and postweaning folic acid supplementation on mammary tumor risk in the offspring. *Cancer research.* 2011;71(3):988-97.

[182] Piyathilake CJ, Macaluso M, Celedonio JE, Badiga S, Bell WC, Grizzle WE. Mandatory fortification with folic acid in the United States appears to have adverse effects on histone methylation in women with pre-cancer but not in women free of pre-cancer. *International journal of women's health.* 2010;1:131-7.

[183] Henderson BE, Bernstein L. The international variation in breast cancer rates: an epidemiological assessment. *Breast cancer research and treatment*. 1991;18 Suppl 1:S11-7.

[184] Korde LA, Wu AH, Fears T, Nomura AM, West DW, Kolonel LN, et al. Childhood soy intake and breast cancer risk in Asian American women. *Cancer epidemiology, biomarkers & prevention : a publication of the American Association for Cancer Research, cosponsored by the American Society of Preventive Oncology*. 2009;18(4):1050-9.

[185] Dolinoy DC, Weidman JR, Waterland RA, Jirtle RL. Maternal genistein alters coat color and protects Avy mouse offspring from obesity by modifying the fetal epigenome. *Environmental health perspectives.* 2006;114(4):567-72.

[186] Klarmann GJ, Decker A, Farrar WL. Epigenetic gene silencing in the Wnt pathway in breast cancer. Epigenetics : *official journal of the DNA Methylation Society*. 2008;3(2):59-63.

[187] Qin W, Zhu W, Shi H, Hewett JE, Ruhlen RL, MacDonald RS, et al. Soy isoflavones have an antiestrogenic effect and alter mammary promoter hypermethylation in healthy premenopausal women. *Nutrition and cancer.* 2009;61(2):238-44.

[188] Welsch CW. Dietary fat, calories, and mammary gland tumorigenesis. *Advances in experimental medicine and biology.* 1992;322:203-22.

[189] MacLennan M, Ma DW. Role of dietary fatty acids in mammary gland development and breast cancer. B*reast cancer research : BCR.* 2010;12(5):211.

[190] Yue S, Cardenas-Mora JM, Chaboub LS, Lelièvre SA, Cheng JX. Label-free analysis of breast tissue polarity by Raman imaging of lipid phase. *Biophysical journal.* 2012;102(5):1215-23.

[191] de Assis S, Wang M, Goel S, Foxworth A, Helferich W, Hilakivi-Clarke L. Excessive weight gain during pregnancy increases carcinogen-induced mammary tumorigenesis in Sprague-Dawley and lean and obese Zucker rats. *The Journal of nutrition.* 2006;136(4):998-1004.

[192] Yenbutr P, Hilakivi-Clarke L, Passaniti A. Hypomethylation of an exon I estrogen receptor CpG island in spontaneous and carcinogen-induced mammary tumorigenesis in the rat. *Mechanisms of ageing and development.* 1998;106(1-2):93-102.

[193] Hilakivi-Clarke L, Cho E, deAssis S, Olivo S, Ealley E, Bouker KB, et al. Maternal and prepubertal diet, mammary development and breast cancer risk. *The Journal of nutrition.* 2001;131(1):154S-7S.

[194] Ip C, Scimeca JA, Thompson H. Effect of timing and duration of dietary conjugated linoleic acid on mammary cancer prevention. *Nutrition and cancer.* 1995;24(3):241-7.

[195] Vidi PA, Bissell MJ, Lelièvre SA. Three-dimensional culture of human breast epithelial cells: the how and the why. *Methods in molecular biology.* 2013;945:193-219.

[196] Welsh J. Vitamin D and prevention of breast cancer. *Acta pharmacologica Sinica.* 2007;28(9):1373-82.

[197] Matthews D, LaPorta E, Zinser GM, Narvaez CJ, Welsh J. Genomic vitamin D signaling in breast cancer: Insights from animal models and human cells. *The Journal of steroid biochemistry and molecular biology*. 2010;121(1-2):362-7.

[198] Zinser GM, Suckow M, Welsh J. Vitamin D receptor (VDR) ablation alters carcinogen-induced tumorigenesis in mammary gland, epidermis and lymphoid tissues. *The Journal of steroid biochemistry and molecular biology*. 2005;97(1-2):153-64.

[199] King-Batoon A, Leszczynska JM, Klein CB. Modulation of gene methylation by genistein or lycopene in breast cancer cells. *Environmental and molecular mutagenesis*. 2008;49(1):36-45.

[200] Sato R, Helzlsouer KJ, Alberg AJ, Hoffman SC, Norkus EP, Comstock GW. Prospective study of carotenoids, tocopherols, and retinoid concentrations and the risk of breast cancer. *Cancer epidemiology, biomarkers & prevention : a publication of the American Association for Cancer Research, cosponsored by the American Society of Preventive Oncology*. 2002;11(5):451-7.

[201] Kabat GC, Kim M, Adams-Campbell LL, Caan BJ, Chlebowski RT, Neuhouser ML, et al. Longitudinal study of serum carotenoid, retinol, and tocopherol concentrations in relation to breast cancer risk among postmenopausal women. *The American journal of clinical nutrition*. 2009;90(1):162-9.

[202] Grafton MM, Wang L, Vidi PA, Leary J, Lelièvre SA. Breast on-a-chip: mimicry of the channeling system of the breast for development of theranostics. *Integrative biology : quantitative biosciences from nano to macro*. 2011;3(4):451-9.

[203] Lelièvre SA, Hodges KB, Vidi PA. Application of theranostics to measure and treat cell heterogeneity in cancer. In *Cancer Theranostics*, Eds Shawn Chen and Stephen Wong. Elsevier, In Press.

In: Mammary Glands
Editor: Edmund B. Rucker

ISBN: 978-1-62948-853-0

Chapter V

Neoplastic Diseases of the Canine Mammary Gland

Maria Isabel Carvalho[1], Teresa Raposo[1], Helena Rodrigues[1], Isabel Pires[2], Justina Prada[2] and Felisbina L. Queiroga*[1,3,4]

[1]Department of Veterinary Sciences,
University of Trás-os-Montes and Alto Douro; Vila Real, Portugal
[2]CECAV, Department of Veterinary Sciences,
University of Trás-os-Montes and Alto Douro, Vila Real, Portugal
[3]Center for Research and Thecnology of Agro-Environment and Biological Sciences (CITAB), University of Trás-os-Montes and Alto Douro, Vila Real, Portugal
[4]Center for the study of Animal Sciences (CECA),
University of Porto, Porto, Portugal

Abstract

Neoplastic diseases are the most frequent clinical occurrence in the mammary gland of the female dogs. Clinically, canine mammary tumors

* Corresponding author: Tel.: 00351 91 782 69 82. Email address: fqueirog@utad.pt (F.L. Queiroga).

(CMT) appear spontaneously and are more frequent in older dogs. The etiology is predominantly hormonal but also of genetic and immunologic origin. At clinical examination, an abnormal growth is detected in the abdominal region; however, the diagnosis can only be confirmed by histopathologic analysis. Current classification of CMT is based on 1999 WHO (World Health Organization) guidelines. Tumours are divided into benign or malignant types according to their histological origin (epithelial or mesenchymal tissue). Briefly, benign tumors are classified as: adenoma, fibroadenoma, benign mixed tumors and ductal papilloma. In turn, malignant tumors are subdivided into various types: complex, simple and special types of carcinomas, sarcomas or carcinosarcomas. The prognosis is usually established in agreement with the tumour aggressiveness and additional characteristics like ulceration, tumour size and lymph node involvement. In recent years, there has been an increasing effort to apply new prognostic factors besides the classic clinicopathological variables.

Introduction

The development of the mammary gland is a puzzling phenomenon and the research on this field has been focused mostly on the carcinogenesis, with a less goal-oriented concern in basic histology. Canine mammary tumours (CMT) represent a serious problem in veterinary medicine (Queiroga et al., 2011). Clinically, these tumours share many similar features with human breast cancer in terms of histopathology, biological behavior, hormone dependence, risk factors and genetic alterations. These similarities have led to a proposed canine model for the study of breast cancer in women (Kumaraguruparan et al., 2006; Paoloni and Khanna, 2007; Sorenmo et al., 2009; Uva et al., 2009).

Mammary Gland Development

The mammary gland is a modified apocrine sweat gland present in the subcutaneous connective tissue, containing a nipple and consisting of a network of ducts surrounded by a fibrovascular and adipocyte-rich stroma. Mammary development can first be recognized during the embryonic stages by the appearance of 2 ventral ridges of ectoderm, which cover the mesodermic regions from the axillary to the inguinal area. The ectodermal cells migrate along each milk line and coalesce in a complex interaction with the mesenchymal cells to form a placode, which eventually becomes an individual mammary gland (Sorenmo et al., 2011). At birth, the mammary gland is not fully developed. Its development continues at puberty, and throughout reproductive life the gland undergoes a morphogenetic process controlled by its hormonal environment. This involves complex interactions between ovarian steroid and polypeptide hormones and growth factors produced in successive oestrous cycles. The last stages of development of the mammary gland occur in the adult female only during pregnancy, with the proliferation of the ductal tissue, differentiation into milk-producing acini, secretion of milk by the acinar cells, and, at the end of lactation, involution of the secretory component of the gland with preservation of the ductal structures (Santos et al., 2010; Sorenmo et al., 2011).

Mammary Gland Anatomy and Blood Supply

Most dogs develop 5 pairs of mammary glands, although 4 or 6 pairs have been found in a few animals. There are 2 thoracic (M1 and M2), 2 abdominal (M3 and M4), and 1 inguinal (M5) pair of mammary glands (Silver, 1966; Evans and Christensen, 1979; Ettinger and Feldman, 2010). The blood supply in canine mammary glands derives from the sternal branches of the internal and lateral thoracic artery, intercostal, the cranial and caudal superficial epigastric arteries, deep cranial epigastric, abdominal segmented and deep iliac circumflex. Venous drainage of the glands is similar to the arterial supply, though small veins may cross the midline between the right and left mammary glands (Evans and Christensen, 1979; Slatter, 1998).

Lymph Drainage of the Mammary Gland

By convention, most malignant epithelial neoplasms (carcinomas) metastasize via the lymphatic system, whereas malignant mesenchymal neoplasms (sarcomas) metastasize via capillaries and veins. Patsikas and colleagues have methodically examined the lymph drainage of CMT located in each of the mammary glands (Patsikas et al., 2006) (Figure 1).

Mammary Gland	**Normal Lymphatic Drainage** (Patsikas and Dessiris, 1996a, b)	**Neoplastic Lymphatic Drainage** (Patsikas et al., 2006)
M1, cranial thoracic	Axillary LN	Axillary LN, sternal LN
M2, caudal thoracic	Axillary LN	Axillary LN, sternal LN
M3, cranial abdominal	Axillary LN, Superficial Inguinal LN	Axillary LN, superficial inguinal LN, medial iliac LN
M4, caudal abdominal	Superficial Inguinal LN	Superficial inguinal LN, axillary LN
M5, inguinal	Superficial Inguinal LN	Superficial inguinal LN, popliteal LN

Figure 1. Lymphatic drainage of normal and neoplastic canine mammary gland. LN, lymph node.

The lymph drainage of the fourth and fifth neoplastic mammary glands is directed to the ipsilateral superficial inguinal lymph nodes as sentinel lymph nodes of the fourth and fifth healthy mammary glands, whereas the two most cranial neoplastic mammary glands generally drain to the axillary lymph nodes. These authors also strength the clinician's notion that mammary carcinomas occurring in the inguinal (M5) gland may show retrograde metastasis via the lymphatic plexus in the subcutis of the inner thigh and to the popliteal lymph nodes. Retrograde metastatic spread is a rare event, but mammary carcinoma metastases to the vagina have been reported in bitches (Roszel, 1974; Gorisek et al., 2000). In normal healthy dogs, lymphatic fluids drain into the ipsilateral lymph nodes. There is no drainage to the contralateral gland or lymph node, but drainage may be altered in cases of mammary neoplasia (Sorenmo et al., 2011).

Lymphatic vessels can also cross the abdominal midline and in doing so pass through the abdominal and thoracic walls. The axillary lymph node collects lymph from thoracic mammary glands, while the superficial inguinal lymph node collects lymph from the abdominal mammary glands. Generally, the lymphatic drainage of the third mammary gland occurs cranially to the axillary lymph node, but deviation is possible to the inguinal drainage region

(Evans and Christensen, 1979; Slatter, 1998). The dual drainage system of this mammary gland is explained by the formation of plexiform lymphatic connections in between the abdominal and caudal thoracic mammary glands (Patsikas and Dessiris, 1996b,a; Patsikas et al., 2006).

Canine Mammary Tumours (CMT)

A General Approach

The investigations of mammary tumours in dog are of particular interest because they constitute an excellent model for the study of breast cancer in women. In fact mammary tumours are very common in the population of domestic dogs and show remarkable clinical, histopathological, and even genetic and molecular similarities with women breast cancer (Uva et al., 2009).

The recent sequencing of the canine genome and the evidence of its similarity to the human genome has emphasized the dog as an attractive alternative model for cancer research (Lindblad-Toh et al., 2005; Joy et al., 2006). In addition, dogs have a considerable body size, genetic variability similar to humans, and develop spontaneous tumors in the context of a natural immune system. Moreover, unlike laboratory animals, these species share the same environment and are exposed to the same carcinogens; however, they develop tumours in shorter time, due to their shorter longevity compared with the humans (Owen, 1979; Lee et al., 2004; Uva et al., 2009; Thamm et al., 2010; Singer et al., 2012). In the future it's possible that this comparative oncology can play a role in translational medicine, making early clinical applications from knowledge obtained from this model (Porrello et al., 2006).

In bitches, mammary tumours are the most common type of cancer, with a high incidence in geographic regions where ovariohysterectomy is not commonly practiced (Sorenmo, 2003). When both sexes are considered, breast tumours are the most common non-cutaneous tumours (Dorn, 1967). As in humans, there is a marked sexual predisposition, males have a risk of developing breast tumours equal or less than 1% (Todorova, 2006; Saba et al., 2007). Studies conducted over the past decade reveal that in dogs diagnosed with cancer, 56% have mammary tumours (Vascellari et al., 2009) and the incidence rate is 205/100,000 cases per year (Dobson et al., 2002).

Predisposing Factors

The incidence of CMT increases with age (Sonnenschein et al., 1991; Egenvall et al., 2005), with middle-aged and older bitches mostly affected (Hellmen, 2005). The mean age of incidence is approximately 10 years; however, the risk of mammary tumours is increased in dogs over 6 years of age (Benjamin et al., 1999; Perez Alenza et al., 2000). Animals younger than 4 years are rarely affected by this condition (Todorova, 2006). The existence of a racial predisposition is a matter of disagreement among authors. Different breeds have been identified as predisposed to the development of these tumours: English springer spaniel, Doberman, Boxer (Egenvall et al., 2005), and also Cocker Spaniel, Dachshund (Moe, 2001) and Bouvier Bernois (Bronden et al., 2010). One study performed in 101 bitches reveals a lower incidence and a smaller dimension of malignant mammary tumours in small breeds (Itoh et al., 2005). This divergence between authors is possibly caused by the different contribution of each breed to the sample size under study. According to some researchers, obesity and type of diet influence the risk of developing mammary tumours in dogs, similar to what happens in humans (Antuofermo et al., 2007).

In women, particularly during menopause, obesity is associated with increased development of breast cancer (Sonnenschein et al., 1991; Sorenmo, 2003; Stephenson and Rose, 2003; Cappellani et al., 2012) and epidemiological studies have shown that consumption of high fat diets is positively correlated with mortality rates caused by this type of cancer (Shofer et al., 1989). The low prevalence of mammary tumours in herbivores leaves us tempted to assume that a diet low in fat and high in vegetable fiber is beneficial. This is contrary to what happens in dogs, who feed mainly on meat (high fat and a tiny amount of fiber) and have a high prevalence of mammary cancer (Munson and Moresco, 2007). In dogs, obesity at a young age, as well as a diet based mostly on red meat and homemade food, appear to be factors potentially associated with a higher risk to develop mammary tumours and dysplasias (Perez Alenza et al., 1998).

Aetiology

The development of a neoplasia is a complex process resulting from various carcinogenic factors, such as ionizing radiation, chemical compounds and oncogenic viruses. The impact of several endogenous factors, genetic, immune and hormonal, is of irrefutable importance and deserves special attention (Todorova, 2006). Hormonal factors have been thoroughly studied and play a fundamental role in canine mammary carcinogenesis (Novosad, 2003; Queiroga et al., 2005b; Queiroga et al., 2008). The development and growth of the mammary gland is influenced by ovarian hormones (e.g., estrogen and progesterone) and the functional contribution of these hormones has been acknowledged in various physiologic and pathologic situations (Munson and Moresco, 2007). As for the genesis of canine mammary gland neoplasia, the role of these hormones has been well established (Rutteman, 1990; van Garderen et al., 1997; Munson and Moresco, 2007). The first observation of the hormonal contribution in mammary carcinogenesis arose in the late 70s, when the effect of administering progestogen inhibitors of the oestrous cycle was first described (Frank et al., 1979). This hypothesis is further supported by evidence of the protective effect of ovariohysterectomy (OVH) in the development of mammary tumours, especially when it occurs at an early age, since the source of hormones is surgically removed (Sonnenschein et al., 1991; Novosad, 2003; Todorova, 2006). It has been reported that mammary tumour incidence rises sharply whenever the OVH is performed following the second oestrous cycle. When compared with female dogs spayed before the first oestrous cycle, those spayed after the first and second oestrous cycle present an 8% and 26% increased risk of developing mammary tumours, respectively (Schneider, 1970).

Analysis of steroid hormone participation in the acquisition of malignancy has shown a loss of estrogen receptors during the neoplastic progression, which suggests a hormone independence at stages of higher tumour aggressiveness (Rutteman et al., 1988). However, conducting an OVH as a therapeutic measure after the initiation of cancer progression does not seem to have a significant beneficial effect in the course of the neoplastic disease (Yamagami et al., 1996a). In fact, CMT appear to be clearly dependent on steroid hormones (estrogen and progesterone) and therefore, the expression of estrogen and progesterone receptors constitutes additional evidence of the endocrine component in mammary neoplasia (Geraldes et al., 2000; Nieto et al., 2000).

Presently, other hormones are also known to be involved in mammary carcinogenesis. During CMT development, changes are found in the production of pituitary hormones, prolactin (PRL) (Queiroga et al., 2005b) and growth hormone (GH), have a specific function in mammary tumourigenesis (Queiroga et al., 2008). Malignant CMTs produce greater amounts of prolactin compared with benign CMTs, and these also produce more prolactin that normal mammary glands. Prolactin and steroid hormones are produced in the mammary gland, functioning in an autocrine-paracrine mode as local growth factors, favouring the progression of malignant mammary tumours (Queiroga et al., 2005b). Concerning GH, excessive production induced by endogenous or exogenous progestagens might promote mammary tumourigenesis while stimulating the proliferation of susceptible mammary epithelium cells (van Garderen et al., 1997). GH tissue levels in malignant CMTs were also astoundingly augmented in relation to benign CMTs (Queiroga et al., 2008). Over the last decade, some studies point out the existence of other factors intervening in canine mammary carcinogenesis, such as insulin-like growth factor I (IGF-1) (Queiroga et al., 2008) epidermal growth factor (EGF) (Queiroga et al., 2009) and epidermal growth factor receptor (EGFR) (Gama et al., 2009).

Besides endocrine factors, genetic mutations are crucial in the development and progression of tumours. The first to occur is the initiation step, an initial lesion that will evolve under the influence of promoting factors until the later stages of invasion and metastasis unfold. Among several genes participating in mammary carcinogenesis, p53, p27 and c-erB-2 or HER2/neu are worth mentioning for the research conducted throughout the last decade (Lee and Kweon, 2002; Gama et al., 2008; Klopfleisch et al., 2010). The *p53* gene is a major regulator of tumour suppression, inducing the apoptosis of cells bearing damaged, irreparable DNA such as neoplastic cells. *p53* gene mutations have been reported in 30-35% of CMTs (Chu et al., 1998; Veldhoen et al., 1999; Lee and Kweon, 2002). Not only do malignant and metastatic tumours bear *p53* mutations, but also benign CMTs, which might indicate this is an early event in mammary carcinogenesis (Muto et al., 2000).

The *p27* gene, an inhibitor of cyclin dependent kinases, hampers the transition to the cell cycle replicative phase. Primary carcinomas and lymph node metastasis have a reduced expression of p27 mRNA, suggesting a preponderant role in tumourigenesis (Klopfleisch et al., 2010).

HER2/neu is an oncogene frequently mutated in human breast cancers, as the encoded receptor is targeted in clinical application by the drug Herceptin. The involvement of this gene as a prognostic marker in CMTs is yet to be well established, but the expression of HER2/neu in tumour biopsies, coupled with other molecular markers (e.g., estrogen receptors, p63 and CK5) is useful in determining a molecular phenotype which, similarly to what has been observed in the human counterpart, presents a relationship with a worse prognosis (Gama et al., 2008). The environmental aetiology has already been suggested, but hitherto not proven true. It is possible that anti-parasitic drugs containing pyrethroid substances accumulate in the peri-mammary adipose tissue and sensitize epithelial cells to proliferation (Andrade et al., 2010).

Diagnosis and Clinical Management

CMTs may present as solitary or multiple masses. The caudal mammary glands are more affected than cranial glands, probably due to their larger size. Clinical signs that indicate a malignant lesion include the observation of the rapid growth of a mass not circumscribed, invasiveness, adherence to the skin or surrounding tissues, and ulceration. However the absence of these signs does not mean that it is excluded as malignant lesion (Perez Alenza et al., 2000). Similarly, large lesions can merely mean that the search for veterinary care was delayed (Sorenmo, 2003). Mammary tumours are staged according to the World Health Organization (WHO) TNM system or a modification of this system (Owens, 1980; Rutteman et al., 2001) (Figure 2).

T: primary tumour	**Stages**
T1: <3 cm maximum diameter	
T2: 3–5 cm maximum diameter	**Stage I - T1, N0, M0**
T3: >5 cm maximum diameter	
N: regional lymph node status	**Stage II - T2, N0, M0**
N0: no metastasis	**Stage III - T3, N0, M0**
N1: metastasis	
M: distant metastasis	**Stage IV - Any T, N1, M0**
M0: absent	**Stage V - Any T, Any N, M1**
M1: present	

Figure 2. Canine mammary tumour staging - modified WHO (Rutteman et al., 2001).

To stage the mammary gland tumors in a dog, information regarding tumor size, lymph node status, and presence of metastasis needs to be collected and verified. The largest malignant tumour in dogs with more than one tumour should be considered in the stage assignment. The lymph nodes should be identified, and if they are clinically enlarged, fine-needle aspirates for cytological evaluation must be performed. Dogs with malignant mammary tumours would also be evaluated for metastatic disease. Three-view thoracic radiographs remain the standard diagnostic method for evaluating veterinary patients for the presence of metastasis (Sorenmo, 2003; Sorenmo et al., 2011), since the lungs are the most common site for distant metastasis (Fidler and Brodey, 1967a, b). However, additional staging tests, including abdominal ultrasound, skeletal radiographs, or other imaging modalities, may be indicated if clinical examination identifies other sites suspicious for metastasis.

On physical examination, clinical signs suggestive of breast cancer are easily identified; however, definitive diagnosis of CMT is reached only after a histopathological study of the sample obtained by biopsy. The cytology by fine needle aspiration, despite being a minimally invasive methodology and easy to perform, is not reliable in the diagnosis of mammary tumors in female dogs due to the high variability and pleomorphism that the same histological tumour can present. Despite the limitations in diagnostic, cytology is a good method to dispose of some differential diagnoses and to determine the nodal disease (Simon et al., 2009).

For neoplastic lesions of the mammary gland in dogs, the classification recommended by the World Health Organization (WHO), published in 1999, is commonly accepted (Misdorp, 1999). The breast neoplasms are divided into benign or malignant, and they may have their origin in epithelial, myoepithelial or mesenchymal tissue. Most mammary gland tumors are of epithelial origin. Some, however, can have mixed histology consisting of both epithelial and myoepithelial tissue, with areas of cartilage and bone, and a few tumors are of purely mesenchymal origin (Sorenmo, 2003).

The term inflammatory carcinoma is not included in WHO classification and is a distinct clinical entity in dogs, characterized histologically by the presence of emboli in dermal lymphatic vessels which is responsible for the severe regional edema observed in most cases (Pena et al., 2003; Lana et al., 2007). Recently, a new proposed classification of canine mammary gland lesions covers the inflammatory carcinoma as a special kind of carcinoma (Goldschmidt et al., 2011).

During embryonic development of the mammary gland, there is a close relationship between the epithelium and mesenchyme. Therefore, in tumoural development of complex adenomas there are combinations of epithelial and myoepithelial components, with mixed mammary tumours presenting cartilage and bone (Sorenmo et al., 2011). CMTs have a complex histogenesis which is not yet completely understood. Stem cells of ductolobular terminal units are identified as a possible origin of many dysplasic and tumoural lesions of the mammary gland (Misdorp, 2002). The application of immunohistochemical techniques, creation of cell lines, and transplant assays has deepened the analysis of mammary tumours histogenesis. In complex adenomas and benign mixed tumours, there is a demonstrated involvement of epithelial and myoepithelial components, as shown from the immunohistochemistry of specific molecular markers CK5 and p63, respectively (Gama et al., 2003; Ramalho et al., 2006).

In canine mammary tumours, it is a relatively common occurrence to have multiple tumour masses. This fact has been overlooked as several different types of tumours are consistently considered as independent primary tumours, isolated and inaccessible to signalling from other tumours in the same organism. Recent studies have nevertheless pointed to an increased risk for the development of malignancies after a first diagnosis of mammary cancer (Sorenmo et al., 2011).

Recent data also reveals that CMTs begin as benign tumours and progress through successive histological types of aggression. This development culminates in the formation of malignant tumours, showing similarities with the process of carcinogenesis in human breast cancer (Sorenmo et al., 2009). The proportion of malignant CMTs is 50% (Gilbertson et al., 1983), and approximately 50% of breast carcinomas metastasize to regional lymph nodes and lungs (Gilbertson et al., 1983; Rosol et al., 2003). The risk of metastasis is influenced by tumor histological type, histological grade of malignancy and several prognostic factors.

Histological Classification of Canine Mammary Tumours: World Health Organization Guidelines (Misdorp, 1999)

The most recent studies conducted in CMT have been based on the classification proposed by the World Health Organization (WHO) (Queiroga et al., 2008; Carvalho et al., 2011; Raposo et al., 2012). This classification system combines histogenic and descriptive morphologic parameters, also incorporating histologic prognostic features that have been associated with an increasing malignancy.

Figure 3 presents all histological types and the reader is encouraged to consult the bibliographic source where can find a detailed description of each tumour type. The most common types of malignant CMTs are presented in Figure 4 in an increasing order of malignancy.

Malignant tumours	Benign tumours
Non-infiltrating (in situ) carcinoma	**Adenoma**
Complex carcinoma	Simple adenoma
	Complex adenoma
	Basaloid adenoma
Simple carcinoma	**Fibroadenoma**
Tubulopapillary carcinoma	High-cellularity fibroadenoma
Solid carcinoma	Low-cellularity fibroadenoma
Anaplastic carcinoma	
Special type of carcinomas	**Benign mixed tumour**
Spindle cell carcinoma	**Duct papilloma**
Squamous cell carcinoma	
Mucinous carcinoma	
Lipid-rich carcinoma	
Sarcoma	
Fibrosarcoma	
Osteosarcoma	
Other sarcomas	
Carcinosarcoma	
Carcinoma or sarcoma in benign tumor	

Figure 3. Histological Classification – WHO (Misdorp, 1999).

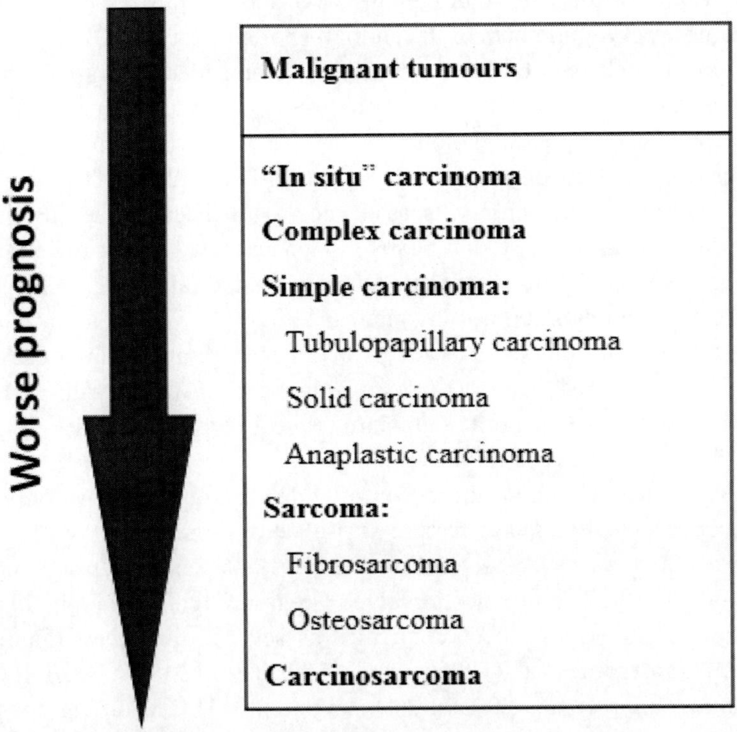

Figure 4. Prognosis of malignant CMT (Misdorp, 1999).

Prognostic Factors

Due to the heterogeneity of pathological types and clinical presentations of CMTs, the histological evidence of malignancy does not necessarily imply a malignant clinical course of the disease (Okamura et al., 2004); therefore, in Veterinary Medicine, the meticulous search and communication of a reliable prognostic factors in a short period of time is an urgent task for the veterinary clinician. A determined characteristic or feature of the dog or the tumour itself is considered as a prognostic factor when it is capable of providing reliable information that allows predicting the onset of recurrence and metastasis after clinical remission. For this reason, in prospective clinical studies, the characteristics with prognostic value should be evaluated based on their ability to predict disease-free survival (DFS, time from the date of the surgery till the occurrence of recurrence and/or metastasis) and overall survival time (ST, time from surgery until death of the animal) (Sorenmo et al., 2011).

As mentioned previously, the presence of considerable variations in the biological behavior, within series of histologically malignant mammary tumours, makes it impossible to obtain a precise prognosis, using no more than the microscopic histopathologic analysis (Sarli et al., 2002). The age of the animal at the time of surgery is associated with disease free survival and overall survival in some studies, where older animals show a lower survival rate when compared with young animals (Hellmen et al., 1993; Perez Alenza et al., 2000; Sorenmo, 2003; Marconato et al., 2008). The rapid and invasive growth rate of the tumour, as well as a larger size, are clinical parameters classically associated with a worse prognosis in dogs with malignant mammary tumours (Misdorp and Hart, 1976; Perez Alenza et al., 1997; Misdorp, 2002; Santos et al., 2013).

The presence of tumour ulceration provides valuable information because it is a clinicopathological feature correlated significantly with tumour malignancy and poor survival (Hellmen et al., 1993; Perez Alenza et al.,1997; Pena et al., 1998). The prognostic value of regional lymph node involvement at the time of surgery has been confirmed by several researchers (Hellmen et al., 1993; Yamagami et al., 1996b; Perez Alenza et al., 1997; Misdorp, 2002; Karayannopoulou et al., 2005; Santos et al., 2013). According to several researchers, mitotic index, nuclear grade, and distant metastases show a statistically significant association with disease-free survival and/or overall survival, and are also considered as prognostic factors (Perez Alenza et al., 1997; Pena et al., 1998).

Although in the context of CMTs a range of clinical and pathological factors with reliable prognostic value have already been identified, it is evident that a complete understanding of tumour behavior is still years away. With the relentless pursuit of understanding this highly complex and dramatically incident phenomenon, the scientific community is focusing on the molecular level to uncover how the tumour processes unfold. In addition, the identification of molecular markers allows for the identification of new therapeutic targets.

Currently, molecular markers for CMTs have been identified that have a prognostic sustained interest which include: PCNA, Ki67, p53, Cox-2, EGFR, tumour-associated macrophages (MAC387), and tumour infiltrating lymphocytes (CD3, CD4, CD8) (Lee et al., 2004; Queiroga et al., 2005a; Gama et al., 2009; Estrela-Lima et al., 2010; Carvalho et al., 2011; Raposo et al., 2012; Santos et al., 2013). Ki67 and PCNA are cell proliferation markers and are correlated with tumour histological grade, nuclear grade, presence of metastases, death by cancer, and shorter disease-free survival after surgery (Pena et al., 1998; Kadthur et al., 2011; Santos et al., 2013). The nuclear expression of p53 protein, resulting from the mutation of the p53 gene, also showed CMT prognostic value in being correlated with shorter survival and increased tumour recurrence (Veldhoen et al., 1999; Lee et al., 2004).

In CMTs, some studies demonstrated an association between COX-2 expression and angiogenesis, the development of distant metastases, a poor prognosis, and shorter survival periods (Queiroga et al., 2005a; Millanta et al., 2006; Lavalle et al., 2009). With respect to EGFR, there was a tendency toward a shorter disease-free survival and overall survival in dogs with positive EGFR expression (Gama et al., 2009). Tumour-associated macrophages revealed a significant association with the decrease in overall survival (Raposo et al., 2012).

In canine malignant mammary tumors, abundant lymphocyte infiltrates are frequently found and animals with high proportions of CD4+ and low CD8+ T-cells have lower survival rates (Estrela-Lima et al., 2010). In addition, there is a tendency for a higher number of CD3+ tumour-infiltrating T-lymphocytes and a shorter overall survival. Interestingly, a statistically significant relationship was observed only for CD3+ T-lymphocytes in the adnexal non-tumoural mammary gland, with a higher number of lymphocytes conferring a reduced overall survival (Carvalho et al., 2011). Figure 5 summarizes the most significant CMT prognostic factors. Despite substantial scientific advances in the area of CMT prognosis, there remains an incessant need to expand our knowledge in order to better understand the biological behavior of these tumours.

Good prognosis	Poor prognosis	Indifferent
o <3cm in diameter	o >3cm in diameter	o Breed
o Well circumscribed	o Invasive, ulcerated	o OVH at time of surgery
o Lymph node: Negative	o Lymph node: Positive	o Type of surgery
o Ulceration absent	o Index of proliferation	o Number of tumours
o Index of proliferation:	Ki-67: high	o Glands involved
Ki-67: low	PCNA: high	
PCNA: low	o High Cox-2	
o Low Cox-2	o p53 gene mutation	

Figure 5. Summary of CMT prognostic factors.

Treatment

Given an animal with a breast tumour, the primary treatment of choice is still surgery (Novosad, 2003), excluding cases of animals with inflammatory tumours of the mammary gland (such as inflammatory carcinoma), or distant metastases (Lana et al., 2007; Sorenmo et al., 2011). The selection of the type of surgery is dependent on the extent of the tumour. Lumpectomy or nodulectomy is recommended for superficial and non-adherent masses smaller than 0.5 cm, which generally have a benign behavior. For 1 cm or larger lesions located at a deeper level and with adhesions, regional or radical mastectomy is recommended (Lana et al., 2007). A prospective clinical study demonstrated that after regional mastectomy, 58% of cases had recurrence of a new tumour in the mammary gland remains of the ipsilateral mammary chain (Stratmann et al., 2008).

Strategies for treatments in addition to surgery have not been well-established yet (Sorenmo, 2003), and the use of chemotherapy or radiotherapy is limited due to their high cost. It becomes necessary to distinguish those animals with breast tumours that may most effectively benefit from the application of these treatments. Although adjuvant chemotherapy is a standard treatment in human breast cancer, limited information exists about its effectiveness in breast tumours in dogs. Routine use in the treatment of these tumours is not recommended because of its ineffectiveness compared to other types of neoplasms (Lana et al., 2007). Nevertheless, chemotherapy may be useful as an adjuvant therapy to the surgical excision of tumours with a probable metastasis or recurrence. There are some studies in CMTs which indicate the relationship of certain types of chemotherapeutic agents (e.g., a combination of 5-fluoroucil, cyclophosphamide and doxorubicin) and an increase in survival of animals (Hershey et al., 1999; Karayannopoulou et al., 2001). Although the impact of these studies is relatively low since they are based on a small sample of animals, they are proof-in-principle that the use of adjuvant chemotherapy may be required in some cases. However, additional well-controlled studies must be performed in order to determine the most appropriate chemotherapeutic agents to treat malignant CMTs. Regarding radiotherapy, the scarcity of studies is evident and the results reveal unattractive effects for this therapeutic modality (Sorenmo, 2003).

In CMTs, exogenous hormonal treatment is indicated in tumours exhibiting estrogen, progesterone, or prolactin receptors (Lana et al., 2007). In human medicine, the use of hormonal manipulation is a common practice. Tamoxifen Citrate is a selective inhibitor of estrogen receptors in the mammary gland and is largely used in human breast cancer treatment strategies. In dogs, due to the high risk of developing pyometra, it is recommended that the administration of tamoxifen is limited to sterilized animals. Moreover, since there is no difference in side effects between higher and lower doses, clinicians should opt for the administration of the highest dose of the drug to increase the chances of therapeutic success (Tavares et al., 2010). Immunotherapy is at the forefront of therapeutic modalities to treat CMTs. In one study, researchers used a vaccinal oncolytic virus (GLV-1h68) in the treatment of CMT. The virus was used to infect and kill canine mammary adenomas cell lines, as well as inhibit tumour proliferation and decrease tumour size in xenotransplants (Gentschev et al., 2009).

Recently, selective COX-2 inhibitors have been used in several studies to strengthen the possibility that these drugs could be used in a prophylactic or as adjuvant therapy in mammary tumours (Ashok et al., 2011). In dogs, clinical trials based on selective COX-2 inhibitors showed success in reducing clinical signs in transitional cell carcinoma of the bladder (Knapp et al., 1994; Mohammed et al., 2002; Mohammed et al., 2003). Recent studies in CMTs revealed a relationship between COX-2 expression and more aggressive tumour phenotypes (Heller et al., 2005; Queiroga et al., 2007; Dias Pereira et al., 2009; Queiroga et al., 2010). These findings emphasize the need for additional studies with selective COX-2 inhibitors in order to verify their true clinical effectiveness.

In canine inflammatory carcinomas, piroxicam (a nonselective inhibitor of COX-2) therapy showed an improvement of the clinical status *in vivo* (de M. Souza et al., 2009) and significant cytotoxic effects were obtained *in vitro* using piroxicam and deracoxib against canine mammary carcinoma cells. This suggests that COX-2 inhibitors can be an attractive approach for the treatment of canine mammary carcinoma (Ustun Alkan et al., 2012). The importance of Cox-2 has been recognized by clinicians in human and veterinary medicine and the increasing use of Cox-2 selective inhibitors. In human medicine, promising results are already evident in published studies based on case series and randomized clinical trials (Ferrandina et al, 2003, Martin et al, 2011). Given the complexity of tumoural development, therapeutic modalities will be constantly updated and refined, which is essential in the evaluation of combined and customized treatments.

Conclusion

Mammary tumours are presumed to be the oncological class which most often plagues female dogs, with approximately 50% of the malignant tumours metastasizing to distant organs. Therapeutic modalities available to treat malignant cases are mainly based in surgery and classical chemotherapic drugs, which affects both normal and neoplastic cells (Queiroga et al., 2011). However, animals with lymph node metastasis and/or metastatic disease pose a challenge to clinicians since no single chemotherapy protocol has been reported to be as effective as adjuvant therapy (Simon et al., 2006). Improvements in this area based on clinical trials, focusing on the establishment of combined and customized treatments, are still necessary in order to aid clinicians in improving the life quality of dogs with mammary cancer.

References

Andrade, F.H., Figueiroa, F.C., Bersano, P.R., Bissacot, D.Z., Rocha, N.S., 2010. Malignant mammary tumor in female dogs: environmental contaminants. *Diagn Pathol* 5, 45.

Antuofermo, E., Miller, M.A., Pirino, S., Xie, J., Badve, S., Mohammed, S.I., 2007. Spontaneous mammary intraepithelial lesions in dogs--a model of breast cancer. *Cancer Epidemiol Biomarkers Prev* 16, 2247-2256.

Ashok, V., Dash, C., Rohan, T.E., Sprafka, J.M., Terry, P.D., 2011. Selective cyclooxygenase-2 (COX-2) inhibitors and breast cancer risk. *Breast* 20, 66-70.

Benjamin, S.A., Lee, A.C., Saunders, W.J., 1999. Classification and behavior of canine mammary epithelial neoplasms based on life-span observations in beagles. *Vet Pathol* 36, 423-436.

Bronden, L.B., Nielsen, S.S., Toft, N., Kristensen, A.T., 2010. Data from the Danish veterinary cancer registry on the occurrence and distribution of neoplasms in dogs in Denmark. *Vet Rec* 166, 586-590.

Cappellani, A., Di Vita, M., Zanghi, A., Cavallaro, A., Piccolo, G., Veroux, M., et al., 2012. Diet, obesity and breast cancer: an update. *Front Biosci* (Schol Ed) 4, 90-108.

Carvalho, M.I., Pires, I., Prada, J., Queiroga, F.L., 2011. T-lymphocytic infiltrate in canine mammary tumours: clinic and prognostic implications. *In Vivo* 25, 963-969.

Chu, L.L., Rutteman, G.R., Kong, J.M., Ghahremani, M., Schmeing, M., Misdorp, W., et al., 1998. Genomic organization of the canine p53 gene and its mutational status in canine mammary neoplasia. *Breast Cancer Res Treat* 50, 11-25.

de M. Souza, C.H., Toledo-Piza, E., Amorin, R., Barboza, A., Tobias, K.M., 2009. Inflammatory mammary carcinoma in 12 dogs: clinical features, cyclooxygenase-2 expression, and response to piroxicam treatment. *Can Vet J* 50, 506-510.

Dias Pereira, P., Lopes, C.C., Matos, A.J., Santos, M., Gartner, F., Medeiros, R., et al., 2009. COX-2 expression in canine normal and neoplastic mammary gland. *J Comp Pathol* 140, 247-253.

Dobson, J.M., Samuel, S., Milstein, H., Rogers, K., Wood, J.L., 2002. Canine neoplasia in the UK: estimates of incidence rates from a population of insured dogs. *J Small Anim Pract* 43, 240-246.

Dorn, C.R., 1967. The epidemiology of cancer in animals. *Calif Med* 107, 481-489.

Egenvall, A., Bonnett, B.N., Ohagen, P., Olson, P., Hedhammar, A., von Euler, H., 2005. Incidence of and survival after mammary tumors in a population of over 80,000 insured female dogs in Sweden from 1995 to 2002. *Prev Vet Med* 69, 109-127.

Estrela-Lima, A., Araujo, M.S., Costa-Neto, J.M., Teixeira-Carvalho, A., Barrouin-Melo, S.M., Cardoso, S.V., et al., 2010. Immunophenotypic features of tumor infiltrating lymphocytes from mammary carcinomas in female dogs associated with prognostic factors and survival rates. *BMC Cancer* 10, 256.

Ettinger, S., Feldman, E., 2010. Urogenital and mammary gland tumors.*Textbook of Veterinary Internal Medicine.* In Ettinger SJ, Feldman EC (Eds.). Missouri: Saunders Elsevier. v.2., 2211-2212.

Evans, H., Christensen, G., 1979. *Miller's Anatomy of lhe Dog. 2nd ed.* W.B.Saunders, Philadelphia.

Fidler, I.J., Brodey, R.S., 1967a. The biological behavior of canine mammary neoplasms. *J Am Vet Med Assoc* 151, 1311-1318.

Fidler, I.J., Brodey, R.S., 1967b. A necropsy study of canine malignant mammary neoplasms. *J Am Vet Med Assoc 1*51, 710-715.

Frank, D.W., Kirton, K.T., Murchison, T.E., Quinlan, W.J., Coleman, M.E., Gilbertson, T.J., et al., 1979. Mammary tumors and serum hormones in the bitch treated with medroxyprogesterone acetate or progesterone for four years. *Fertil Steril* 31, 340-346.

Gama, A., Alves, A., Gartner, F., Schmitt, F., 2003. p63: a novel myoepithelial cell marker in canine mammary tissues. *Vet Pathol* 40, 412-420.

Gama, A., Alves, A., Schmitt, F., 2008. Identification of molecular phenotypes in canine mammary carcinomas with clinical implications: application of the human classification. *Virchows Arch* 453, 123-132.

Gama, A., Gartner, F., Alves, A., Schmitt, F., 2009. Immunohistochemical expression of Epidermal Growth Factor Receptor (EGFR) in canine mammary tissues. *Res Vet Sci* 87, 432-437.

Gentschev, I., Stritzker, J., Hofmann, E., Weibel, S., Yu, Y.A., Chen, N., et al., 2009. Use of an oncolytic vaccinia virus for the treatment of canine breast cancer in nude mice: preclinical development of a therapeutic agent. *Cancer Gene Ther* 16, 320-328.

Geraldes, M., Gartner, F., Schmitt, F., 2000. Immunohistochemical study of hormonal receptors and cell proliferation in normal canine mammary glands and spontaneous mammary tumours. *Vet Rec* 146, 403-406.

Gilbertson, S.R., Kurzman, I.D., Zachrau, R.E., Hurvitz, A.I., Black, M.M., 1983. Canine mammary epithelial neoplasms: biologic implications of morphologic characteristics assessed in 232 dogs. *Vet Pathol* 20, 127-142.

Goldschmidt, M., Pena, L., Rasotto, R., Zappulli, V., 2011. Classification and grading of canine mammary tumors. *Vet Pathol* 48, 117-131.

Gorisek, B., Zegura, B., Kavalar, R., But, I., Krajnc, I., 2000. *Primary breast cancer of the vulva: a case report and review of the literature.* Wien Klin Wochenschr 112, 855-858.

Heller, D.A., Clifford, C.A., Goldschmidt, M.H., Holt, D.E., Shofer, F.S., Smith, A., et al., 2005. Cyclooxygenase-2 expression is associated with histologic tumor type in canine mammary carcinoma. *Vet Pathol* 42, 776-780.

Hellmen, E., 2005. Complex mammary tumours in the female dog: a review. *J Dairy Res* 72 Spec No, 90-97.

Hellmen, E., Bergstrom, R., Holmberg, L., Spangberg, I.B., Hansson, K., Lindgren, A., 1993. Prognostic factors in canine mammary tumors: a multivariate study of 202 consecutive cases. *Vet Pathol* 30, 20-27.

Hershey, A.E., Kurzman, I.D., Forrest, L.J., Bohling, C.A., Stonerook, M., Placke, M.E., et al., 1999. Inhalation chemotherapy for macroscopic primary or metastatic lung tumors: proof of principle using dogs with spontaneously occurring tumors as a model. *Clin Cancer Res* 5, 2653-2659.

Itoh, T., Uchida, K., Ishikawa, K., Kushima, K., Kushima, E., Tamada, H., et al., 2005. Clinicopathological survey of 101 canine mammary gland tumors: differences between small-breed dogs and others. *J Vet Med Sci* 67, 345-347.

Joy, F., Basak, S., Gupta, S.K., Das, P.J., Ghosh, S.K., Ghosh, T.C., 2006. Compositional correlations in canine genome reflects similarity with human genes. *J Biochem Mol Biol* 39, 240-246.

Kadthur, J.C., Rao, S., Sonnahallipura, B.M., Thimmanahalli, D.S., Laxmikanth, S.M., 2011. Prognostic value of Ki-67 proliferation antigen in canine malignant mammary gland tumours. *Braz J Vet Pathol*. 4, 36-40.

Karayannopoulou, M., Kaldrymidou, E., Constantinidis, T.C., Dessiris, A., 2001. Adjuvant post-operative chemotherapy in bitches with mammary cancer. *J Vet Med A Physiol Pathol Clin Med* 48, 85-96.

Karayannopoulou, M., Kaldrymidou, E., Constantinidis, T.C., Dessiris, A., 2005. Histological grading and prognosis in dogs with mammary carcinomas: application of a human grading method. *J Comp Pathol* 133, 246-252.

Klopfleisch, R., Schutze, M., Gruber, A.D., 2010. Loss of p27 expression in canine mammary tumors and their metastases. *Res Vet Sci* 88, 300-303.

Knapp, D.W., Richardson, R.C., Chan, T.C., Bottoms, G.D., Widmer, W.R., DeNicola, D.B., et al., 1994. Piroxicam therapy in 34 dogs with transitional cell carcinoma of the urinary bladder. *J Vet Intern Med* 8, 273-278.

Kumaraguruparan, R., Prathiba, D., Nagini, S., 2006. Of humans and canines: Immunohistochemical analysis of PCNA, Bcl-2, p53, cytokeratin and ER in mammary tumours. *Res Vet Sci* 81, 218-224.

Lana, S., Rutteman, G., Withrow, S., 2007. Tumors of the Mammary Gland. In: Withrow, S.J., Vail, D.M., eds. Withrow and MacEwen's *Small Animal Clinical Oncology. 4º ed.* Missouri, E.U.A: Saunders Elsevier, 619-635.

Lavalle, G.E., Bertagnolli, A.C., Tavares, W.L., Cassali, G.D., 2009. Cox-2 expression in canine mammary carcinomas: correlation with angiogenesis and overall survival. *Vet Pathol* 46, 1275-1280.

Lee, C.H., Kim, W.H., Lim, J.H., Kang, M.S., Kim, D.Y., Kweon, O.K., 2004. Mutation and overexpression of p53 as a prognostic factor in canine mammary tumors. *J Vet Sci* 5, 63-69.

Lee, C.H., Kweon, O.K., 2002. Mutations of p53 tumor suppressor gene in spontaneous canine mammary tumors. *J Vet Sci* 3, 321-325.

Lindblad-Toh, K., Wade, C.M., Mikkelsen, T.S., Karlsson, E.K., Jaffe, D.B., Kamal, M., et al., 2005. Genome sequence, comparative analysis and haplotype structure of the domestic dog. *Nature* 438, 803-819.

Marconato, L., Lorenzo, R.M., Abramo, F., Ratto, A., Zini, E., 2008. Adjuvant gemcitabine after surgical removal of aggressive malignant mammary tumours in dogs. *Vet Comp Oncol* 6, 90-101.

Millanta, F., Citi, S., Della Santa, D., Porciani, M., Poli, A., 2006. COX-2 expression in canine and feline invasive mammary carcinomas: correlation with clinicopathological features and prognostic molecular markers. *Breast Cancer Res Treat* 98, 115-120.

Misdorp, W., 1999. *Histological classification of mammary tumors of the dog and the cat. Washington*: Armed Forces Institute of Pathology in cooperation with the American Registry of Pathology and the World Health Organization Collaborating Center for Worldwide Reference on Comparative Oncology.

Misdorp, W., 2002. Tumors of the Mammary Gland. In *Tumors in Domestic Animals,* edited by D. J. Meuten: Iowa State Press, 575-606.

Misdorp, W., Hart, A.A., 1976. Prognostic factors in canine mammary cancer. *J Natl Cancer Inst* 56, 779-786.

Moe, L., 2001. Population-based incidence of mammary tumours in some dog breeds. *J Reprod Fertil Suppl* 57, 439-443.

Mohammed, S.I., Bennett, P.F., Craig, B.A., Glickman, N.W., Mutsaers, A.J., Snyder, P.W., et al., 2002. Effects of the cyclooxygenase inhibitor, piroxicam, on tumor response, apoptosis, and angiogenesis in a canine model of human invasive urinary bladder cancer. *Cancer Res* 62, 356-358.

Mohammed, S.I., Craig, B.A., Mutsaers, A.J., Glickman, N.W., Snyder, P.W., deGortari, A.E., et al., 2003. Effects of the cyclooxygenase inhibitor, piroxicam, in combination with chemotherapy on tumor response, apoptosis, and angiogenesis in a canine model of human invasive urinary bladder cancer. *Mol Cancer Ther* 2, 183-188.

Munson, L., Moresco, A., 2007. Comparative pathology of mammary gland cancers in domestic and wild animals. *Breast Dis* 28, 7-21.

Muto, T., Wakui, S., Takahashi, H., Maekawa, S., Masaoka, T., Ushigome, S., et al., 2000. p53 gene mutations occurring in spontaneous benign and malignant mammary tumors of the dog. *Vet Pathol* 37, 248-253.

Nieto, A., Pena, L., Perez-Alenza, M.D., Sanchez, M.A., Flores, J.M., Castano, M., 2000. Immunohistologic detection of estrogen receptor alpha in canine mammary tumors: clinical and pathologic associations and prognostic significance. *Vet Pathol* 37, 239-247.

Novosad, C.A., 2003. Principles of treatment for mammary gland tumors. *Clin Tech Small Anim Pract* 18, 107-109.

Okamura, Y., Haraguchi, T., Morimoto, M., Okuda, M., Une, S., Nakaichi, M., et al., 2004. Expression of a tumor-associated antigen, RCAS1, in canine mammary tumors. *J Vet Med Sci* 66, 651-658.

Owen, L.N., 1979. A comparative study of canine and human breast cancer. *Invest Cell Pathol* 2, 257-275.

Owens, L., 1980. *Classification of Tumors in Domestic Animals, 1st ed.* World Health Organization, Geneva, Switzerland.

Paoloni, M.C., Khanna, C., 2007. Comparative oncology today. *Vet Clin North Am Small Anim Pract* 37, 1023-1032; v.

Patsikas, M.N., Dessiris, A., 1996a. The lymph drainage of the mammary glands in the bitch: a lymphographic study. Part I: The 1st, 2nd, 4th and 5th mammary glands. *Anat Histol Embryol* 25, 131-138.

Patsikas, M.N., Dessiris, A., 1996b. The lymph drainage of the mammary glands in the Bitch: a lymphographic study. Part II: The 3rd mammary gland. *Anat Histol Embryol* 25, 139-143.

Patsikas, M.N., Karayannopoulou, M., Kaldrymidoy, E., Papazoglou, L.G., Papadopoulou, P.L., Tzegas, S.I., et al., 2006. The lymph drainage of the neoplastic mammary glands in the bitch: a lymphographic study. *Anat Histol Embryol* 35, 228-234.

Pena, L., Perez-Alenza, M.D., Rodriguez-Bertos, A., Nieto, A., 2003. Canine inflammatory mammary carcinoma: histopathology, immunohistochemistry and clinical implications of 21 cases. *Breast Cancer Res Treat* 78, 141-148.

Pena, L.L., Nieto, A.I., Perez-Alenza, D., Cuesta, P., Castano, M., 1998. Immunohistochemical detection of Ki-67 and PCNA in canine mammary tumors: relationship to clinical and pathologic variables. *J Vet Diagn Invest* 10, 237-246.

Perez Alenza, D., Rutteman, G.R., Pena, L., Beynen, A.C., Cuesta, P., 1998. Relation between habitual diet and canine mammary tumors in a case-control study. *J Vet Intern Med* 12, 132-139.

Perez Alenza, M.D., Pena, L., del Castillo, N., Nieto, A.I., 2000. Factors influencing the incidence and prognosis of canine mammary tumours. *J Small Anim Pract* 41, 287-291.

Perez Alenza, M.D., Pena, L., Nieto, A.I., Castano, M., 1997. Clinical and pathological prognostic factors in canine mammary tumors. *Ann Ist Super Sanita* 33, 581-585.

Porrello, A., Cardelli, P., Spugnini, E.P., 2006. Oncology of companion animals as a model for humans. an overview of tumor histotypes. *J Exp Clin Cancer Res* 25, 97-105.

Queiroga, F.L., Alves, A., Pires, I., Lopes, C., 2007. Expression of Cox-1 and Cox-2 in canine mammary tumours. *J Comp Pathol* 136, 177-185.

Queiroga, F.L., Perez-Alenza, D., Silvan, G., Pena, L., Illera, J.C., 2009. Positive correlation of steroid hormones and EGF in canine mammary cancer. *J Steroid Biochem Mol Biol* 115, 9-13.

Queiroga, F.L., Perez-Alenza, M.D., Silvan, G., Pena, L., Lopes, C., Illera, J.C., 2005a. Cox-2 levels in canine mammary tumors, including inflammatory mammary carcinoma: clinicopathological features and prognostic significance. *Anticancer Res* 25, 4269-4275.

Queiroga, F.L., Perez-Alenza, M.D., Silvan, G., Pena, L., Lopes, C., Illera, J.C., 2005b. Role of steroid hormones and prolactin in canine mammary cancer. *J Steroid Biochem Mol Biol* 94, 181-187.

Queiroga, F.L., Perez-Alenza, M.D., Silvan, G., Pena, L., Lopes, C.S., Illera, J.C., 2008. Crosstalk between GH/IGF-I axis and steroid hormones (progesterone, 17beta-estradiol) in canine mammary tumours. *J Steroid Biochem Mol Biol* 110, 76-82.

Queiroga, F.L., Pires, I., Lobo, L., Lopes, C.S., 2010. The role of Cox-2 expression in the prognosis of dogs with malignant mammary tumours. *Res Vet Sci* 88, 441-445.

Queiroga, F.L., Raposo, T., Carvalho, M.I., Prada, J., Pires, I., 2011. Canine mammary tumours as a model to study human breast cancer: most recent findings. *In Vivo* 25, 455-465.

Ramalho, L.N., Ribeiro-Silva, A., Cassali, G.D., Zucoloto, S., 2006. The expression of p63 and cytokeratin 5 in mixed tumors of the canine mammary gland provides new insights into the histogenesis of these neoplasms. *Vet Pathol* 43, 424-429.

Raposo, T., Gregorio, H., Pires, I., Prada, J., Queiroga, F.L., 2012. Prognostic value of tumour-associated macrophages in canine mammary tumours. *Vet Comp Oncol.*

Rosol, T.J., Tannehill-Gregg, S.H., LeRoy, B.E., Mandl, S., Contag, C.H., 2003. Animal models of bone metastasis. *Cancer* 97, 748-757.

Roszel, J.F., 1974. Canine metastatic mammary carcinoma cells in smears from genital epithelium. *Vet Pathol* 11, 20-28.

Rutteman, G., Withrow, S., MacEwen, E., 2001. Tumors of the mammary gland. In: *Small Animal Clinical Oncology,* ed. SJ Withrow, EG MacEwen, 3rd ed., pp. 455–477. WB Saunders, Philadelphia, PA.

Rutteman, G.R., 1990. Hormones and mammary tumour disease in the female dog: an update. *In Vivo* 4, 33-40.

Rutteman, G.R., Misdorp, W., Blankenstein, M.A., van den Brom, W.E., 1988. Oestrogen (ER) and progestin receptors (PR) in mammary tissue of the female dog: different receptor profile in non-malignant and malignant states. *Br J Cancer* 58, 594-599.

Saba, C.F., Rogers, K.S., Newman, S.J., Mauldin, G.E., Vail, D.M., 2007. Mammary gland tumors in male dogs. *J Vet Intern Med* 21, 1056-1059.

Santos, A.A., Lopes, C.C., Ribeiro, J.R., Martins, L.R., Santos, J.C., Amorim, I.F., et al., 2013. Identification of prognostic factors in canine mammary malignant tumours: a multivariable survival study. *BMC Vet Res* 9, 1.

Santos, M., Marcos, R., Faustino, A.M., 2010. Histological study of canine mammary gland during the oestrous cycle. *Reprod Domest Anim* 45, e146-154.

Sarli, G., Preziosi, R., Benazzi, C., Castellani, G., Marcato, P.S., 2002. Prognostic value of histologic stage and proliferative activity in canine malignant mammary tumors. *J Vet Diagn Invest* 14, 25-34.

Schneider, R., 1970. Comparison of age, sex, and incidence rates in human and canine breast cancer. *Cancer* 26, 419-426.

Shofer, F.S., Sonnenschein, E.G., Goldschmidt, M.H., Laster, L.L., Glickman, L.T., 1989. Histopathologic and dietary prognostic factors for canine mammary carcinoma. *Breast Cancer Res Treat* 13, 49-60.

Silver, I.A., 1966. The anatomy of the mammary gland of the dog and cat. *J Small Anim Pract* 7, 689-696.

Simon, D., Schoenrock, D., Baumgartner, W., Nolte, I., 2006. Postoperative adjuvant treatment of invasive malignant mammary gland tumors in dogs with doxorubicin and docetaxel. *J Vet Intern Med* 20, 1184-1190.

Simon, D., Schoenrock, D., Nolte, I., Baumgartner, W., Barron, R., Mischke, R., 2009. Cytologic examination of fine-needle aspirates from mammary gland tumors in the dog: diagnostic accuracy with comparison to histopathology and association with postoperative outcome. *Vet Clin Pathol* 38, 521-528.

Singer, J., Weichselbaumer, M., Stockner, T., Mechtcheriakova, D., Sobanov, Y., Bajna, E., et al., 2012. Comparative oncology: ErbB-1 and ErbB-2 homologues in canine cancer are susceptible to cetuximab and trastuzumab targeting. *Mol Immunol* 50, 200-209.

Slatter, D., 1998. *Manual de cirurgia de pequenos animais. 2. ed.* SãoPaulo: Ed. Manole.

Sonnenschein, E.G., Glickman, L.T., Goldschmidt, M.H., McKee, L.J., 1991. Body conformation, diet, and risk of breast cancer in pet dogs: a case-control study. *Am J Epidemiol* 133, 694-703.

Sorenmo, K., 2003. Canine mammary gland tumors. *Vet Clin North Am Small Anim Pract* 33, 573-596.

Sorenmo, K.U., Kristiansen, V.M., Cofone, M.A., Shofer, F.S., Breen, A.M., Langeland, M., et al., 2009. Canine mammary gland tumours; a histological continuum from benign to malignant; clinical and histopathological evidence. *Vet Comp Oncol* 7, 162-172.

Sorenmo, K.U., Rasotto, R., Zappulli, V., Goldschmidt, M.H., 2011. Development, anatomy, histology, lymphatic drainage, clinical features, and cell differentiation markers of canine mammary gland neoplasms. *Vet Pathol* 48, 85-97.

Stephenson, G.D., Rose, D.P., 2003. Breast cancer and obesity: an update. *Nutr Cancer* 45, 1-16.

Stratmann, N., Failing, K., Richter, A., Wehrend, A., 2008. Mammary tumor recurrence in bitches after regional mastectomy. *Vet Surg* 37, 82-86.

Tavares, W.L., Lavalle, G.E., Figueiredo, M.S., Souza, A.G., Bertagnolli, A.C., Viana, F.A., et al., 2010. Evaluation of adverse effects in tamoxifen exposed healthy female dogs. *Acta Vet Scand* 52, 67.

Thamm, D.H., Kurzman, I.D., Clark, M.A., Ehrhart, E.J., 3rd, Kraft, S.L., Gustafson, D.L., et al., 2010. Preclinical investigation of PEGylated tumor necrosis factor alpha in dogs with spontaneous tumors: phase I evaluation. *Clin Cancer Res* 16, 1498-1508.

Todorova, I., 2006. Prevalence and etiology of the most common malignant tumours in dogs and cats. *Bulgarian Journal of Veterinary Medicine* 9, 85-98.

Ustun Alkan, F., Ustuner, O., Bakirel, T., Cinar, S., Erten, G., Deniz, G., 2012. The effects of piroxicam and deracoxib on canine mammary tumour cell line. *ScientificWorldJournal* 2012, 976740.

Uva, P., Aurisicchio, L., Watters, J., Loboda, A., Kulkarni, A., Castle, J., et al., 2009. Comparative expression pathway analysis of human and canine mammary tumors. *BMC Genomics* 10, 135.

van Garderen, E., de Wit, M., Voorhout, W.F., Rutteman, G.R., Mol, J.A., Nederbragt, H., et al., 1997. Expression of growth hormone in canine mammary tissue and mammary tumors. Evidence for a potential autocrine/paracrine stimulatory loop. *Am J Pathol* 150, 1037-1047.

Vascellari, M., Baioni, E., Ru, G., Carminato, A., Mutinelli, F., 2009. Animal tumour registry of two provinces in northern Italy: incidence of spontaneous tumours in dogs and cats. *BMC Vet Res* 5, 39.

Veldhoen, N., Watterson, J., Brash, M., Milner, J., 1999. Identification of tumour-associated and germ line p53 mutations in canine mammary cancer. *Br J Cancer* 81, 409-415.

Yamagami, T., Kobayashi, T., Takahashi, K., Sugiyama, M., 1996a. Influence of ovariectomy at the time of mastectomy on the prognosis for canine malignant mammary tumours. *J Small Anim Pract* 37, 462-464.

Yamagami, T., Kobayashi, T., Takahashi, K., Sugiyama, M., 1996b. Prognosis for canine malignant mammary tumors based on TNM and histologic classification. *J Vet Med Sci* 58, 1079-1083.

In: Mammary Glands
Editor: Edmund B. Rucker

ISBN: 978-1-62948-853-0

Chapter VI

Infection of the Lactating Mammary Gland: Current Status on the Molecular Biology of Mastitis

Koen Breyne* and Evelyne Meyer
Laboratory of Biochemistry, Department of Pharmacology, Toxicology and Biochemistry, Faculty of Veterinary Medicine, Merelbeke, Ghent University, Belgium

Mastitis, an Inflammatory Disease Affecting Mammals

The Post-Natal Mammary Gland has a Transient Morphology in Mammals

Lactation is a mammalian hallmark wherein neonates are nourished postpartum through a very effective and adaptable organ [1]. Hundred millions

* Correspondence: Breyne Koen, MSc., Laboratory of Biochemistry, Department of Pharmacology, Toxicology and Biochemistry, Faculty of Veterinary Medicine, Salisburylaan 133, 9820 Merelbeke, Ghent University, Belgium. Tel: 0032(0)92647356. Email: Koen.Breyne@Ugent.be.

of years ago, evolutionary reprogramming of apocrine cutaneous glands associated with either hair follicles or evolutionary merging of different skin glands, resulted in a new excretion organ to support altricial offspring [2, 3]. The Eutherian mammary gland is rudimental at birth and develops further into a post-pubertal quiescent gland [5]. During the post-natal period the fat pad (FP) expands its primitive epithelial ductal system at the terminal end buds (TEB, Figure 1A, B) in mice, called terminal ductal lobular units in cows and humans. Branching of the ductal architecture coincides with the start of the estrous cycle forming alveolar buds embedded in adipose tissue [6].

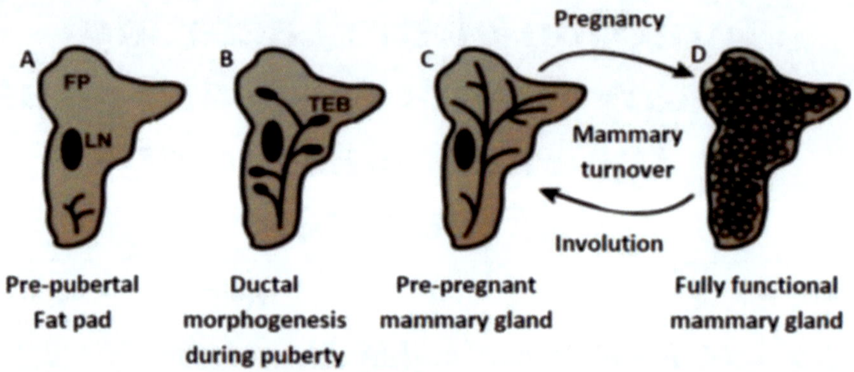

Figure 1. Morphological stages of the development of the post-natal murine mammary gland. The post-natal fat pad (FP) has a distinct lymph node (LN) embedded in the mammary adipose tissue, close to a small epithelial entity that develops through puberty. (A) The forthcoming mammary gland exposes an extensive epithelial branching due to the growth at the terminal end buds (TEB). (B) It further enlarges during pregnancy and finally contains a completely functional alveo-lobular structure able to produce milk. When the milk production stops, the lactating gland regresses in a programmed cell death process called involution (C-D) (Image adapted from [4]).

At the onset of lactation, the slumber state of the exocrine gland differentiates with parturition due to female sex hormonal signalling [7]. Morphologically, the mammary gland generally enlarges due to extensive branching of ducts and alveolar formation (Figure 1C). Once fully functional, lactogenesis is initiated and sustained in the galactopoietic stage. Alveolar secretion starts with the highly protein- and fat-rich colostrum leading to the production of copious mature milk with a relative stable constitution under the influence of prolactin [8]. Mammary secretions contain a diversity of constituents synthesized and secreted by several cellular pathways. Milk proteins such as casein are produced in the endoplasmic reticulum and are guided by the Golgi system to the cellular membrane. Budding of this membrane results in micelles loaded with proteins encoded in the mammary epithelial cells and is perceived as a mildly invasive apocrine secretion method. These membrane remnants, together with both *de novo* mammary triglyceride formation related to the fatty acid synthase activity and *ex novo* liver or diet lipids locally released by capillary associated lipoprotein lipase activity, render milk its characteristic fatty nature [9]. Milk saccharides such as lactose are also produced by the mammary cell compartment, while minerals such as calcium ions can be released through transepithelial transport from the bloodstream. The latter have important implications creating a hormonally-regulated osmotic gradient and eventually fluid excretion [10]. In animals that lack milking stimuli, regression of the complete mammary gland to its state prior to pregnancy is introduced either through weaning of the litter or through entering the dry-off period (Figure 1C, D). This involution process involves programmed cell death programs of specific epithelial cell populations and is reversible at its onset. Dead mammary cells are first discarded from their originating epithelial layer (anoikis) and subsequently released in the alveolar lumen [11].

In each state (embryonic, prepregnant, fully functional gestational and involutional) the mammary gland is compartmentalized in a parenchymal and a stromal portion. The ductal parenchym of pseudo-stratified cuboidal architecture consists of contractile myoepithelial cells and encircles another layer of epithelial cells that encloses the lumen. The alveolar parenchyma concentrated in lobuli has a similar structure consisting of the same cell types. These different cell layers can be identified by means of their specific cytokeratin expression [12]. The luminal mammary epithelial cells have a secretory potential which depends on the mammary stage. When alveoli are full of secretion, the myoepithelial cells contract and guide the milk through the ducts which collects in sinuses towards the orifice, where it gets released. Embedded in both layers of epithelia from this alveo-lobular structure, reside stem cells responsible for the morphological dynamicity of the post-natal mammary gland. These two layers contain several functionally distinct subpopulations, including stem, progenitor and differentiated cells [4].

This complex cellular framework is supported by an elaborate stromal compartment called the extra-cellular matrix (ECM). Based on its position in the gland, the ECM is subdivided in basal lamina, intra- and inter-lobular stroma and fibrous connective tissue [13]. These ECM molecules actively participate in the organization of the complex mammary gland architecture and furthermore in cell functions including adhesion, survival, apoptosis, proliferation and differentiation of the mammary gland [14]. Although they are not yet fully understood, alterations in ECM constituents likely have implications in mammary gland diseases due to their influence on internalization of bacteria in host' epithelia following an mammary infection [15, 16], on infiltration and activation of immune cells and on tumor development [17].

The Mammary Immune System and Mammary Gland Diseases

Based on phylogenetic tree data, scientists discovered mammary glands as organs that have evolved from originally antimicrobial glands into milk-producing entities. More specifically, many milk nutrients are now considered as an evolutionary bypass of these original antimicrobial molecules. This remarkable modification has been most explicitly documented for the transition of lysozyme into α-lactalbumin. Whereas α-lactalbumin is a prototypical mammalian protein that enables lactose production in the mammary gland, lysozyme is an anti-bacterial peptide producing enzyme that dates back already to non-vertebrate species. Despite their functional differences, both proteins share a 40% amino acid identity and have a nearly identical three-dimensional structure [18]. These data illustrate the important bactericidal function of mammary glands, which is further emphasized below.

Indeed, the mammary gland displays on the one hand a humoral defence system comprising an array of antibacterial proteins consisting - besides lysozymes - of lactoferrins and β-defensins [19], of oligosaccharides [20], fatty acids [21], mucins [22] and secreted milk antibodies such as immunoglobulins (Igs) [23]. On the other hand, the immunobiology of the mammary gland also contains an extensive cellular component as reviewed concisely in the following paragraphs. Although the numerical values of immune cells in bovine milk haven been reported by differentiating the somatic cell count (SCC) in normal cows and mastitic cases, to our knowledge no such data are available for mice [24].

Lymphocytes

In general, the prevailing leukocyte populations of a healthy mammary gland consist of both acquired and innate immune cells i.e., lymphocytes and macrophages, respectively. Lymphocytes are organized in LNs (Figure 1) and are part of an elaborate lymphatic system [25]. T-lymphocytes get activated in these mammary-associated LNs by antigens captured either by mammary dendrocytes or by LN resident B-lymphocytes and other antigen-presenting cells (APC) such as macrophages. However, some specific aspects of the mammary cell panel organization are species-dependent. For example, dairy cow udders do not have mammary LN but are drained by retro-mammary LNs and contain a Furstenberg's Rosette where lymphocytes are numerous. Moreover, bovine lymphocytes are predominantly cytotoxic T cells ($CD8^+$) compared to a lower number of T-helper cells ($CD4^+$). Both these subtypes are released in different ratios in milk depending on the lactational stage [26, 27]. Overall, lymphocytes have important implications for all mammals in the mammary defence against exogenous agents [28], protection of the milk-fed offspring [29] and even in breast cancer metastasis as more recently recognized [30].

The number of lymphocytes increases following bacterial infection of the mammary gland [31]. Interaction with antigens such as *Staphylococcus aureus* (*S. aureus*) enterotoxins induces T-lymphocyte activation, immunosuppression (i.e., decreased T-cell proliferation) or influences cell viability [32-34]. Activated T-lymphocytes secrete specific pro-inflammatory cytokines aiding the efficient clearance of bacteria [35, 36]. This potential makes them key players in chronic mammary gland infections and therefore suggests innovative prevention perspectives in the context of staphylococcal mastitis vaccination [37].

In humans, maternal milk protects infants against pathogenic infections, primes their immunity, aids in there immuno-tolerance against allergens and in the development of a competent mucosal immune system [38, 39]. All these aspects are dependent on the milk Ig content. Indeed, mammary lymphocytes release IgA into milk and are highly efficient in targeting infectious agents in the newborn. This IgA is also known to enable antigenic stimulation of mucosa-associated lymphoid tissue in both the gut and airways of the offspring. Consequently, infants are temporarily protected against infections allowing them to acquire their own immune system [40]. Again marked species-differences exist as IgG1 and IgG2 rather than IgA are the main antibodies defending against pathogens in cow milk [41].

As for breast tumors, these mostly initiate from the mammary epithelial layer [42]. Tumor cells eventually penetrate the mammary gland barrier as progressive invasiveness is gained in response to signals emitted by the epithelial as well as by various stromal ECM cells [43]. Breast cancer models demonstrated that $CD4^+$ T-cells indirectly promote invasion and subsequent lung metastasis of mammary adenocarcinomas [44]. Interestingly, this pro-tumorigenic property of $CD4^{+}$ effector cells is believed to originate from their ability to regulate tumor-associated macrophages [44, 45].

Macrophages

During mammary gland inflammation, the function of macrophages is not restricted to that of APC for T-cells. Additionally, macrophages act as professional phagocytes against invading microorganisms and further trigger the innate immune response through prostaglandin-, leukotriene- and cytokine-mediated signalling [46].

Moreover, these macrophage-derived chemokines partly guide polymorphonuclear neutrophils which either nullify or at least weaken bouts of microbial agents [47]. This statement is further elaborated by the possibility of inducing mammary inflammation with a cell wall component derived of gram-negative bacteria, where macrophages are proven to be responsible for neutrophil infiltration. Upon an inflammatory insult, macrophages also neutralize leukocytes, dead cells and debris that form a potential pro-inflammatory threat. Dead cells generally expose extracellular phosphatidylserine, efficiently recognized as an “eat me” signal to phagocytize cellular remains [48]. Through this elegant strategy, dead immune cells decompose safely, a crucial process supporting homeostasis.

Macrophages are also essential for the proper development of the post-pubertal and lactating gland [49]. This pleiotropic epithelial modulating capacity renders them tumor-developing properties. In brief, macrophages alter programmed cell death and enhance proliferation of epithelial cells. While interacting in a paracrine manner with the surrounding adipose tissue, they remodel the mammary gland ECM, facilitating metastasis and promoting angiogenesis by the secretion of chemoattractants and of stimulating factors.

Polymorphonuclear Neutrophilic Leukocytes (Neutrophils)

In FPs and healthy functional mammary glands, other leukocytes than macrophages and lymphocytes are relatively rare. Nevertheless, they rapidly become the principal innate immune cell type found in infected mammary tissue and in its secretions. Neutrophils are non-specific leukocytes and are actively recruited to the site of infection. At this site an environmental niche is orchestrated by the resident Toll like receptor (TLR)-containing cells through a cocktail of inflammatory mediators. Furthermore, local endothelial cells get stimulated and fenestrated so that blood neutrophils can leak in the infected mammary tissue guided by chemoattractants. Once in the presence of pathogens, neutrophils again use phagocytosis which is complemented by potent bactericidal means (both oxygen-dependent as mediated by the respiratory burst and oxygen-independent via small antibacterial molecules like cathepsins and calpains) to eliminate the bacterial hazard as rapidly as possible [50].

Mammary Epithelial Cells (MEC)

The most prominent cell type in the mammary gland clearly is the epithelial cell. The main purpose of these cells was producing nutrition for the young during the lactation phase of the mammary gland. More recently, they started to be perceived as an imminent part of the mammary gland immune system [51].

As the mammary gland regresses fastly during the involution phase post-weaning, there is a scary accumulation of dead cells in the lumen at that time (Figure 1C, D). These might expose their intracellular compounds and thus imply an inflammatory danger [52]. Therefore, mammary epithelial cells also can act as (non-professional) phagocytes and engulf either partly damaged or already dead cells to resolve or prevent such undesired inflammatory conditions. Although less efficient in this elimination function than the professional macrophages, they also utilize specific receptors such as the phosphatidylserine receptor, CD36, vitronectin receptor and CD91 to scavenge the vast lumen for damaged cells. Upon the detection hereof they respond by excreting anti-inflammatory mediators like transforming growth factor (TGF)-β1, while reducing the amounts of pro-inflammatory mediators like tumor necrosis factor (TNF)-α and macrophage inflammatory protein (MIP)-2 thus bridging the critical time frame before massive influx of immune cells occurs [51]. Mammary epithelial cells indeed should be considered as non-professional immune cells as they even express TLRs embedded in their membrane, which enable them not only to sense exogenous bacterial ligands but moreover to react against this threat as an essential part of the innate immunity [53].

What Is Mastitis?

Until recently, mastitis was only recognized as a relevant pathological process in food producing animals because it has a substantial economic and animal welfare impact especially on the dairy industry. In its most simple way it could therefore be defined as an inflammatory - infectious - disease of the (lactating) udder in ruminant species [54, 55]. In the bovine species, mastitis is characterized by typical changes which can be either directly observed (i.e., clinical symptoms of udder tissue inflammation and organoleptic loss of milk quality) or indirectly diagnosed (i.e., subclinical inflammation confirmed after counting the number of somatic cells in milk above a well-defined threshold). However, since a few years, an increasing number of researchers from veterinary and human medicine have intensified the sharing of their knowledge on mammary gland inflammation. This interdisciplinary communication resulted in a major added value for the field of mastitis research. Consequently, the now accepted concept is that probably all mammals and certainly also humans suffer from mammary gland inflammation [55]. Moreover, the cell types described in the previous section are common between mammals and thus participate in the host' (innate) immune response during mammary gland diseases.

Nevertheless, it remains difficult to define in a general species-independent manner the complex syndrome called "mastitis" because the molecular biology is only partly elucidated. Indeed, as reviewed by Contreras and Rodriguez [55], non-infectious mastitis instead of its typically infectious counterpart in ruminants has been frequently described in breastfeeding women. Only after culture of milk samples, it became clear that also in humans milk fluid is not sterile and often contains (pathogenic) bacteria. Besides the variation in etiology, also the diagnosis and clinical presentation may vary substantially between mammals. With the substantial growth in interest to better understand the molecular mechanisms of mastitis for different species including humans, the use of *in vivo* mouse models has become a more accepted strategy for this purpose. Both gram-negative and -positive pathogens can thus be inoculated. Of note, the recognized but not yet unravelled presence of the non-contagious CNS bacteria in the bovine udder might be relevant for breastfeeding women too [56]. Indeed, the CNS strain *S. epidermidis* is a largely underrated cause of human mastitis [55].

In Vitro and *In Vivo* Models Contribute to Novel Mastitis Insights

To study the molecular mechanism of mastitis and in order to improve therapies, different experimental-induced infection models systems and approaches have been developed.

Pros and Cons of Mastitis Models

Dairy cows have been genetically selected for their unique linked or pleiotropic traits to achieve high production efficiency. However, the heritability for these milk producing traits brings along a negative energy balance as body reserves are in a major part being used for milk component anabolism. Although these features are very convenient for milk yield, they generally affect other highly energy-dependent anabolism and more specifically also the animals' immunity [54]. It is well recognized that a high milk yield concomitant with high milk management predisposes dairy cows to mastitis by impairing the cow's defence system [47].

Milk contains a variety of nutrients and the host produces a wide range of potent growth inhibitors and opsonic proteins to control undesired micro-organisms in milk [57]. Nevertheless, it has been increasingly reported that a number of mastitic pathogens have adapted to grow in the milky environment despite the presence of these antibacterial biomolecules such as carbohydrates, lipids, enzymes (i.e., lactoferrin, lysozyme, lactoperoxidase, xanthine oxido-reductase, etc.) [57], complement component 3 and antibodies [58, 59]. For example, mastitic *Escherichia coli* (*E. coli*) strains grown in milk are known to up- and down-regulate hundreds of proteins in contrast to the same strains grown in conventional culture media [60]. This observation highlights the possibility that mastitic bacteria - contrary to other strains of the same bacterial species - adapted to their niche allowing them to replicate faster and circumvent their rapid clearance from milk. Although proper confirmation of this hypothesis is still lacking and certainly warrants in-depth research, the term "MPEC" was introduced suggesting the existence of distinct *E. coli* with specific mammary pathogenicity and inherent local inflammatory potential [61]. Interestingly, similar indications are also accumulating for *S. aureus* mastitis strains. It is known that the mastitic *S. aureus*-suppressing activity of antibiotics in milk cultures is lower than in broth cultures [62]. These data again highlight that the adaptability of the bacterial species is probably not only niche-dependent but also host-dependent [63].

In summary, dairy cows contain particular genetic traits that make them vulnerable to fastidious germs that have in turn adapted to the unique environment of the lactating udder. Both arguments imply that confirmatory mastitis studies should always be finally performed within the target-species. Nevertheless, such experiments are severely limited by research tools and infrastructure, are also very expensive and labor-intensive. As a result, *in vitro* culture models and *in vivo* mouse models have been developed to tackle these major drawbacks. *In vitro* models culture isolated udder cells but are hampered by the limited number of cell types that can be included in a single analysis and their lack of dynamism. During an inflammation process in the udder, there is a constant change of cells that influence one another, which cannot be addressed by the *in vitro* experimental approach. In parallel, researchers therefore utilize preclinical *in vivo* models which mimic ruminant udder infections with mastitic bacteria isolated from field cases. Unlike *in vitro* models, the latter models do include a dynamic multicellular system yet in another genetic background. As mice are homologous to other mammals, these mammary gland inflammation data can at least partly be extrapolated to cows and also to breastfeeding women. Nevertheless, some aspects of both the physiology and the specific traits of udders or breasts differ with those of the murine mammary glands. Therefore, care should be taken when attempting to extrapolate results from the mouse to other mammals as the pathogenicity of some inflammatory agents and the acquired host response can be species-dependent. However, this will be hardly the case for the innate immunity aspects of the mammary gland biology, which is highly conserved between all mammals.

In Vitro Infection Models

Udder tissue can elegantly be harvested *in vivo* through endoscopically guided biopsies and subsequently cultured [64]. Discarding unwanted stromal cells from proteolytically dissociated udder tissue enables selective culturing of bovine MEC (bMEC). These primary mammary gland cells are then exposed to either live or heat-killed or attenuated mastitic pathogens, to bacterial components such as toxins, or to a wide range of inflammatory mediators and their subsequent response is monitored. Alternatively to the labor-intensive and non-heterogeneous mammary isolated cells, primary bovine epithelial cells can be transformed into a continuous cell line by introducing the SV-40 large T-antigen such as in the MAC-T cell line [65]. Although this elegant tool facilitates research, it is generally considered to be less relevant for the *in vivo* situation than data obtained from primary isolated cells. In analogy to human breast or murine mammary gland epithelia, the bovine udder epithelium is not built up as clonal cell line [66]. As also described in the first section, it is constructed as a tissue with an extensive mammary cell hierarchy which can be phenotyped by different extracellular markers in cows, but even more so in mice and humans [67].

Broad-spectrum analyses such as transcriptome studies can be performed on infected bMEC, pinpointing up- or down-regulated genes that are critically involved in the hosts' immune defence [68]. To fine-tune which part of the bacterium interacts with a pattern recognition receptor (PRR), and which specific reaction is induced in the epithelium, cells can be stimulated with microbial-associated molecular patterns (MAMP). These bacterial agonists e.g., lipopolysaccharide (LPS), lipotheichoic acid (LTA) and flagellin elicit a specific response that is typically characterized by PCR at the mRNA expression level or by ELISA at the protein level [69]. The importance of host factors identified in screening studies can further be evaluated with genetically modified mammary epithelial cells, either lacking specific genes or overexpressing transfected transgenes. For example, the role of NF-κB in bMEC was elucidated by gene expression studies in genetically engineered cells. As seen in infected udders, bMEC exposed to MAMP or bacteria display a transiently enhanced IL-8 mRNA expression. IL-8 is a neutrophil chemoattractant induced by nuclear factor-kappa B (NF-κB) [70, 71]. The latter transcription factor is a dimer that needs proper activation and nuclear translocation to interact with κB-sites in the responsive promoter of the IL-8 gene [72]. Immunoprecipitation analysis revealed that p65 is constitutively present on the IL-8 promoter in untreated epithelia, while p50 is quickly recruited only following pathogen exposure. The transcriptional activity of NF-κB following its recruitment to the IL-8 promoter was verified with expression vectors for p65 and/or p50 transgenes which were co-transfected into bMEC with an IL-8 reporter construct. Unexpectedly, this analysis showed that p65/p50 heterodimers completely abolish IL-8 transcription, while p65/p65 and p50/p50 homodimers also repress IL-8 transcription albeit only in a concentration-dependent manner. Interestingly, this negative regulation of IL-8 transcription was overridden by co-transfecting with another transcription factor i.e., C/EBPβ, which also binds the IL-8 promoter region. Moreover, single expression of C/EBPβ activated IL-8 transcription again in a concentration-dependent manner [73]. Therefore, the authors conclude that both a shift from NF-κB heterodimers to homodimers and C/EBPβ are required for IL-8 transcription following infection in wT bMECs. Moreover, their concentration and interplay probably explain the transient character (IL-8 peak) of this activation. In summary, the versatility of co-transfected bMEC allowed to elucidate how complex dynamic molecular systems work in the mammary gland.

These bMEC can also be exposed to cytokines. For example, mammary epithelia respond to *E. coli* by the production of TNF-α. To verify the host' response induced by TNF-α signalling, bMEC were cultured with TNF-α and this resulted in a shift from p65/p65 homodimers to p65/p50 heterodimers at the κB-sites, concomitant with IL-8 secretion specifically in the mucosal compartment [74].

Finally, studies with other mammary or inflammatory cells can aid to unravel their function in mastitis. Blood neutrophils or macrophages can easily be harvested and stimulated with mastitic bacteria to monitor their response. Mammary-resident immune cells in healthy udders can be extracted either through milk collection or through biopsies [75, 76].

Although *in vitro* data are crucial to gain understanding in the cell type specific interactions, findings always have to be confirmed *in vivo*. To illustrate this, a recent paper compared their infected bMEC results with those obtained in isolated mRNA from infected udder tissue and came to different conclusions [53].

Experimental Induction of Mastitis Pathogens in the Murine Mammary Gland

The cross-talk and interaction between mastitic pathogens and the surrounding mammary stroma, the ECM and infiltrating cells of the immune system constantly modulate the hosts' inflammatory response. This complex multi-factorial process is impossible to address with conventional *in vitro* models. Therefore *in vivo* approaches, such as mouse mastitis models have been widely used and adapted over the years. Generally, mouse models are extensively investigated for a whole array of human diseases. They provide easily accessible tools that can simulate specific pathologies. As such, these latter models have made major contributions to the understanding of disease pathogenesis, highlighting diagnostic and treatment possibilities.

Albeit sample collection or experiments on dairy cows are ethically more accepted compared to those on humans or primates, they have some similar drawbacks e.g., labor- and cost intensity, genetic diversity. Moreover, far less immunological reagents are available for bovine compared to murine research. To address mastitis in a more convenient way for the study of the molecular biology and key signalling pathways in the mammary gland, experimental mouse models were first developed and characterized already in the 1970s [77-80]. Although the overall physiology of cow udders and mice mammary glands shows differences, they both have glands in the inguinal region. In mice, the fourth inguinal gland pair is the biggest and therefore preferred one for suckling by the pups. The litter is nursed by the mother for about 10 to 14 days. During this lactation period the mammary gland is fully functional and can expand to about seven-fold its original volume. Consequently, the teat canal ducts become easily accessible for experimental infection.

Introduction Methods of Mastitic Germs in the Murine Mammary Gland

There are several methods to mimic bovine mastitis in lactating mice with bovine mastitis isolates. The introduction method - as well as the choice of mastitic pathogen - greatly influences the inflammation process in these mouse models.

The first method consists of simply dropping a pathogen-dense inoculum on top of the nipple, enabling bacteria to descend through the duct orifice into the mammary gland. With this non-invasive procedure, that probably best reflects the natural infection route, the number of bacteria that infect the gland is however not controllable. Inter-animal differences are consequently very high. Therefore, other techniques were developed that focused on introducing the concentrated bacterial load directly into the teat orifice. For this purpose researchers tried to optimize the pipetting of the bacterial suspension into the ducts through the use of smaller tips, illumination fibers, microscopes and micro-manipulators.

This second method was successfully achieved when small volumes were reproducibly introduced with the help of pediatric blunted needles (> 30 Gauge). The point of entry can optionally be enlarged by an additional minimal cut in the nipple top. The needle is then positioned at an angle of about 180 degrees can thus enter the primary duct fluently when performed by an experienced researcher (Figure 2A). The released volume spreads out through the accessible lactating lobules as visualized by Chinese ink administration or even more elegantly with *in vivo* imaging of luminescent bacteria (Figure 2B, C), and subsequently interacts with the host' tissue. The latter intraductal (or intramammary) injection technique is superior to the first strategy as the infection rate is about 100% when the mammary glands are fully lactating and thus have become easily accessible. When the inoculum is administered correctly - demanding experience from the researcher - the CFU can be as low as 10 CFU/injection and still induce mastitis. Nevertheless, higher inocula have the advantage of lower inter-animal variation. It should be remarked that the small incision implicates a low-grade induction of inflammation. Therefore, sham-inoculated mammary glands should always be included in these experiments [81].

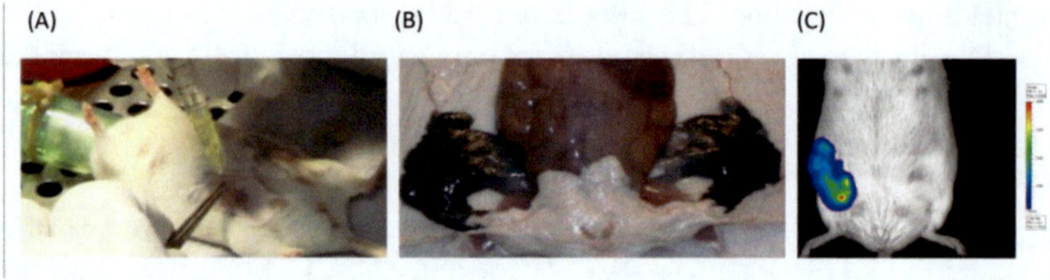

Figure 2. Experimental induction of mastitis pathogens in the murine mammary gland. Mastitis isolates or bacterial toxins or even mammary tumor cells (Breyne et al., *unpubl. data)* can be intraductally introduced in anesthetized lactating mice by means of a blunted pediatric needle to infect the murine mammary gland simulating either bovine mastitis or breast cancer. (A) These intramammarily injected cells or molecules remain local, as visualized with Chinese ink in both glands of the fourth pair, and can multiply in the mammary gland while eliciting an inflammatory host response both locally and systemically (B). Bioluminescent *E. coli* bacteria injected in the right mammary gland of the fourth pair can be tracked through *in vivo* imaging and remain local in a time-lapse of 24 hours (C).

The mouse model has been successfully used with different mastitic bacteria including *E. coli*, *S. aureus* and *S. uberis*, but still needs to be tested for others such as coagulase-negative Staphylococci (CNS). Similarly to *in vitro* models, mammary gland inflammation can alternatively be induced by intramammary injection of multiple exogenous factors in either genetically modified or wild-type mice. These intramammary introduced molecules vary from host factors (such as cytokines) to MAMP (toxins, wall fragments, etc.) which all aided in unravelling the molecular pathways involved in this complex disease mechanism.

Mastitis mouse models downsize the number of animals used to achieve a statistically conclusive result and also facilitate mastitis experiments because experimentally used mice strains have the same genotype, have - in contrary to cows - far less natural bacterial mammary flora, are easily housed and/or managed. Besides these practical issues, they open up a wide panel of research possibilities that are very difficult or even impossible to perform in cow mastitis experiments. One has to keep in mind that these models are mainly relevant for highly evolutionary conserved processes in Mammalia especially regarding the innate immune system. As stated before, dairy cattle has been genetically selected for milk production hampering other energy costing processes such as the immune system and mastitic germs have adapted to the anti-bacterial defence in the milky udder environment [82]. Milk composition is species-dependent due to the diet preference and the specific catabolism of the different mammals such as the presence of butyric acid in ruminant milk resulting from rumen fermentation [83]. Therefore, it can be speculated that cow mastitic germs prefer to tide in the bovine udders rather than in mouse mammary glands. This working hypothesis remains to be investigated.

Unique Applications of Murine Models to Study the Molecular Biology of Mastitis

As mouse models have been employed for decades to study a vast number of pathologies, a plethora of molecular tools came available to study them.

The contribution of a selected gene can be verified through the lack, the adaptable expression, the overexpression, or the presence of an additional gene in that host. Consequently, researchers have engineered mice with modern biotechnological techniques to study the effect of an underlining genotype in a pathology model. Mastitis research greatly benefited from the use of these genetically modified mouse models. Transgenic mice have also aided, albeit in a relatively modest number, to unravel key features of the early pathophysiological process of mastitis (Table 1).

Table 1. Overview of the types of transgenic mice that have been employed to study the molecular biology of mastitis

Genetically modified mouse model	Intramammarily injected agents	Reference
TLR4 KO	*E. coli*	[93] [94]
TLR2 KO	*E. coli*; LPS, Pam3CSK4	[82]
IL-1R KO	*E. coli*; LPS	[79] [95]
LAO KO	*S. aureus*	[87]
IL-8R KO	*E. coli*; LPS	[93]
iNOS KO	*E. coli*; LPS	[93] [95]
TNF-α KO	*E. coli*, LPS	[93]
Caspase-1 KO	*E. coli*	[79]
NF-κB luciferase	*E. coli*, LPS	[80]
CX3CR1 GFP/+	*E. coli*	[94]

S. aureus = *Staphylococcus aureus*; *E. coli* = *Escherichia coli*, LPS = lipopolysaccharide, Pam3CSK4 = synthetic bacterial lipopeptide, a Toll-like receptor (TLR) 2 agonist; IL = interleukin, LOA = L-amino acid oxidase, TNF-α = tumor necrosis factor-α, iNOS = inducible nitric oxide synthase, NF-κB = nuclear factor-kappa B, CX3CR1 GFP = CX3C chemokine receptor 1 green fluorescent protein.

As bacteria are sensed by host receptors enabling transcription and/or activation of cytokines to guide an elaborate local innate immune response (described in detail below), TLR knock-out (KO) mice were tested following intramammary mastitic pathogen exposure [84].

It has been observed that LPS-induced mammary gland inflammation is abolished by TLR4 KO and that it can be reversed through the introduction of wild-type macrophages, although a potential contribution of MEC in this process cannot be completely ruled out [71]. The proper influx of neutrophils in this elegant model is guided by cytokines such as TNF-α (primordially macrophage-dependent response), IL-1 (primordially neutrophil- dependent response), IL-8 (mice KC and MIP-2 are orthologous to IL-8 in cows), and inducible nitric oxide synthase (iNOS); each mechanism being proven by the use of TNF-α KO, IL-1R KO, IL-8R KO or iNOS KO mice, respectively [46] (Figure 3).

Unfortunately, live MPEC infections are far more elaborate than the simple LPS inflammations models used for the latter study. Comparable to a LPS injection, MPEC infection in mice also induces transcription of similar cytokines induced by the transcription factor NF-κB as demonstrated elegantly with *in vivo* imaging in reporter mice [71] and described in the *in vitro* studies section. However, in marked contrast to LPS, the latter signalling is not fully triggered by TLR4 on macrophages [71]. A mammary MPEC infection has multiple MAMP and can still induce either a neutrophil influx or a cytokine response when either TLR4 (using TLR4 KO) or macrophages are lacking. Also in contrast to the observations in wT infected mice, the mastitic pathogens invade the mammary epithelia and form intracellular colonies in the absence of either TLR4 (again using TLR4 KO) or of macrophages. This colonization process is mediated by iNOS and IL-1 (as indicated by the use of iNOS KO and IL-1R KO mice, respectively). Upon neutrophil depletion instead of the previously described macrophage depletion, such an MPEC infection becomes lethal for the mice, proving the necessity of a neutrophil influx to resolve the bacterial mammary infection [85]. A similar observation has also been reported post-infection with coliform mastitis germs in cows that were made neutropenic with equine anti-bovine leukocyte serum compared to normal cows [86].

In contrast to LPS-induced mammary inflammation, an MPEC infection elicits a far more complex host response implicating that several MAMP are responsible for a proper neutrophil influx into the mammary gland. Synthetic analogues mimicking triacylated lipoproteins present on the cell membrane of gram-negative bacteria have been used in the mouse mastitis model, showing that these molecules facilitate the essential neutrophil influx. While they activate neutrophil influx following their injection in wT mice, they do not do so in TLR2 KO mice. Interestingly, MPEC inoculation induces neutrophil influx even in the absence of TLR2 signalling (using TLR2 KO). The latter signalling pathway is macrophage-independent and also restricts MPECs from invading the mammary tissue [87].

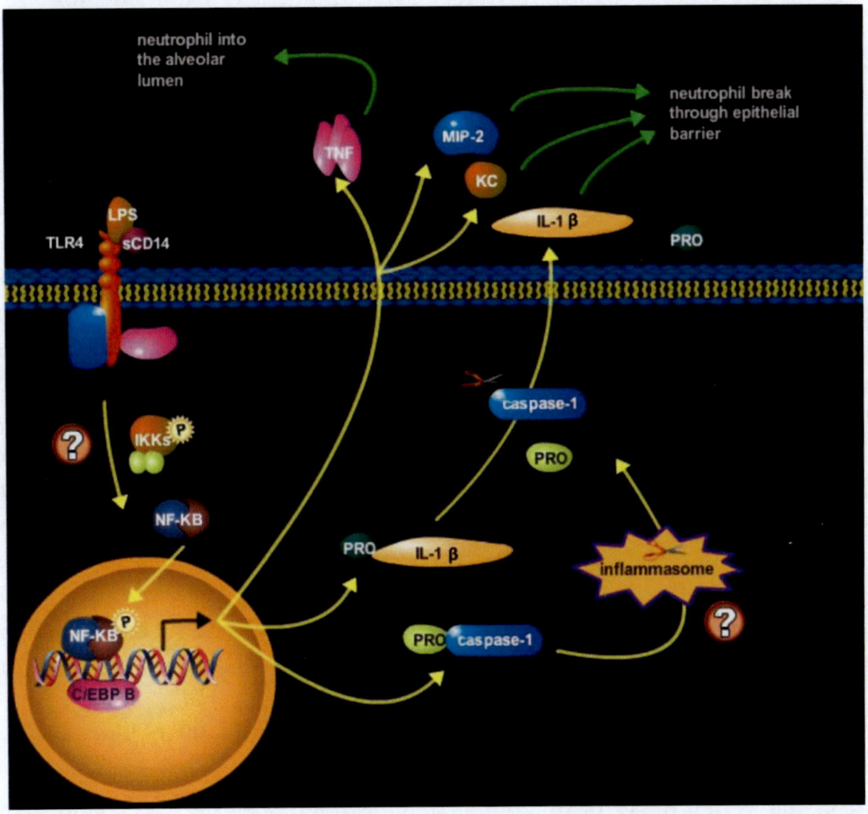

Figure 3. Schematic *E. coli*-induced inflammatory signalling in mammary cells based on mouse mastitis experiments with transgenic mice. *E. coli* triggers many TLRs on a multitude of cell types. Induction of mammary inflammation through TLR4 signalling is primarily a macrophage response, while the TLR2 response is macrophage unrelated. The question marks indicate areas of investigation as discussed in the future prospects section (made with software from www.proteinlounge.com).

Mastitis models have also been developed to improve treatments, or test novel identified molecular targets for new treatments. Antimicrobial treatment is the most frequently therapeutic strategy for mastitis in dairy cows. Over the past decades this curative strategy has succeeded to significantly decrease the prevalence and incidence of this infectious disease and positively affected animal health and milk productivity [56]. Nevertheless, in recent years, both pathogen adaptation to the udder and misuse/abuse of the current antibiotics has resulted in a need to further improve the treatment of mastitis. Antimicrobial testing of putative new substances is primarily screened *in vitro* by exposing pathogens to a library of compounds. Minimal inhibitory concentration (MIC) tests define the lowest concentration of an antimicrobial substance that kills or inhibits any visible growth of a bovine mastitic isolate. These dilution-based culture methods describe the susceptibility of mastitic pathogens to antibiotic molecules which aids the selection of an optimal therapy. Although this *in vitro* research provides very valuable data, the effective dose (ED) of an antibiotic substance can differ from the MIC value and influences the clinical outcome. The optimal drug concentration *in vitro* differs from that *in vivo* due to several factors including the dosing regimen, the host-pathogen inflammatory interaction and species-differences. Therefore, mouse mastitis models can extend the MIC data of potential antibiotic treatments before going into clinical trials with in udder-infected cows [88, 89]. These preclinical models provide a platform that mimics the pathogen properties such as the exponential growth of bacteria in a very dense mammary gland compartment, the formation of biofilms and the expression of bacterial toxins, in addition to host-related factors such as multicellular interactions, infiltration of (innate) inflammatory cells and milk antibacterial factors. In these set-ups the selected live pathogens are intramammarily inoculated and an intramammary injection with an antibiotic is subsequently performed. The use of mice has the advantage that different conditions can be compared.

As such the efficacy of one compound can be validated by a dose-response control. The lower the concentration of the candidate novel antibiotic agent the better it performs compared to a reference test compound taken along in the set-up. Additionally, the compound effectiveness can be further improved by changing the excipient [90].

This model has been validated for this screening purpose using commercial antibiotics as well as novel substances and this for multiple mastitic strains [91]. An innovative application was achieved by engineering a fusion protein attaching the streptococcal endolysin endopeptidase domain to the staphylococcal cell wall binding domain from the staphylococcal phage K endolysin. This newly bioengineered molecule was intramammarily injected in mice post-infection with *S. aureus* mastitis. It was able to significantly reduce the mammary CFU load and this effect was enhanced when co-injected with bacterial lysostaphin [92].

It must be remarked that all these candidate antibiotic treatments, similar to their existing commercialized counterparts, may lead in time to undesirable selection of drug-resistant bacteria. As an alternative strategy, inadequate - but accessible - host mediators which boost the immune system and protect the animal, can be administered preventively rather than curatively. A lactating mammary gland contains already antibacterial mechanisms protecting the host and its offspring from disease spread through milk residing pathogens. Transgenic murine models were developed to protect the host by up- or down-regulating one of these genes of interest. This promising concept may in time be used either for better clearance of pathogens by local or systemic administration of this factor or for vaccination purposes.

A first example of an immuno-modulating host factor that holds promise is L-amino acid oxidase (LAO), an antibacterial enzyme present in mouse milk during the first 10 days of lactation. Its antibacterial function is considered to occur through the production of H_2O_2 by oxidative processing of milk L-amino acids. Researchers generated LAO KO mice and introduced *S. aureus* mastitis pathogens intramammarily in these genetically modified animals. After 24 hours (h), an exudate was observed in the inguinal region concomitant with a 30-fold higher local bacterial growth compared to wild-type animals.

The gene had also severe systemic consequences for the host, as the LAO KO-infected animals were far more susceptible to the *S. aureus* toxicity. The effect could be partly reversed by administering wild-type whey to these infected KO mice [93].

A second example is an immuno-modulating host factor derived from the knowledge that ligand binding with plasma membrane associated TLRs is facilitated through scavenger receptors such as CD14 [94]. In an attempt to enhance the clearance of bacteria during mastitis, MPEC were co-injected with the soluble CD14 (sCD14) co-receptor. The sCD14 opsonizes bacteria and sensitizes the mammary gland for an upcoming bacterial hazard [95]. This enhanced alertness of the mammary gland by sCD14 brings along a subtle immune reaction. The latter was demonstrated by the occurrence of lower local TNF-α levels and proved to be more effective, as a lower number of mammary CFU was observed compared to the non-sCD14 pre-treated specimen [96]. The preclinical effect was extrapolated to dairy cows and an udder injection of MPEC together with sCD14 elicited also lower TNF-α and IL-8 levels concomitant with a more rapid decline of bacterial CFU due to a faster neutrophil influx [97]. In analogy with this sCD14 treatment, new therapies focusing on the host immunity rather than on antibacterial substances are now rapidly emerging and are first tested with the preclinical mastitis models. One of these reported anti-inflammatory compounds is helenalin acting as an NF-κB inhibitor which upon i.p. injection reduced mammary *S. aureus* proliferation and leukocyte infiltration in the mammary glands following *S. aureus* inoculation [98].

How Will Murine Models Further Advance Our Understanding of Mammary Gland Inflammatory Diseases?

Mastitis remains a major infectious disease in cattle that costs the dairy industry billions of dollars on a yearly basis worldwide. The inherent excessive and/or injudicious use of antimicrobials potentially promotes the development of antimicrobial resistance against both veterinary and human pathogens. To improve the cow's welfare and support the adequate control measures associated with this public health threat several bovine but also murine models were developed to aid in better understanding mammary gland inflammation.

In these mouse models, bovine mastitis isolates are orthotopically introduced and thus elicit a fast neutrophil influx concomitant with the local growth of the infecting bacteria within less than 24h. The small timeframe of disease progression, which involves in a major part the innate immune system, and the elaborate molecular tools available for mice in contrast to cows, entail that the *in vivo* murine model is very suitable for fundamental mastitis research. Also for human mammary diseases, preclinical mammary gland inflammation models are very valuable [100]. It allows the discovery of novel therapeutic targets and precedes the development of new treatment strategies. Nevertheless, it remains mandatory that these findings in mice are confirmed in the target species. The inflamed murine mammary gland can simulate udder infections with various strains of mastitic pathogens that prefer growth in a milky anti-microbial environment. These bacteria either display or produce a panel of MAMP that stimulate different TLR-expressing mammary cells. In response, inflammatory signalling is activated and the corresponding cytokine response induces the influx of immune cells to clear the bacterial hazard. Schematic molecular pathways have been proposed to provide the hypothetic innate signalling explaining this complex phenomenon [101] (Figure 3). Through transgenic mice models lacking specific genes this signalling scheme can be verified and if required, adjusted accordingly. The thus generated novel insights will allow to detect mastitis cases in an earlier stage and to ameliorate therapy significantly, either curatively or even preferably by boosting the host' (innate) immune system which holds promise for more effective vaccination strategies. As future prospect, the employment of even more performant technologies such as broad proteomics that simultaneously assess a panel of cytokines is envisaged with preclinical *in vivo* models. When such state-of-the-art technology is made available for application in cow blood or even better in milk samples, it could be provide the ultimate diagnostic tool for early mastitis detection. Indeed, in contrast to single cytokine detection, cytokine profiles are believed to be pathogen-specific [101]. Based on this multifactorial information an appropriate treatment could be pinpointed more easily, clearance of the infectious hazard could be achieved faster, the therapeutic costs could be downgraded and the inherent risk of developing multidrug-resistant bacteria could be reduced.

Mice models will be increasingly and flexibly adapted in order to reveal either the lack or the overproduction of a detected target associated with a mammary gland inflammation. If inappropriately low concentrations of such a host factor are associated with the pathogenicity, this factor might be boosted by injecting an agonist of the relevant signalling pathway or by administering the suited biomolecule [93, 96]. On the other hand, excessive levels of host factors can overstimulate the inflammation process and damage the mammary structure. Ideal therapeutic agents reducing this severe inflammation can still clear the germs but induce a milder, less acute syndrome [98]. A yet unexplored domain for mastitis vaccination and treatment purposes is inflammasome-related [102] (Figure 3). Similarly as in a large number of inflammatory diseases NF-κB, IL-1β and caspase-1 involvement has been implicated by our research group in the context of mastitis [76, 103, 104]. In these former diseases PRR-containing cells respond to so called "danger signals" that activate NF-κB, which is responsible for proIL-1β transcription. ProIL-1β maturation into its active IL-1β can be the consequence of procaspase-1 activation in multi-protein complexes called inflammasomes [105]. In essence, inflammasomes are highly controlled signalling nodules whose activity is responsible for cytokine release. When inflammasome activity is modulated by caspase-1 inhibitors, NF-κB inhibitors or sIL-1R, inflammation progression can be adjusted. Novel candidate host targets such as the inflammasome may be altered to treat mastitis and hypothetically this strategy may even entail a plausible vaccination opportunity [106]. Vaccination can also be ensued through IL-17A, which is a mediator between immune system and various epithelial tissues, stimulating various defensive mechanisms to bacterial infections [107].

Mouse models will also continue to be used for the evaluation of new anti-bacterial strategies against mastitic germs, identifying targets on the microbe instead of the host which enable mastitis bacteria to grow and infect the host. By transforming mastitic isolates into less pathogenic strains through site-specific mutagenesis, or by injecting a single pathogenic factor into the host, immunity can be raised against the original pathogenic germ [108, 109]. This strategy would also identify virulence factors that enable pathogens to invade host' tissue and display their pathogenicity as a target for specific treatment by facilitating bacterial clearance by the host [109]. Instead of transforming mastitis germs to prime the host inflammatory system, udder bacteria with beneficial properties can be inoculated in mice prior to a pathogenic infection. As CNS bacteria have pro-biotic properties they would be a suitable species to evaluate this treatment possibility [110, 111].

Last but not least, mouse mammary gland inflammation models can help us in our general understanding of other mammary gland disorders than mastitis. Indeed, early mammary gland involution occurs in a pro-inflammatory environment characterized by mastitis signalling such as NF-κB and TNF-α [112]. Although this initial inflammation becomes rapidly balanced by ensuing anti-inflammatory pathways, common characteristics of wound healing may well promote tumor progression in mice and humans. Moreover, a remarkable resemblance is observed when comparing gene-expression profiles during involution and inflammation of the mammary gland. Although there are no pathogens in a non-infected gland, the mammary cells of importance during the pathogenesis of mastitis have also essential functions in mammary tumor development. It is believed that epigenetic alterations in stromal cells might be initiated by chronic inflammation thereby resulting in an abnormal microenvironment and increased risk of tumor initiation [43]. Moreover, an excessive form of mammary inflammation can lead to inflammatory carcinomas, an aggressive form of breast cancer [113]. Additionally, lesions of non-bacterial inflammatory breast disease resembling breast carcinomas have been injected in mice. Post-injection of these carcinomas, the mice experienced a similar clinical and pathological manifestation [114]. Those recent studies underscore the relevance of ongoing research where bacteria or their toxins are intraductally injected together with murine mammary tumor cells in an attempt to bridge mouse mastitis research and the inflammatory process associated with different types of breast cancer /mammary tumors [115].

Acknowledgment

The authors would like to thank Dr. Pierre Germon (INRA, France) for his critical comments and helpful suggestions.

References

[1] Kuruppath, S., et al., Monotremes and marsupials: comparative models to better understand the function of milk. *J Biosci,* 2012. 37(4): p. 581-8.

[2] Capuco, A.V. and R.M. Akers, The origin and evolution of lactation. *J Biol,* 2009. 8(4): p. 37.

[3] Oftedal, O.T., The mammary gland and its origin during synapsid evolution. *J Mammary Gland Biol Neoplasia,* 2002. 7(3): p. 225-52.

[4] Smith, B.A., A.L. Welm, and B.E. Welm, On the shoulders of giants: a historical perspective of unique experimental methods in mammary gland research. *Semin Cell Dev Biol*, 2012. 23(5): p. 583-90.

[5] Lombardi, J., *Comparative vertebrate reproduction*. 1998: Kluwer Academic Pub.

[6] Richert, M.M., et al., An atlas of mouse mammary gland development. *J Mammary Gland Biol Neoplasia,* 2000. 5(2): p. 227-41.

[7] Lamote, I., et al., Sex steroids and growth factors in the regulation of mammary gland proliferation, differentiation, and involution. *Steroids*, 2004. 69(3): p. 145-59.

[8] Lacasse, P., et al., New developments on the galactopoietic role of prolactin in dairy ruminants. *Domest Anim Endocrinol,* 2012. 43(2): p. 154-60.

[9] Neville, M.C., Classic studies of mammary development and milk secretion: 1945 - 1980. *J Mammary Gland Biol Neoplasia*, 2009. 14(3): p. 193-7.

[10] Anantamongkol, U., et al., Prolactin and dexamethasone regulate second messenger-stimulated cl (-) secretion in mammary epithelia. *J Signal Transduct*, 2012. 2012: p. 192142.

[11] Watson, C.J. and P.A. Kreuzaler, Remodeling mechanisms of the mammary gland during involution. *Int J Dev Biol*, 2011. 55(7-9): p. 757-62.

[12] Sleeman, K.E., et al., CD24 staining of mouse mammary gland cells defines luminal epithelial, myoepithelial/basal and non-epithelial cells. *Breast Cancer Res,* 2006. 8(1): p. R7.

[13] Maller, O., H. Martinson, and P. Schedin, Extracellular Matrix Composition Reveals Complex and Dynamic Stromal-Epithelial Interactions in the Mammary Gland. *Journal of Mammary Gland Biology and Neoplasia,* 2010. 15(3): p. 301-318.

[14] Brownfield, D.G., et al., Patterned collagen fibers orient branching mammary epithelium through distinct signaling modules. *Curr Biol,* 2013. 23(8): p. 703-9.

[15] Dziewanowska, K., et al., *Staphylococcal* fibronectin binding protein interacts with heat shock protein 60 and integrins: Role in internalization by epithelial cells. *Infection and Immunity,* 2000. 68(11): p. 6321-6328.

[16] Dziewanowska, K., et al., Fibronectin binding protein and host cell tyrosine kinase are required for internalization of *Staphylococcus aureus* by epithelial cells. *Infection and Immunity,* 1999. 67(9): p. 4673-4678.

[17] Lochter, A. and M.J. Bissell, Involvement of extracellular matrix constituents in breast cancer. *Semin Cancer Biol,* 1995. 6(3): p. 165-73.

[18] Irwin, D.M., J.M. Biegel, and C.B. Stewart, Evolution of the mammalian lysozyme gene family. *BMC Evol Biol*, 2011. 11: p. 166.

[19] Huang, Y.Q., et al., Differential immunolocalization between lingual antimicrobial peptide and lactoferrin in mammary gland of dairy cows. *Vet Immunol Immunopathol,* 2012. 145(1-2): p. 499-504.

[20] Moon, J.S., et al., The antibacterial and immunostimulative effect of chitosan-oligosaccharides against infection by *Staphylococcus aureus* isolated from bovine mastitis. *Appl Microbiol Biotechnol*, 2007. 75(5): p. 989-98.

[21] Batovska, D.I., et al., Antibacterial study of the medium chain fatty acids and their 1-monoglycerides: individual effects and synergistic relationships. *Pol J Microbiol,* 2009. 58(1): p. 43-7.

[22] Sando, L., et al., Bovine Muc1 is a highly polymorphic gene encoding an extensively glycosylated mucin that binds bacteria. *J Dairy Sci*, 2009. 92(10): p. 5276-91.

[23] Boumahrou, N., et al., An increase in milk IgA correlates with both pIgR expression and IgA plasma cell accumulation in the lactating mammary gland of PRM/Alf mice. *J Reprod Immunol*, 2012. 96(1-2): p. 25-33.

[24] Schwarz, D., et al., Flow cytometric differential cell counts in milk for the evaluation of inflammatory reactions in clinically healthy and subclinically infected bovine mammary glands. *J Dairy Sci*, 2011. 94(10): p. 5033-44.

[25] Van den Broeck, W., A. Derore, and P. Simoens, Anatomy and nomenclature of murine lymph nodes: Descriptive study and nomenclatory standardization in BALB/cAnNCrl mice. *J Immunol Methods*, 2006. 312(1-2): p. 12-9.

[26] Taylor, B.C., et al., Bovine milk lymphocytes display the phenotype of memory T cells and are predominantly CD8+. *Cell Immunol*, 1994. 156(1): p. 245-53.

[27] Asai, K.-i., et al., Variation in $CD4^{+/T}$ and $CD8^{+/T}$ lymphocyte subpopulations in bovine mammary gland secretions during lactating and non-lactating periods. *Veterinary immunology and immunopathology*, 1998. 65(1): p. 51-61.

[28] Denis, M., et al., *Streptococcus uberis*-specific T cells are present in mammary gland secretions of cows and can be activated to kill *S. uberis*. *Vet Res Commun*, 2011. 35(3): p. 145-56.

[29] Sabbaj, S., C.C. Ibegbu, and A.P. Kourtis, Cellular immunity in breast milk: implications for postnatal transmission of HIV-1 to the infant. *Adv Exp Med Biol*, 2012. 743: p. 161-9.

[30] Tan, W., et al., Tumour-infiltrating regulatory T cells stimulate mammary cancer metastasis through RANKL-RANK signalling. *Nature*, 2011. 470(7335): p. 548-53.

[31] Cao, D., et al., Dynamics of CD4+ Lymphocytes in Mouse Mammary Gland Challenged with *Staphylococcus aureus*. *Asian Journal of Animal and Veterinary Advances,* 2012. 7(10): p. 1041-1048.

[32] Slama, P., et al., Effect of *Staphylococcus aureus* and *Streptococcus uberis* on apoptosis of bovine mammary gland lymphocytes. *Res Vet Sci,* 2009. 87(2): p. 233-8.

[33] Park, Y.H., et al., Suppression of proliferative response of BoCD4+ T lymphocytes by activated BoCD8+ T lymphocytes in the mammary gland of cows with *Staphylococcus aureus* mastitis. *Vet Immunol Immunopathol,* 1993. 36(2): p. 137-51.

[34] Webb, S.R. and N.R. Gascoigne, T-cell activation by superantigens. *Curr Opin Immunol,* 1994. 6(3): p. 467-75.

[35] Riollet, C., et al., Determination and characterization of bovine interleukin-17 cDNA. *Journal of interferon & cytokine research*, 2006. 26(3): p. 141-149.

[36] Persson Waller, K., et al., Cytokines in mammary lymph and milk during endotoxin-induced bovine mastitis. *Res Vet Sci,* 2003. 74(1): p. 31-6.

[37] Wallemacq, H., et al., CD40 triggering induces strong cytotoxic T lymphocyte responses to heat-killed *Staphylococcus aureus* immunization in mice: A new vaccine strategy for staphylococcal mastitis. *Vaccine*, 2012. 30(12): p. 2116-2124.

[38] Liu, B. and D.S. Newburg, Human Milk Glycoproteins Protect Infants Against Human Pathogens. *Breastfeeding Medicine*, 2013. 8(4): p. 354-362.

[39] Ismail, I.H., et al., Relationship between breast milk sCD14, TGF-beta 1 and total IgA in the first month and development of eczema during infancy. *Pediatric Allergy and Immunology*, 2013. 24(4): p. 352-360.

[40] Brandtzaeg, P., The mucosal immune system and its integration with the mammary glands. *The Journal of pediatrics*, 2010. 156(2): p. S8-S15.

[41] Farrell, H.M., Jr., et al., Nomenclature of the proteins of cows' milk--sixth revision. *J Dairy Sci*, 2004. 87(6): p. 1641-74.

[42] Leung, C.T. and J.S. Brugge, Outgrowth of single oncogene-expressing cells from suppressive epithelial environments. *Nature*, 2012. 482(7385): p. 410-3.

[43] Polyak, K. and R. Kalluri, The role of the microenvironment in mammary gland development and cancer. *Cold Spring Harb Perspect Biol*, 2010. 2(11): p. a003244.

[44] Pardoll, D., Metastasis-Promoting Immunity: When T Cells Turn to the Dark Side. *Cancer Cell*, 2009. 16(2): p. 81-82.

[45] DeNardo, D.G., et al., CD4 (+) T cells regulate pulmonary metastasis of mammary carcinomas by enhancing protumor properties of macrophages. *Cancer Cell,* 2009. 16(2): p. 91-102.

[46] Elazar, S., et al., Neutrophil recruitment in endotoxin-induced murine mastitis is strictly dependent on mammary alveolar macrophages. *Vet Res,* 2010. 41(1): p. 10.

[47] Sordillo, L.M. and K.L. Streicher, Mammary gland immunity and mastitis susceptibility. *J Mammary Gland Biol Neoplasia*, 2002. 7(2): p. 135-46.

[48] Schwertfeger, K.L., J.M. Rosen, and D.A. Cohen, Mammary gland macrophages: pleiotropic functions in mammary development. *J Mammary Gland Biol Neoplasia***,** 2006. 11(3-4): p. 229-38.

[49] O'Brien, J., et al., Macrophages are crucial for epithelial cell death and adipocyte repopulation during mammary gland involution. *Development*, 2012. 139(2): p. 269-75.
[50] Paape, M., et al., Defence of the bovine mammary gland by polymorphonuclear neutrophil leukocytes. *J Mammary Gland Biol Neoplasia*, 2002. 7(2): p. 109-21.
[51] Monks, J., et al., Epithelial cells as phagocytes: apoptotic epithelial cells are engulfed by mammary alveolar epithelial cells and repress inflammatory mediator release. *Cell Death Differ*, 2005. 12(2): p. 107-14.
[52] Monks, J., et al., Epithelial cells remove apoptotic epithelial cells during post-lactation involution of the mouse mammary gland. *Biol Reprod*, 2008. 78(4): p. 586-94.
[53] Gunther, J., et al., Assessment of the immune capacity of mammary epithelial cells: comparison with mammary tissue after challenge with *Escherichia coli*. *Vet Res*, 2009. 40(4): p. 31.
[54] Rauw, W.M., et al., Undesirable side effects of selection for high production efficiency in farm animals: a review. *Livestock Production Science*, 1998. 56(1): p. 15-33.
[55] Contreras, G.A. and J.M. Rodriguez, Mastitis: comparative etiology and epidemiology. *J Mammary Gland Biol Neoplasia*, 2011. 16(4): p. 339-56.
[56] Piepers, S., et al., Prevalence and distribution of mastitis pathogens in subclinically infected dairy cows in Flanders, Belgium. *Journal of Dairy Research*, 2007. 74(4): p. 478-483.
[57] Benkerroum, N., Antimicrobial peptides generated from milk proteins: a survey and prospects for application in the food industry. *A review. International Journal of Dairy Technology*, 2010. 63(3): p. 320-338.
[58] Barrio, M.B., P. Rainard, and B. Poutrel, Milk complement and the opsonophagocytosis and killing of *Staphylococcus aureus* mastitis isolates by bovine neutrophils. *Microb Pathog*, 2003. 34(1): p. 1-9.
[59] Rainard, P., The complement in milk and defence of the bovine mammary gland against infections. *Vet Res,* 2003. 34(5): p. 647-70.
[60] Lippolis, J.D., D.O. Bayles, and T.A. Reinhardt, Proteomic changes in *Escherichia coli* when grown in fresh milk versus laboratory media. *J Proteome Res,* 2009. 8(1): p. 149-58.
[61] Shpigel, N.Y., S. Elazar, and I. Rosenshine, Mammary pathogenic *Escherichia coli*. *Curr Opin Microbiol,* 2008. 11(1): p. 60-5.

[62] Louhi, M., et al., Relevance of sensitivity testings (MIC) of *S. aureus* to predict the antibacterial action in milk. *Zentralbl Veterinarmed B,* 1992. 39(4): p. 253-62.

[63] Le Marechal, C., et al., *Staphylococcus aureus* seroproteomes discriminate ruminant isolates causing mild or severe mastitis. *Vet Res,* 2011. 42(1): p. 35.

[64] Vangroenweghe, F., et al., Endoscopic examination and tissue sampling of the bovine teat and udder cistern. *J Dairy Sci,* 2006. 89(5): p. 1516-24.

[65] Huynh, H.T., G. Robitaille, and J.D. Turner, Establishment of bovine mammary epithelial cells (MAC-T): an *in vitro* model for bovine lactation. *Exp Cell Res,* 1991. 197(2): p. 191-9.

[66] Sharma, N. and D.K. Jeong, Stem Cell Research: A Novel Boulevard towards Improved Bovine Mastitis Management. *Int J Biol Sci,* 2013. 9(8): p. 818-29.

[67] Rauner, G. and I. Barash, Cell hierarchy and lineage commitment in the bovine mammary gland. *PLoS One*, 2012. 7(1): p. e30113.

[68] Swanson, K.M., et al., Transcriptome profiling of Streptococcus uberis-induced mastitis reveals fundamental differences between immune gene expression in the mammary gland and in a primary cell culture model. *J Dairy Sci,* 2009. 92(1): p. 117-29.

[69] Porcherie, A., et al., Repertoire of *Escherichia coli* agonists sensed by innate immunity receptors of the bovine udder and mammary epithelial cells. *Vet Res*, 2012. 43(1): p. 14.

[70] Strandberg, Y., et al., Lipopolysaccharide and lipoteichoic acid induce different innate immune responses in bovine mammary epithelial cells. *Cytokine*, 2005. 31(1): p. 72-86.

[71] Gonen, E., et al., Toll-like receptor 4 is needed to restrict the invasion of *Escherichia coli* P4 into mammary gland epithelial cells in a murine model of acute mastitis. *Cell Microbiol,* 2007. 9(12): p. 2826-38.

[72] Perkins, N.D., et al., Distinct Combinations of Nf-Kappa-B-Subunits Determine the Specificity of Transcriptional Activation. *Proceedings of the National Academy of Sciences of the United States of America*, 1992. 89(5): p. 1529-1533.

[73] Liu, S., et al., Lingual antimicrobial peptide and IL-8 expression are oppositely regulated by the antagonistic effects of NF-kappaB p65 and C/EBPbeta in mammary epithelial cells. *Mol Immunol*, 2011. 48(6-7): p. 895-908.

[74] Fitzgerald, D.C., et al., Tumour necrosis factor-alpha (TNF-alpha) increases nuclear factor kappa B (NF kappa B) activity in and interleukin-8 (IL-8) release from bovine mammary epithelial cells. *Veterinary Immunology and Immunopathology,* 2007. 116(1-2): p. 59-68.

[75] Notebaert, S., L. Duchateau, and E. Meyer, NF-kappaB inhibition accelerates apoptosis of bovine neutrophils. *Vet Res*, 2005. 36(2): p. 229-40.

[76] Demeyere, K., et al., *Escherichia coli* induces bovine neutrophil cell death independent from caspase-3/-7/-1, but with phosphatidylserine exposure prior to membrane rupture. *Vet Immunol Immunopathol,* 2013. 153(1-2): p. 45-56.

[77] Chandler, R.L., Preliminary report on the production of experimental mastitis in the mouse. *Vet Rec*, 1969. 84(26): p. 671-2.

[78] Chandler, R.L., Ultrastructural pathology of mastitis in the mouse. A study of experimental staphylococcal and streptococcal infections. *Br J Exp Pathol,* 1970. 51(6): p. 639-45.

[79] Chandler, R.L., Experimental bacterial mastitis in the mouse. *J Med Microbiol,* 1970. 3(2): p. 273-82.

[80] Chandler, R.L., Studies on experimental mouse mastitis relative to the assessment of pharmaceutical substances. *J Comp Pathol*, 1971. 81(4): p. 507-14.

[81] Barham, W., et al., Intraductal injection of LPS as a mouse model of mastitis: signaling visualized via an NF-kappaB reporter transgenic. *J Vis Exp*, 2012(67): p. e4030.

[82] van Knegsel, A.T., et al., Natural antibodies related to energy balance in early lactation dairy cows. *J Dairy Sci,* 2007. 90(12): p. 5490-8.

[83] Neville, M.C. and M.F. Picciano, Regulation of milk lipid secretion and composition. *Annu Rev Nutr*, 1997. 17: p. 159-83.

[84] De Schepper, S., et al., The toll-like receptor-4 (TLR-4) pathway and its possible role in the pathogenesis of *Escherichia coli* mastitis in dairy cattle. *Vet Res*, 2008. 39(1): p. 5.

[85] Elazar, S., et al., Essential role of neutrophils but not mammary alveolar macrophages in a murine model of acute *Escherichia coli* mastitis. *Veterinary Research*, 2010. 41(4).

[86] Jain, N.C., O.W. Schalm, and J. Lasmanis, Experimentally induced coliform (*Aerobacter aerogenes*) mastitis in normal cows and in cows made neutropenic by an equine anti-bovine leukocyte serum. *Am J Vet Res*, 1971. 32(12): p. 1929-35.

[87] Mintz, M., et al., Pam3CSK4/TLR2 signaling elicits neutrophil recruitment and restricts invasion of *Escherichia coli* P4 into mammary gland epithelial cells in a murine mastitis model. *Vet Immunol Immunopathol*, 2013. 152(1-2): p. 168-75.

[88] Brouillette, E., et al., Mouse mastitis model of infection for antimicrobial compound efficacy studies against intracellular and extracellular forms of *Staphylococcus aureus. Veterinary Microbiology,* 2004. 101(4): p. 253-262.

[89] Brouillette, E., et al., Inflammatory cell infiltration as an indicator of *Staphylococcus aureus* infection and therapeutic efficacy in experimental mouse mastitis. *Veterinary Immunology and Immunopathology*, 2005. 104(3-4): p. 163-169.

[90] Demon, D., et al., The intramammary efficacy of first generation cephalosporins against *Staphylococcus aureus* mastitis in mice. *Veterinary Microbiology*, 2012. 160(1-2): p. 141-150.

[91] Demon, D., et al., Short communication: Antimicrobial efficacy of intramammary treatment with a novel biphenomycin compound against *Staphylococcus aureus*, *Streptococcus uberis*, and *Escherichia coli*-induced mouse mastitis. *Journal of Dairy Science*, (0).

[92] Schmelcher, M., et al., Chimeric Phage Lysins Act Synergistically with Lysostaphin To Kill Mastitis-Causing *Staphylococcus aureus* in Murine Mammary Glands. *Applied and Environmental Microbiology*, 2012. 78(7): p. 2297-2305.

[93] Nagaoka, K., et al., L-amino acid oxidase plays a crucial role in host defence in the mammary glands. *FASEB J*, 2009. 23(8): p. 2514-20.

[94] Zanoni, I. and F. Granucci, Role of CD14 in host protection against infections and in metabolism regulation. *Front Cell Infect Microbiol*, 2013. 3: p. 32.

[95] Wang, Y., et al., Recombinant bovine soluble CD14 sensitizes the mammary gland to lipopolysaccharide. *Veterinary Immunology and Immunopathology*, 2002. 86(1-2): p. 115-124.

[96] Lee, J.W., M.J. Paape, and X. Zhao, Recombinant bovine soluble CD14 reduces severity of experimental *Escherichia coli* mastitis in mice. *Veterinary Research*, 2003. 34(3): p. 307-316.

[97] Lee, J.W., et al., Recombinant soluble CD14 reduces severity of intramammary infection by *Escherichia coli. Infection and Immunity*, 2003. 71(7): p. 4034-4039.

[98] Boulanger, D., et al., Helenalin reduces *Staphylococcus aureus* infection *in vitro* and *in vivo*. *Veterinary Microbiology*, 2007. 119(2-4): p. 330-338.

[99] Notebaert, S., et al., *In vivo* imaging of NF-kappaB activity during *Escherichia coli*-induced mammary gland infection. *Cell Microbiol*, 2008. 10(6): p. 1249-58.

[100] Cauwels, A., B. Vandendriessche, and P. Brouckaert, Of mice, men, and inflammation. *Proc Natl Acad Sci U S A*, 2013. 110(34): p. E3150.

[101] Gunther, J., et al., Comparative kinetics of *Escherichia coli*- and *Staphylococcus aureus*-specific activation of key immune pathways in mammary epithelial cells demonstrates that *S. aureus* elicits a delayed response dominated by interleukin-6 (IL-6) but not by IL-1A or tumor necrosis factor alpha. *Infect Immun*, 2011. 79(2): p. 695-707.

[102] Dostert, C., K. Ludigs, and G. Guarda, Innate and adaptive effects of inflammasomes on T cell responses. *Curr Opin Immunol*, 2013. 25(3): p. 359-65.

[103] Becker, C.E. and L.A.J. O'Neill, Inflammasomes in inflammatory disorders: The role of TLRs and their interactions with NLRs. *Seminars in Immunopathology*, 2007. 29(3): p. 239-248.

[104] Notebaert, S., et al., Inflammatory mediators in *Escherichia coli*-induced mastitis in mice. *Comp Immunol Microbiol Infect Dis*, 2008. 31(6): p. 551-65.

[105] Lamkanfi, M. and V.M. Dixit, Inflammasomes and their roles in health and disease. *Annu Rev Cell Dev Biol*, 2012. 28: p. 137-61.

[106] Brade, L., S. Hensen, and H. Brade, Evaluation of a LPS-based glycoconjugate vaccine against bovine *Escherichia coli* mastitis: Formation of LPS Abs in cows after immunization with *E. coli* core oligosaccharides conjugated to hemocyanine. *Innate Immun,* 2013. 19(4): p. 368-77.

[107] Bougarn, S., et al., *Staphylococcal*-associated molecular patterns enhance expression of immune defence genes induced by IL-17 in mammary epithelial cells. *Cytokine*, 2011. 56(3): p. 749-59.

[108] Chen, L., et al., Protective effect of recombinant staphylococcal enterotoxin A entrapped in polylactic-co-glycolic acid microspheres against *Staphylococcus aureus* infection. *Vet Res,* 2012. 43(1): p. 20.

[109] Bramley, A.J., et al., Roles of alpha-toxin and beta-toxin in virulence of *Staphylococcus aureus* for the mouse mammary gland. *Infect Immun*, 1989. 57(8): p. 2489-94.

[110] Braem, G., *Exploration of antibacterial activities by CNS bovine teat apex skin in view of their inhibitory effect on mastitis-related pathogens.* 2012, VUB.

[111] De Vliegher, S., et al., Invited review: Mastitis in dairy heifers: Nature of the disease, potential impact, prevention, and control. *Journal of Dairy Science*, 2012. 95(3): p. 1025-1040.

[112] Lyons, T.R., et al., Postpartum mammary gland involution drives progression of ductal carcinoma *in situ* through collagen and COX-2. *Nature Medicine*, 2011. 17(9): p. 1109-U116.

[113] Uematsu, T., MRI findings of inflammatory breast cancer, locally advanced breast cancer, and acute mastitis: T2-weighted images can increase the specificity of inflammatory breast cancer. *Breast Cancer,* 2012. 19(4): p. 289-94.

[114] Yu, J.J., et al., Mouse model of plasma cell mastitis. *Journal of Translational Medicine,* 2012. 10.

[115] Breyne K. et al., *Flow cytometric immunophenotyping of the bacterially infected mammary gland, abstract GRC mammary gland biology conference*, 2012.

In: Mammary Glands
Editor: Edmund B. Rucker

ISBN: 978-1-62948-853-0

Chapter VII

Mastitis Resistance

Mayumi Sugimoto
National Livestock Breeding Center, Odakura, Nishigo, Fukushima, Japan

Abstract

Mastitis, a mammary gland inflammation in response to bacterial infection, is a major problem in the dairy industry. Recent scanning of the whole genome of cows (*Bos taurus*) that were susceptible or resistant to mastitis in the half-sib families has revealed that *forebrain embryonic zinc finger-like* (*FEZL)* and *insulin-like growth factor 1 receptor* (*IGF1R*) were responsible genes for mastitis resistance. Originally FEZL has been known as a transcription factor with a role in neuronal development. However, cows susceptible to mastitis had a three-base insertion in a glycine coding stretch of the gene for FEZL, which makes FEZL containing 13 glycines (13G) instead of 12 glycines (12G). Mastitis-induced *FEZL* expression in mammary glands and enhanced FEZL promoted expression of the axon-attracting molecule semaphorin (SEMA) 5A through a GCAG sequence. *SEMA5A* expression in susceptible cattle carrying 13G FEZL were lower than in resistant cattle carrying 12G FEZL. Enhanced SEMA5A induced expression of at least 9 genes related to the host's immune response including *tumor necrosis factor* α and *interleukin-8*. Susceptibility to mastitis results from an impaired immune response due to the lower transcription activity of 13G

FEZL. Thus, FEZL and SEMA5A play unexpected roles in immune response in addition to in neuronal development.

Further investigation of the whole genome of cows that were susceptible or resistant to mastitis identified that susceptible cows had a relatively long stretch of cytosine residues (C stretch) in the 5' untranslated region of *IGF1R*. Surprisingly, FEZL bound the C stretch of *IGF1R*. In contrast with *SEMA5A* expression, 13G FEZL and the longer C stretch of *IGF1R* together enhanced expression of IGF1R. IGF1R controls autophagy in conjunction with changes in nutrient levels through phosphatidylinositol 3-kinase and target of rapamycin signaling. As expected, an increase of IGF1R inhibited autophagy in response to *Streptococcus agalactiae*, which is one of the major bacteria causing mastitis, invasion of mammary epithelial cells. On the other hand, treatment with rapamycin, a known inducer of autophagy, rescued mammary epithelial cells from its invasion. Cows carrying 13G FEZL and the longer C stretch of *IGF1R* might be more susceptible to mastitis due to impaired autophagy. Taken together, FEZL and IGF1R could control innate immunity and serve as a potential tool for preventing mastitis.

Introduction

Mastitis is a common infectious disease of the mammary gland and a major problem in the dairy industry. It generates annual total losses of over 69 billion yen in Japan [1] and 2 billion dollars in US [2] by reducing milk quantity/quality and increasing the health costs. Just as current selective breeding programs based on population genetics have successfully increased milk yield, genetic selection for mastitis resistance could potentially be practiced, not only to reduce the cost of producing milk but also to improve the health and well-being of dairy cows. Recently Wall et al. [3] produced transgenic cows resistant to infection by inducing the cells of the mammary gland to secrete an antibacterial protein. However, the public may not quickly accept milk from transgenic animals despite the improved health of dairy herds [4].

On the other hand, several groups have begun quantitative trait locus (QTL) mapping using a granddaughter design to identify genes influencing mastitis resistance [5, 6, 7, 8, 9, 10, 11, 12, 13]. QTL mapping is designed to find naturally occurring mutations affecting phenotype in the population. Thus it will improve health of dairy herds based on genetic selection rather than transgenic technology, which might be acceptable to the public. Nevertheless, the drawback of this method is a large cost to genotype many samples because a granddaughter design is an analysis using genotypes determined on sons of heterozygous sires and phenotypes measured on daughters of the sons [14].

Alternatively, other groups performed QTL mapping based on selective genotyping [2, 15, 16]. Selective genotyping is an analysis using mastitis-resistant and mastitis-susceptible daughters, which reduces the number of samples genotyped. The function of a gene carrying a putative polymorphism positionally identified should significantly influence the phenotype. This chapter shows two successful examples using selective genotyping for detecting genes responsible for mastitis resistance, which turned out to play unexpected roles in immune function in mammary gland.

An SCS Locus is Linked to FEZL

To determine QTL influencing mastitis resistance, 6 half-sib families derived from the grandsire, Walkway Chef Mark, were chosen because they were large families consisted of a total of 6,561 daughters in the Tokachi county area, Hokkaido, Japan. Samples were collected in this specific area to minimize possible environmental variations. Since there is a strong genetic correlation between somatic cell score (SCS) and mastitis [17, 18], the average SCS ($\log_2$ (somatic cell count /100) +3) during the first lactation period was used as a phenotype parameter. Somatic cell count in milk did not normally distribute while SCS did (skewness = 0.93, kurtosis = -0.42). Among 6,561 samples, mastitis-susceptible daughters whose average SCS was more than 4 and resistant daughters whose average SCS was less than 2 were collected for selective genotyping. The resulting families consisted of 181 daughters with high SCS of 4.82 and 297 daughters with low SCS of 0.65.

After isolating genomic DNA from blood of these 478 samples, a whole-genome scan of 29 autosomal chromosomes was conducted by typing 272 microsatellite markers selected from Shirakawa-USDA genetic map [19]. The analysis using the DISMULT program of the DISEQ package [20], which is suitable for a multi-point analysis of selective genotyping data, revealed significant linkage of SCS loci to *Bos taurus* autosomal chromosomes (BTA) 21 and 22 with a likelihood of odds (LOD) score of more than 5. Further analysis with an additional 64 markers in BTA22 supported the linkage, although the LOD scores by DISEQ are likely overestimates because all pedigrees were related.

The significant linkage at the 1% genome-wide level was also confirmed as an F-statistic of 4.45 in a total of 6,561 daughters of the families using QTL express [21], which was developed for the analysis of QTL from outbred populations and able to include the phenotype information of untyped samples. Next the critical region for SCS harboring the 6.2-centimorgan (cM) interval with a LOD score of more than 18 by DISEQ was constructed from a bacterial artificial chromosome (BAC) contig based on screening the bovine CHORI-240, RPCI-42, and Wagyu BAC libraries [22, 23] using polymerase chain reaction (PCR). Partial sequencing of the contig indicated that the 6.2-cM region was equivalent to *Homo sapiens* autosomal chromosome 3p14.2, where 6 known genes were assigned [24].

Sequencing exons of these six genes identified neither nonsense nor missense mutations except for a three base insertion in forebrain embryonic zinc finger-like (FEZL) [25]. FEZL contains 6 C2H2 type zinc-finger domains and a glycine stretch where the insertion resulted in an extension of 12 glycines (12G) to 13 glycines (13G). Although the possibility that one or more of the other five genes may affect SCS cannot be excluded, it is valuable to examine whether the polymorphism in FEZL affects SCS.

Mastitis Induces FEZL

FEZL controls the development of monoaminergic neurons [26]. Hirata et al. [27] reported that FEZL-deficient mice display hyperactive behavior, suggesting that FEZL has a role in neuronal development. Consistent with a role for FEZL as a transcription factor that regulates forebrain development, real-time PCR revealed that bovine *FEZL* was expressed strongly in brain and weakly in mammary gland.

Nevertheless, among mammary glands, *FEZL* expression was greater in the quarter affected with mastitis, confirmed by the California Mastitis Test, than in the cured quarter of the same cattle. Because it is possible that infection enhances *FEZL* expression in the mammary gland, FEZL might have an important role in antimicrobial response and the polymorphism described here might affect its function.

FEZL Binds GCAG

To elucidate the effect of the polymorphism on function, V5-tagged FEZL was transfected into monkey kidney COS-7 cells or human breast cancer-derived OCUB-M cells. Immunofluorescence using fluorescein isothiocyanate-conjugated V5 antibody demonstrated that both 12G and 13G FEZL localized to the nucleus, indicating that the polymorphism does not affect protein localization.

In many transcription factors, the zinc fingers mediate binding to promoter elements of their target genes [28]. To determine the optimal binding sequences for the FEZL protein, chromatin immunoprecipitation (ChIP) assays of cells transfected with His-tagged FEZL was performed. Comparison of the selected sequences by anti-His antibody yielded an optimal binding site of GCAG and there was no difference between the 12G and 13G FEZL consensus in COS-7 and OCUB-M cells. Gel mobility shift and competition experiments showed that binding was abolished by co-incubation with unlabeled consensus but not by AP2 in either COS-7 cells transfected with 12G FEZL or 13G FEZL, demonstrating that DNA binding activities of 12G and 13G FEZL are similar.

FEZL Activates SEMA5A

Androgen receptors contain a glycine stretch and its complete deletion reduces trans-activation *in vitro* [29], suggesting that the length of the glycine stretch in FEZL might affect its transcription activity. To compare 12G and 13G FEZL transcription activities, the first (1) and second (2) introns of Semaphorin (SEMA) 5A were selected as binding sequences obtained from the ChIP assays and fused into reporter construsts. Luciferase assays by cotransfecting FEZL and SEMA5A reporter constructs revealed that 12G FEZL induced both the SEMA5A1 and SEMA5A2 reporters to higher levels than 13G FEZL. Moreover real-time PCR using OCUB-M cells transfected with FEZL indicated that 12G FEZL stimulated greater *SEMA5A* expression than 13G FEZL. Conversely, transfection of small interfering RNA (siRNA) targeting *FEZL* reduced *SEMA5A* expression. Additionally *SEMA5A* expression was greater in 12G/13G FEZL cattle than in 13G/13G FEZL cattle, indicating that SEMA5A is the target of FEZL *in vivo*. Furthermore, mastitis induced *SEMA5A* expression, demonstrating that infection enhances SEMA5A through FEZL *in vivo*. Thus, the glycine stretch in FEZL appeared to influence transcription activity of SEMA5A after infection.

FEZL Induces TNFα and IL-8 through SEMA5A

SEMA5A, an axon guidance cue [30], belongs to the semaphorin family characterized by functionally conserved roles in neuronal development [31]. Recent studies, however, revealed the existence of crosstalk between neuronal development and immunity. The neuronal repellent Slit regulates both neuronal and leukocyte migration [32]. The semaphorin family members SEMA4A and SEMA4D activate T cells [33] and enhance B cell responses [34], respectively. Kumanogoh called them "immune semaphorins" although it is not known if SEMA5A is an immune semaphorin.

To investigate potential genes that might be induced by SEMA5A, OCUB-M cells transfected with SEMA5A were screened by microarray analysis. The candidate genes induced by SEMA5A included 9 genes related to chemotaxis and inflammatory/immune response. The induction of two of the 9 genes, *tumor necrosis factor* (*TNF*) α and *interleukin* (*IL*) *8*, was also confirmed by real-time PCR. In addition, 12G FEZL induced greater *TNF*α and *IL-8* expression than 13G FEZL. In contrast, siRNA targeting *FEZL* or *SEMA5A* reduced *TNF*α and *IL-8* expression. Impaired *TNF*α and *IL-8* expression controlled by FEZL and SEMA5A could explain susceptibility of 13G FEZL cattle to mastitis.

Infection Induces FEZL through TRIF

Escherichia coli causes 13.9% of mastitis [1]. To build a model of mammary glands infected by gram-negative bacteria, real-time PCR using OCUB-M cells after lipopolysaccharide (LPS) treatment was conducted. Consistent with the results in bovine mammary gland, treatment with 10 μg/ml LPS from *E. coli* induced both *FEZL* and *SEMA5A* expression in OCUB-M cells. The maximum induction was achieved at 6 h, suggesting that FEZL-SEMA5A signaling is involved in the late phase of the infection. LPS facilitates the myeloid differentiation primary-response protein 88 (MyD88)-

dependent response in the early phase and the MyD88-independent response in the late phase through toll-like receptor (TLR) 4 [35]. RNA interference experiments targeting MyD88, toll/IL-1-receptor-domain-containing adapter protein-inducing interferon-β (TRIF), and interferon-regulatory factor (IRF) 3 revealed that both siRNAs targeting TRIF and IRF3 reduce *FEZL* and *SEMA5A* expressions 6 h after LPS treatment while siRNA targeting MyD88 does not. These observations indicated that LPS activates *FEZL* expression in a MyD88-independent manner through the late phase of infection mediated by TLR4, TRIF, and IRF3.

Impact of FEZL

As shown above, *FEZL* was mapped as a gene influencing SCS in a large family derived from a specific sire, Walkway Chief Mark. The effects of FEZL on SCS and the incidence of mastitis, however, must be confirmed among randomly collected samples before genetic selection based on this gene can be implemented in the dairy industry. To determine the impact of 12G FEZL on resistance to mastitis, a total of 918 DNA samples from commercially available sires in Japan and a total of 41,431 clinical mastitis records in 162,655 lactation periods of daughters derived from these sires were collected [36].

FEZL typing of these 918 sires revealed that 97 sires had 12G/13G FEZL while 821 sires had 13G/13G FEZL. In daughters younger than 3 years old, 2,136 (18.9 %) among 11,283 daughters derived from sires carrying 12G/13G FEZL were affected, while 12,691 (20.1 %) among 63,165 daughters derived from sires carrying 13G/13G FEZL were affected. Fisher's exact test [37] indicated a difference (p = 0.004) between these two groups. In daughters older than 3 years old, the proportion of affected daughters derived from sires carrying 12G/13G FEZL was significantly lower than that of affected daughters derived from sires carrying 13G/13G FEZL [36]. These findings confirmed that FEZL impacts the incidence of mastitis as well as SCS.

An SCS Locus Is Linked to IGF1R

To identify the genes that influence susceptibility to mastitis in addition to FEZL on BTA22, 478 cows from 6 half-sib families were further analyzed with an additional 161 microsatellite markers on BTA21. QTL express [21] detected the QTL effect of SCS on 4 cM of BTA21 at the 5 % chromosome-wide level. Because FEZL helps modulate the innate immune response [16], the F-statistic for BTA21 was computed by weighting with the genotype of FEZL to evaluate whether this transcription factor affected linkage in the chromosome. Surprisingly, the F-statistic for BTA21 by weighting with FEZL was increased and the QTL was significant at the 5% genome-wide level. These observations suggested a potential interrelationship between FEZL and the candidate genes on BTA21.

FEZL is a transcription factor and 12G FEZL and 13G FEZL have different effects on the expression of SEMA5A [16]. Therefore, a gene influencing susceptibility to mastitis on BTA21 should fulfill the following criteria. First, the gene of interest should be located in the critical region for SCS harboring the 8-cM interval between 2 and 10 cM of BTA21 based on the 5% chromosome-wide significance by QTL express [21]. Second, the expression of the gene of interest should be controlled by FEZL. Third, 12G FEZL and 13G FEZL should have different effects on the expression of the gene of interest. Fourth, the gene of interest should carry a polymorphism that differs between alleles in resistant and susceptible animals. Fifth and finally, 13G FEZL should differentially affect the expression of the gene of interest depending on the polymorphic alleles.

With respect to the first criterion, the Bos_taurus_UMD_3.1/bosTau6 assembly (http://www.hgsc.bcm.tmc.edu/projects/bovine/) identified 11 genes located in the critical region. To test whether these genes fulfilled the second and third criteria, real-time PCR of bovine mammary epithelial cells (BMECs) [38] transfected with FEZL were conducted and verified that FEZL did not affect the expression of any of the 11 genes except for *insulin-like growth factor 1 receptor* (*IGF1R*). 13G FEZL enhanced the expression of *IGF1R* more than 12G FEZL, implying that *IGF1R* fulfilled the second and third criteria. In regard to the fourth criterion, polymorphisms of *IGF1R* that were carried by susceptible and resistant cows derived from the half-sib families were searched and found different length of a stretch of cytosine residues (C stretch) on the 5' untranslated region (5'UTR). To test whether *IGF1R* fulfilled the fifth criterion, luciferase assays were performed using COS-7 cells co-transfected with FEZL and luciferase vectors encoding the 5'UTR of *IGF1R* with different alleles. Consistent with the results of real-time PCR of BMECs transfected with FEZL, 13G FEZL enhanced the luciferase activity of *IGF1R* with a long C stretch. Based on the fulfillment of these five criteria, *IGF1R* appeared to be the most promising candidate gene.

FEZL Binds the C stretch

The optimal binding sequence of FEZL was GCAG — not the C stretch — based on ChIP assays and sequencing [16]. Characterizations of transcription factor targets tend to be biased if DNA microarrays are not used [39]. Thus, FEZL might bind to the C stretch of *IGF1R*, and the different effects of the C stretch might have been due to their different binding abilities. To test this hypothesis, a gel mobility-shift assay using COS-7 cells transfected with FEZL was performed. As expected, FEZL bound to the 5'UTR of *IGF1R* and the specificity of binding was confirmed by gel supershift assays using the specific antibody. Next the binding ability of the C stretch of *IGF1R* more closely using competitors was assessed, which revealed that a long C stretch, 10C, bound stronger to FEZL than 9C. Taken together, these findings indicate that FEZL binds to the 5'UTR of *IGF1R* and the length of the C stretch affects the binding ability.

Impact of IGF1R

IGF1R plays a role in insulin/insulin-like growth factor signaling (IIS), an evolutionarily conserved process that controls the lifespan of organisms. Nematodes, flies, and mice with impaired IIS are relatively long-lived [40, 41, 42]. IIS modulates resistance to challenges by heat shock, oxidative stress, ultraviolet damage, and pathogens [43, 44]. Long-lived *daf-2* mutants are resistant to bacterial pathogens including *Pseudomonas aeruginosa*, *Enterococcus faecalis*, and *Staphylococcus aureus* [45]. Therefore, IGF1R might modulate defense against invading bacteria.

Cows carrying 13G/13G FEZL and *IGF1R* with a long C stretch showed greater expression of IGF1R at both the messenger RNA (mRNA) and protein level, demonstrating that the longer C stretch in combination with 13G/13G FEZL enhanced IGF1R *in vivo*. The allelic mRNA ratio determined by SNaPshot also revealed that the level of mRNA from the 10C allele yielded higher than the 9C allele. Enhanced IGF1R might affect resistance to infection in mammals, consistent with the findings of experiments on nematodes that *daf-2* mutants are resistant to bacterial pathogens [45]. Indeed, cows carrying 13G/13G FEZL and *IGF1R* with a longer C stretch had higher SCS among 478 cows from 6 half-sib families, indicating that they are susceptible to mastitis. Furthermore, cows derived from sires carrying 13G/13G FEZL and

IGF1R with a longer C stretch have a greater incidence of clinical mastitis, suggesting that enhanced IGF1R is linked to increased susceptibility to mastitis.

Autophagy and Mastitis Resistance

Autophagy is another evolutionarily conserved process, through which the intracellular contents are digested in order to recover nutrients in response to starvation [46]. IIS controls autophagy in conjunction with changes in nutrient levels through phosphatidylinositol 3-kinase (PI3K) and target of rapamycin (TOR) signaling [47]. An increase of class I PI3K products suppresses autophagy [48]. Inactivation of TOR, which is one of the downstream components of PI3K signaling, induces autophagy [49]. Treatment with rapamycin, an inhibitor of TOR, also induces autophagy in yeast [50]. It has been confirmed that class I PI3K signaling suppresses starvation-induced autophagy, while loss of TOR activity induces autophagy even without starvation in flies [51]. More directly, *daf-2* IGF1R mutants have been reported to show enhanced autophagy in nematodes [52].

Surprisingly, recent studies have revealed that cells also deploy their autophagic machinery as a defense against invading bacteria [53]. When *Streptococcus pyogenes* entered the cytoplasm of nonphagocytic cells, the bacteria were selectively sequestered and killed by autophagy [54]. The induction of autophagy by starvation or treatment by rapamycin suppressed the intracellular survival of *Mycobacterium tuberculosis* [55]. In *C. elegans*, genetic knockdown of autophagy genes abrogates pathogen resistance [56]. Thus, the activation of autophagy, leading to improved defenses against bacteria, might represent a role of IIS in innate immunity in mammals.

To test this hypothesis, BMECs [38] were initially investigated whether infection-induced autophagy was observed. Mammary epithelial cells are the first line of defense in protecting hosts from invading *Streptococcus agalactiae,* which is one of the major pathogens causing 16.9% of mastitis [1]. As expected, infected *S. agalactiae* colocalized with LC3, which is an autophagosome-specific membrane marker [54] in immunostaining of BMECs. Western blotting revealed that starvation as well as infection of *S. agalactiae* in BMECs induced the amount of 16 kD band of LC3-II, which is a molecular form binding to autophagosome [54]. Thus, the BMECs appeared to defend the host against *S. agalactiae* through autophagy.

Next to investigate the effects of IIS on the autophagy of *S. agalactiae* in BMECs, colony forming unit viability assays were conducted. Treatment with IGF1, a ligand of IGF1R, increased the bacterial viability in the BMECs dose-dependently. On the other hand, treatment with rapamycin, an inhibitor of TOR as well as an inducer of autophagy, reduced the bacterial viability. These observations suggested that enhanced IIS repressed infection-induced autophagy in BMECs, and cows carrying 13G/13G FEZL and *IGF1R* with a longer C stretch might thus be more susceptible to mastitis due to impaired autophagy.

Discussion

Multiple lines of evidence have been demonstrated that FEZL is one of the genes responsible for mastitis resistance in cattle. First, the FEZL region was mapped as a QTL on BTA22 using 6 half-sib families having the same grandsire. It is important to note that several studies identified QTLs for SCS and mastitis on BTA22 [5, 13, 15]. Second, the polymorphism of the length of the glycine stretch of FEZL was significantly associated with SCS. Third, the length of the glycine stretch of FEZL impacts its transcription activity, leading to control of cytokine expression. A single glycine insertion into the glycine stretch of FEZL has a large effect on its downstream pathway.

Many studies have documented the importance of neutrophil migration for innate immunity. Neutrophils are highly effective phagocytes for clearing infecting bacterial pathogens from host tissue [57]. The number of neutrophils migrating to the site of infection has been associated with the production of IL-8 [58]. TNFα induces *IL-8* expression in the late phase of infection [59] and the IL-8 receptor is also involved in transepithelial neutrophil migration [60]. Moreover, lung-specific transgenic mice with KC, one of the IL-8 homologues in the mouse, are resistant to *Klebsiella pneumoniae* infection [61]. On the other hand, IL-8 receptor knock-out mice are susceptible to acute experimental pyelonephritis [62]. Thus, the ability of FEZL to promote *TNFα* and *IL-8* expression through SEMA5A triggered by LPS represents a plausible mechanism to explain the enhanced antimicrobial activity of FEZL-expressing cells.

There is accumulating evidence to suggest that lifetime exposure to infectious diseases influences human lifespan [63, 64]; however, the role of IGF1R in innate immunity in mammals has remained unclear, despite its influence on longevity in humans [65, 66, 67] and mice [42]. This linkage study for mastitis resistance provided direct evidence that IGF1R is involved in innate immunity through autophagy in a mammalian species. In *Bos taurus*, a polymorphism in the 5'UTR of IGF1R on BTA21 was associated with mastitis incidence. It is noteworthy that Boichard et al. [8] and Schulman et al. [11] also identified QTLs for SCS on BTA21. The susceptible genotype of *IGF1R* is associated with its elevated expression and enhanced IGF1R inhibited autophagy in response to *S. agalactiae* invasion. Moreover, the polymorphisms in the autophagy genes are linked to genetic susceptibility to the inflammatory bowel disorder, Crohn's disease, in human [68]. Together, these data demonstrate a critical role for IGF1R through autophagy in mediating pathogen resistance in mammals.

How the polymorphism in the 5'UTR of IGF1R works *in vivo* was unknown. However, gel mobility-shift assay and competition assays revealed that FEZL binds to the 5'UTR of *IGF1R* and the length of the C stretch affects the binding ability. The genotype of FEZL and IGF1R influences the expression level of IGF1R. *cis*-Acting polymorphisms would affect transcription, mRNA processing, mRNA stability, and protein translation [69]. Rapamycin has proven to suppress translation of mRNAs which contains an oligopyrimidine tract at their transcriptional start [70]. FEZL might modify the expression level of IGF1R through binding to its 5'UTR together with TOR signaling.

Although it has been confirmed that autophagy protected bovine mammary gland cells from invading *S. agalactiae*, whether autophagy protects mammary gland from other pathogens involved in mastitis such as *S. aureus* should be clarified. It has been known that *S. pyogenes* and *M. tuberculosis* were killed by autophagy whereas *Shigella flexneri* was able to escape from autophagy [54, 55, 71]. Some reported that autophagic degradation was induced against *S. aureus* [72]. On the other hand, others demonstrated that *S. aureus* escaped from autophagy [73]. The role of autophagy for pathogens causative of mastitis in mammary gland other than *S. agalactiae* is yet to be resolved.

It is notable that autophagy is a mechanism for the elimination of damaged cells [53]. Mammary epithelial cells are involved in the phagocytosis of apoptotic cells during involution, and in the regulation of inflammation [74]. Impaired phagocytosis in mammary epithelial cells causes mastitis in mice [75]. Autophagy might thus be an important mechanism in innate immunity, as a line of defense to protect hosts from invading bacteria.

Conclusion

It has been demonstrated here that cows that were susceptible to mastitis had 13G FEZL and/or a long C stretch in the 5'UTR of *IGF1R*. Mastitis enhances FEZL, FEZL promotes SEMA5A, and SEMA5A induces *TNF*α and *IL-8* expression. Because 13G FEZL promotes less *SEMA5A* expression than 12G FEZL, the susceptibility to mastitis might result from impaired immune response. On the other hand, 13G FEZL and the longer C stretch of *IGF1R* together enhanced expression of IGF1R in terms of both mRNA and protein levels. Enhancing IGF1R inhibited autophagy in response to *S. agalactiae* invasion of BMECs, suggesting that the susceptibility to mastitis might result from impaired autophagy. These results thus demonstrated unexpected roles for the FEZL–SEMA5A and FEZL–IGF1R pathways in innate immunity in mammary gland. By identifying two of the mechanisms underlying FEZL-mediated immune function, a potential new method has been discovered for selecting cows in order to improve their health and welfare.

References

[1] Arita, T. (1991). *Mastitis in cattle: Clinical diagnosis and treatment*. (1st edition). Tokyo, JAPAN: Tikusan Press.

[2] Ashwell, M. S., Rexroad, C. E., Jr. Miller, R. H. & VanRaden, P. M. (1996). Mapping economic trait loci for somatic cell score in Holstein cattle using microsatellite markers and selective genotyping. *Anim. Genet*, 27, 235–242.

[3] Wall, R. J., Powell, A. M., Paape, M. J., Kerr, D. E., Bannerman, D. D., Pursel, V. G., Wells, K. D., Talbot, N. & Hawk, H. W. (2005). Genetically enhanced cows resist intramammary *Staphylococcus aureus* infection. *Nat. Biotechnol*, 23, 445–451.

[4] Rainard, P. (2005). Tackling mastitis in dairy cows. *Nat. Biotechnol*, 23, 430–432.

[5] Heyen, D. W., Weller, J. I., Ron, M., Band, M., Beever, J. E., Feldmesser, E., Da, Y., Wiggans, G. R., VanRaden, P. M. & Lewin, H.A. (1999). A genome scan for QTL influencing milk production and health traits in dairy cattle. *Physiol. Genomics*, 1, 165–175.

[6] Schrooten, C., Bovenhuis, H., Coppieters, W. & Van Arendonk, J. A. (2000). Whole genome scan to detect quantitative trait loci for

conformation and functional traits in dairy cattle. *J Dairy Sci*, 83, 795–806.

[7] Van Tassell, C. P., Ashwell, M. S. & Sonstegard, T. S. (2000). Detection of putative loci affecting milk, health, and conformation traits in a US Holstein population using 105 microsatellite markers. *J Dairy Sci*, 83, 1865–1872.

[8] Boichard, D., Grohs, C., Bourgeois, F., Cerqueira, F., Faugeras, R., Neau, A., Rupp, R., Amigues, Y., Boscher, M. Y. & Levéziel, H. (2003). Detection of genes influencing economic traits in three French dairy cattle breeds. *Genet Sel Evol*, 35, 77–101.

[9] Hiendleder, S., Thomsen, H., Reinsch, N., Bennewitz, J., Leyhe-Horn, B., Looft, C., Xu, N., Medjugorac, I., Russ, I., Kühn, C., Brockmann, G. A., Blümel, J., Brenig, B., Reinhardt, F., Reents, R., Averdunk, G., Schwerin, M., Förster, M., Kalm, E. & Erhardt, G. (2003). Mapping of QTL for body conformation and behavior in cattle. *J Hered*, 94, 496–506.

[10] Kühn, Ch., Bennewitz, J., Reinsch, N., Xu, N., Thomsen, H., Looft, C., Brockmann, G. A., Schwerin, M., Weimann, C., Hiendleder, S., Erhardt, G., Medjugorac, I., Förster, M., Brenig, B., Reinhardt, F., Reents, R., Russ, I., Averdunk, G., Blümel, J. & Kalm, E. (2003). Quantitative trait loci mapping of functional traits in the German Holstein cattle population. *J Dairy Sci,* 86, 360–368.

[11] Schulman, N. F., Viitala, S. M., de Koning, D. J., Virta, J., Mäki-Tanila, A. & Vilkki, J. H. (2004). Quantitative trait loci for health traits in Finnish Ayrshire cattle. *J Dairy Sci*, 87, 443–449.

[12] Holmberg, M. & Andersson-Eklund, L. (2004). Quantitative trait loci affecting health traits in Swedish dairy cattle. *J Dairy Sci,* 87, 2653–2659.

[13] Lund, M. S., Guldbrandtsen, B., Buitenhuis, A. J., Thomsen, B. & Bendixen, C. (2008). Detection of quantitative trait loci in Danish Holstein cattle affecting clinical mastitis, somatic cell score, udder conformation traits, and assessment of associated effects on milk yield. *J Dairy Sci*, 91, 4028–4036.

[14] Coppieters, W., Kvasz, A., Farnir, F., Arranz, J. J., Grisart, B., Mackinnon, M. & Georges, M. (1998). A rank-based nonparametric method for mapping quantitative trait loci in outbred half-sib pedigrees: application to milk production in a granddaughter design. *Genetics*, 149, 1547–1555.

[15] Sharma, B. S., Jansen, G. B., Karrow, N. A., Kelton, D., Jiang, Z., Sharma, B. S., Jansen, G. B., Karrow, N. A., Kelton, D. & Jiang Z. (2006). Detection and characterization of amplified fragment length polymorphism markers for clinical mastitis in Canadian Holsteins. *J Dairy Sci,* 89, 3653–3663.

[16] Sugimoto, M., Fujikawa, A., Womack, J. E. & Sugimoto, Y. (2006). Evidence that bovine forebrain embryonic zinc finger-like gene influences immune response associated with mastitis resistance. *Proc. Natl. Acad. Sci. USA,* 103, 6454–6459.

[17] Emanuelson, U., Danell, B. & Philipsson, J. (1988). Genetic parameters for clinical mastitis, somatic cell counts, and milk production estimated by multiple-trait restricted maximum likelihood. *J. Dairy Sci*, 71, 467–476.

[18] Shook, G. E & Schutz, M. M. (1994). Selection on somatic cell score to improve resistance to mastitis in the United States. *J. Dairy Sci*, 77, 648–658.

[19] Ihara, N., Takasuga, A., Mizoshita, A., Takeda, H., Sugimoto, M., Mizoguchi, Y., Reed, K. M., Snelling, W. M., Kappes, S. M., Beattie, C. W., Bennett, G. L. & Sugimoto, Y. (2004). A comprehensive genetic map of the cattle genome based on 3802 microsatellites. *Genome Res,* 14, 1987–1998.

[20] Terwilliger, J. D. (1995). A powerful likelihood method for the analysis of linkage disequilibrium between trait loci and one or more polymorphic marker loci. *Am. J. Hum. Genet*, 56, 777–787.

[21] Seaton, G., Haley, C. S., Knott, S. A., Kearsey, M. & Visscher, P. M. (2002). QTL Express: mapping quantitative trait loci in simple and complex pedigrees. *Bioinformatics*, 18, 339–340.

[22] Warren, W., Smith, T. P., 3rd Rexroad, C. E., Fahrenkrug, S. C., Allison T, Shu, C. L., Catanese, J. & de Jong, P. J. (2000). Construction and characterization of a new bovine bacterial artificial chromosome library with 10 genome-equivalent coverage. *Mamm. Genome*, 11, 662–663.

[23] Fujisaki, S., Mizoguchi, Y., Takahashi, S., Chen, Y. Z., Suzuki, K., Asakawa, S., Soeda, E., Shimizu, N., Sugimoto, Y. & Yasue, H. (2002). Construction of a bovine bacterial artificial chromosome library from fibroblasts used for cloned cattle. *Anim. Genet*, 33, 379–381.

[24] Kent, W. J., Sugnet, C. W., Furey, T. S., Roskin, K. M., Pringle, T. H., Zahler, A. M. & Haussler, D. (2002). The human genome browser at UCSC. *Genome Res,* 12, 996–1006.

[25] Matsuo-Takasaki, M., Lim, J. H., Beanan, M. J., Sato, S. M. & Sargent, T. D. (2000). Cloning and expression of a novel zinc finger gene, Fez, transcribed in the forebrain of Xenopus and mouse embryos. *Mech. Dev,* 93, 201–204.

[26] Levkowitz, G., Zeller, J., Sirotkin, H. I., French, D., Schilbach, S., Hashimoto, H., Hibi, M., Talbot, W. S. & Rosenthal A. (2003). Zinc finger protein too few controls the development of monoaminergic neurons. *Nat. Neurosci*, 6, 28–33.

[27] Hirata, T., Suda, Y., Nakao, K., Narimatsu, M., Hirano, T. & Hibi, M. (2004). Zinc finger gene fez-like functions in the formation of subplate neurons and thalamocortical axons. *Dev. Dyn*, 230, 546–556.

[28] Bieker, J. J. (2001). Krüppel-like factors: three fingers in many pies. *J. Biol. Chem*, 276, 34355–34358.

[29] Lee, D. K. & Chang, C. (2003). Endocrine mechanisms of disease: Expression and degradation of androgen receptor: mechanism and clinical implication. *J. Clin. Endocrinol. Metab,* 88, 4043–4054.

[30] Kantor, D. B., Chivatakarn, O., Peer, K. L., Oster, S. F., Inatani, M., Hansen, M. J., Flanagan, J. G., Yamaguchi, Y., Sretava, D. W., Giger, R. J. & Kolodkin A. L. (2004). Semaphorin 5A is a bifunctional axon guidance cue regulated by heparan and chondroitin sulfate proteoglycans. *Neuron*, 44, 961–975.

[31] Goodman, C. S., Kolodkin, A. L., Luo, Y., Püchel, A. W. & Raper, J. A. (1999). Unified nomenclature for the semaphorins/collapsins. Semaphorin Nomenclature Committee. *Cell*, 97, 551–552.

[32] Wu, J. Y., Feng, L., Park, H. T., Havlioglu, N., Wen, L., Tang, H., Bacon, K. B., Jiang, Z., Zhang, X. & Rao, Y. (2001). The neuronal repellent Slit inhibits leukocyte chemotaxis induced by chemotactic factors. *Nature*, 410, 948–952.

[33] Kumanogoh, A., Marukawa, S., Suzuki, K., Takegahara, N., Watanabe, C., Ch'ng, E., Ishida, I., Fujimura, H., Sakoda, S., Yoshida, K. & Kikutani, H. (2002). Class IV semaphorin Sema4A enhances T-cell activation and interacts with Tim-2. *Nature*, 419, 629–633.

[34] Kumanogoh, A. & Kikutani, H. (2003). Immune semaphorins: a new area of semaphorin research. *J. Cell Sci*, 116, 3463–3470.

[35] Akira, S. & Takeda, K. (2004). Toll-like receptor signalling. *Nature Rev. Immunol,* 4, 499–511.

[36] Sugimoto, M., Itoh, T., Gotoh, Y., Kawahara, T., Moriya, H. Uchimura, Y. & Sugimoto, Y. (2011). Enhanced clinical mastitis resistance in

Holsteins with a FEZL p.Gly105(12_13) polymorphism. *J. Dairy Sci,* 94, 2103–2107.

[37] Agresti, A. (1992). A survey of exact inference for contingency tables. *Stat. Sci*, 7, 131–153.

[38] Rose, M. T., Aso, H., Yonekura, S., Komatsu, T., Hagino, A., Ozutsumi, K. & Obara, Y. (2002). *In vitro* differentiation of a cloned bovine mammary epithelial cell. *J. Dairy Res*, 69, 345–355.

[39] Iyer, V. R., Horak, C. E., Scafe, C. S., Botstein, D., Snyder, M. & Brown, P. O. (2001). Genomic binding sites of the yeast cell-cycle transcription factors SBF and MBF. *Nature*, 409, 533–538.

[40] Kenyon, C., Chang, J., Gensch, E., Rudner, A. & Tabtiang, R. A. (1993). *C. elegans* mutant that lives twice as long as wild type. *Nature*, 366, 461–464.

[41] Clancy, D. J, Gems, D., Harshman, L. G., Oldham, S., Stocker, H. Hafen, E., Leevers, S. J. & Partridge, L. (2001). Extension of life-span by loss of CHICO, a *Drosophila* insulin receptor substrate protein. *Science*, 292, 104–106.

[42] Holzenberger, M., Dupont, J., Ducos, B., Leneuve, P., Géloën, A. Even, P. C., Cervera, P. & Le Bouc, Y. (2003). IGF-1 receptor regulates lifespan and resistance to oxidative stress in mice. *Nature*, 421, 182–187.

[43] Murphy, C. T., McCarroll, S. A., Bargmann, C. I., Fraser, A., Kamath R. S., Ahringer, J., Li, H. & Kenyon, C. (2003). Genes that act downstream of DAF-16 to influence the lifespan of *Caenorhabditis elegans*. *Nature*, 424, 277–283.

[44] Wolf, S., Ma, H., Burch, D., Maciel, G. A., Hunter T. & Dillin A. (2006). SMK-1, an essential regulator of DAF-16-mediated longevity. *Cell*, 124, 1039–1053.

[45] Garsin, D. A., Villanueva, J. M., Begun, J., Kim, D. H., Sifri, C. D., Calderwood, S. B., Ruvkun, G. & Ausubel, F. M. (2003). Long-lived *C. elegans daf-2* mutants are resistant to bacterial pathogens. *Science*, 300, 1921.

[46] Levine, B. & Klionsky, D. J. (2004). Development by self-digestion: Molecular mechanisms and biological functions of autophagy. *Dev. Cell*, 6, 463–477.

[47] Hay, N. & Sonenberg, N. (2004). Upstream and downstream of mTOR. *Genes Dev,* 18, 1926–1945.

[48] Petiot, A., Ogier-Denis, E., Blommaart, E. F., Meijer, A. J. & Codogno, P. (2000). Distinct classes of phosphatidylinositol 3'-kinases are

involved in signaling pathways that control macroautophagy in HT-29 cells. *J. Biol. Chem*, 275, 992–998.

[49] Blommaart, E. F., Luiken, J. J., Blommaart, P. J., van Woerkom G. M. & Meijer, A. J. (1995). Phophorylation of ribosomal protein S6 is inhibitory for autophagy in isolated rat hepatocytes. *J. Biol. Chem*, 270, 2320–2326.

[50] Noda T, & Ohsumi, Y. (1998). Tor, a phosphatidylinositol kinase homologue, controls autophagy in yeast. *J. Biol. Chem*, 273, 3963–3966.

[51] Scott, R. C., Schuldiner, O. & Neufeld, T. P. (2004). Role and regulation of starvation-induced autophagy in the *Drosophila* fat body. *Dev. Cell*, 7, 167–178.

[52] Mèlendez, A., Tallócsy, Z., Seaman, M., Eskelinen, E., Hall, D. H. & Levine, B. (2003). Autophagy genes are essential for dauer development and life-span extension in *C. elegans*. *Science*, 301, 1387–1391.

[53] Levine, B. (2005). Eating oneself and uninvited guests: autophagy-related pathways in cellular defense. *Cell*, 120, 159–162.

[54] Nakagawa, I., Amano, A., Mizushima, N., Yamamoto, A., Yamaguchi, H., Kamimoto, T., Nara, A., Funao, J., Nakata, M., Tsuda, K., Hamada, S. & Yoshimori, T. (2004). Autophagy defends cells against invading group A *Streptococcus*. *Science*, 306, 1037–1040.

[55] Gutierrez, M. G., Master, S. S., Singh, S. B., Taylor, G. A., Colombo, M. I. & Deretic, V. (2004). Autophagy is a defense mechanism inhibiting BCG and *Mycobacterium tuberculosis* survival in infected macrophages. *Cell*, 119, 753–766.

[56] Jia, K., Thomas, C., Akbar, M., Sun, Q., Adams-Huet B. Gilpin, C. & Levine, B. (2009). Autophagy genes protect against *Salmonella typhimurium* infection and mediate insulin signaling-regulated pathogen resistance. *Proc. Natl. Acad. Sci. U S A*, 106, 14564–14569.

[57] Saad, A. M., Concha, C. & Astrom, G. (1989). Alterations in neutrophil phagocytosis and lymphocyte blastogenesis in dairy cows around parturition. *Zentralbl Veterinarmed B*, 36, 337–345.

[58] Agace, W. W., Hedges, S. R., Ceska, M. & Svanborg, C. (1993). Interleukin-8 and the neutrophil response to mucosal gram-negative infection. *J. Clin. Invest*, 92, 780–785.

[59] Lafleur, R. L., Abrahamsen, M. S. & Maheswaran, S. K. (1998). The biphasic mRNA expression pattern of bovine interleukin-8 in *Pasteurella haemolytica* lipopolysaccharide-stimulated alveolar macrophages is primarily due to tumor necrosis factor alpha. *Infect. Immun*, 66, 4087–4092.

[60] Godaly, G., Hang, L., Frendéus, B. & Svanborg, C. (2000). Transepithelial neutrophil migration is CXCR1 dependent in vitro and is defective in IL-8 receptor knockout mice. *J. Immunol*, 165, 5287–5294.

[61] Tsai, W. C., Strieter, R. M., Wilkowski, J. M., Bucknell, K. A, Burdick, M. D., Lora, S. A. & Standiford, T. J. (1998). Lung-specific transgenic expression of KC enhances resistance to *Klebsiella pneumoniae* in mice *J. Immunol,* 161, 2435–2440.

[62] Frendéus, B., Godaly, G., Hang, L., Karpman, D., Lundstedt, A. C. & Svanborg, C. (2000). Interleukin 8 receptor deficiency confers susceptibility to acute experimental pyelonephritis and may have a human counterpart. *J. Exp. Med,* 192, 881–890.

[63] Finch, C. E. & Crimmins, E. M. (2004). Inflammatory exposure and historical changes in human life-spans. *Science*, 305, 1736–1739.

[64] Christensen, K., Johnson, T. E. & Vaupel, J. W. (2006). The quest for genetic determinants of human longevity: challenges and insights. *Nat. Rev. Genet,* 7, 436–448.

[65] Bonafè, M., Barbieri, M., Marchegiani, F., Olivieri, F., Ragno E., Giampieri, C., Mugianesi, E., Centurelli, M., Franceschi, C., & Paolisso, G. (2003). Polymorphic variants of insulin-like growth factor I (IGF-I) receptor and phosphoinositide 3-kinase genes affect IGF-I plasma levels and human longevity: cues for an evolutionarily conserved mechanism of life span control. *J. Clin. Endocrinol. Metab*, 88, 3299–3304.

[66] Kojima, T., Kamei, H., Aizu, T., Arai, Y., Takayama, M., Nakazawa, S., Ebihara, Y., Inagaki, H., Masui, Y., Gondo, Y., Sakaki, Y. & Hirose, N. (2004). Association analysis between longevity in the Japanese population and polymorphic variants of genes involved in insulin and insulin-like growth factor 1 signaling pathways. *Exp. Gerontol,* 39, 1595–1598.

[67] Suh, Y., Atzmon, G., Cho, M. O., Hwang, D., Liu, B., Leahy, D. J., Barzilai, N. & Cohen, P. (2008). Functionally significant insulin-like growth factor I receptor mutations in centenarians. *Proc. Natl. Acad. Sci. U S A,* 105, 3438–3442.

[68] Massey, D. C. & Parkes, M. (2007). Genome-wide association scanning highlights two autophagy genes, *ATG16L1* and *IRGM*, as being significantly associated with Crohn's disease. *Autophagy*, 3, 649–651.

[69] Wittkopp P. J., Haerum B. K. & Clark, A. G. (2004). Evolutionary changes in *cis* and *trans* gene regulation. *Nature*, 430, 85–88.

[70] Jefferies, H. B. J., Fumagalli, S., Dennis, P. B., Reinhard, C., Pearson, R. B. & Thomas G. (1997). Rapamycin suppresses 5'TOP mRNA translation through inhibition of $p70^{s6k}$. *EMBO. J,* 16, 3693–3704.

[71] Ogawa, M., Yoshimori, T., Suzuki, T., Sagawa, H., Mizushima, N. & Sasakawa, C. (2005). Escape from intracellular *Shigella* from autophagy. *Science*, 307, 727-731.

[72] Amano, A., Nakagawa, I. & Yoshimori, T. (2006). Autophagy in innate immunity against intracellular bacteria. *J. Biochem*, 140, 161–166.

[73] Schnaith, A., Kashkar, H., Leggio, S. A., Addicks, K., Krönke, M.& Krut, O. (2007). *Staphylococcus aureus* subvert autophagy for induction of caspase-independent host cell death. *J. Biol. Chem*, 282, 2695–2706.

[74] Monks, J., Rosner, D., Geske, F. J., Lehman, L. Hanson, L. Neville, M. C. & Fadok, V. A. (2005). Epithelial cells as phagocytes: apoptotic epithelial cells are engulfed by mammary alveolar epithelial cells and repress inflammatory mediator release. *Cell Death Differ,* 12, 107–114.

[75] Hanayama, R. & Nagata, S. (2005). Impaired involution of mammary glands in the absence of milk fat globule EGF factor 8. *Proc. Natl. Acad. Sci. USA*, 102, 16886–16891.

In: Mammary Glands
Editor: Edmund B. Rucker

ISBN: 978-1-62948-853-0

Chapter VIII

Indicators of the Mammary Gland Health Status in Dairy Animals

Aneta Brodziak[1], **Jolanta Król**[2], **Piotr Stanek**[1] and **Zygmunt Litwińczuk**[1]*

[1]University of Life Sciences in Lublin, Faculty of Biology and Animal Breeding, Department of Breeding and Protection of Genetic Resources of Cattle, Akademicka Lublin, Poland

[2]University of Life Sciences in Lublin, Faculty of Biology and Animal Breeding, Department of Commodity Science and Processing of Animal Raw Materials, Akademicka Lublin, Poland

Abstract

Mastitis is the most costly and challenging to master with traditional methods of treatment disease of dairy cattle. This results in enormous losses to the economy and constitutes a serious threat to the stability of dairy herds. Losses resulting from mammary gland inflammation are also related to adverse changes in the chemical composition of milk, deterioration of its technological suitability, lower microbiological

* Corresponding author: Email address: aneta.brodziak@up.lublin.pl (A. Brodziak).

quality, diseases and falls of calves fed milk obtained from the unhealthy udder, suspension necessity of deliveries of milk obtained chiefly from the treated heads (the grace period) as well as risk of permanent damage or inactivation of all or part of mammary gland. The difficulties in mastitis control in particular are due to very complex reasons for its occurrence. Genetic differences in susceptibility of cows to mastitis were stated, however, the mechanisms of various animal resistance to this disease have not yet been fully understood because the mastitis occurrence is depended on many genes. In addition, the selection in direction of milk production increase pursuing for many years leads to a systematic decline in mastitis resistance of cows, due to existing antagonism between milk yield and udder health status. Commonly used key indicator of udder health status is the somatic cell count (SCC). The selection aiming at reducing the incidence of mastitis relies on selecting to generation the animals less susceptible to mammary gland inflammation, based on somatic cell count. Unfortunately, it is a very slow process due to a low heritability of this disease. Currently, researchers searching such a tool which allows for faster progress in disease controlling with simultaneous maintaining of high milk production. Numerous authors as reference indicators of inflammation indicate the level of serum albumin in milk (BSA – bovine albumin serum), activity of enzyme exterminating cell membranes of bacteria (N-acetyl-β-D-glucosaminidase – NAG) or lactic acid dehydrogenase (LDH), used in routine mastitis diagnosis (Oliszewski et al., 2002; Pyörälä, 2003; Leitner et al., 2004). Moreover, the exploitable indicators of subclinical mastitis could be lactose concentration and milk conductivity. More specific marker of milk quality than SCC is PMN (polymorphonuclear neutrophilic leukocytes) count – PMNC, which increase is the first signal informing about changes in the health status of the mammary gland. High positive correlation coefficient between PMN antigen and SCC in milk (r=0.94) was obtained (O'Sullivan et al., 1992; Kelly et al., 2000). A potential indicator of milk quality could also be α-lactalbumin (α-LA) which is a component of lactose synthase complex. It plays a crucial role in a regulation of lactose level and indirectly effects on milk yield. The decline in α-LA concentration is correlated with the reduction of milk lactose content during a typical lactation (Bleck et al., 2009). Lesser level of α-LA has also been noticed in cows that have mammary gland infection, coincidence with a decline in lactose concentration.

At the time of initiation of the inflammatory process an increase of antibacterial activity of several milk components, i.e., lactoferrin, lysozyme and lactoperoxidase, is occurred. According to several authors, these compounds could also be used as the indicators of udder health status (Rupp and Boichard, 2003; Wojdak-Maksymiec et al., 2006; Soyeurt et al., 2012). Recent studies indicate the potential use of lactoferrin on a larger scale in an animal breeding programs to augment the accuracy of selection for resistance to mastitis in dairy cows. Furthermore, naturally increasing content of lactoferrin in milk through selection could have a beneficial effect on human health. Genetic markers determining the susceptibility to mastitis (MAS) are also searched. A potential possibility for use of BoLA class II genes and lactoferrin in the selection of cows resistant to mastitis is exist as well.

The aim of authors will be therefore preparing the review chapter with regard to the indicators of mammary gland health status of dairy animals, mostly cows, on the basis of the recent world literature in this field.

Symptoms and Types of Mastitis

Inflammation of the mammary gland reveals as a glandular tissue injury of the udder, which can be caused by invasive or toxigenic microorganisms and their toxins. With the development of inflammation, they predominate due to an imbalance in the microbial population of the mammary gland. Etiological factors that cause mastitis are primarily bacteria, especially S*taphylococci* and *Streptococci*, as well as mycoplasmas, fungi, algae, protozoa and viruses. Inflammation can also develop as a result of physical udder injury or because of the activity of chemical irritants. However, the principal etiological factors inducing the inflammation of mammary gland in cows are bacteria (Sender et al., 2003; Jones and Bailey, 2009).

Depending on the etiological factor (way of infection) two types of mastitis can be distinguished, i.e., caused by contagious and environmental factors. The "contagious" agents (e.g., *Staphylococcus aureus*, *Streptococcus agalactiae* or *Streptococcus dysgalactiae*) are responsible mainly for subclinical and chronic inflammation of the mammary gland. Microorganisms that cause an infectious mastitis exist on the skin of the udder and are well adopted for survival and proliferation in the mammary gland. They are typically spread from animal to animal at or around the time of milking. In contrast, the "environmental" factors, i.e., pathogens living in an environment of animals (e.g., earth, water, bedding), such as the *coli* group (*Escherichia coli* (particularly) or *Klebsiella pneumoniae*), *Streptococcus uberis* or *Enterococci spp.*, are less virulent pathogens. Generally, they are not adapted to survival within the host. Typically they invade, multiply, engender a host immune response and are rapidly eliminated by the immune system (Bergonier et al., 2003; Wernery et al., 2008; Jones and Bailey, 2009; Smulski et al., 2011; Awale et al., 2012).

Cases of contagious mastitis are classified as subclinical, clinical or chronic, depending on the severity of the infection, what, in turn, is conditioned by the immunity of the host (animal). These three types differ from each in course, symptoms and difficulty in diagnosis.

Subclinical mastitis is a type of disease which is characterized by the lack of visible symptoms, i.e., udder and milk seem to be normal. However, in the fact there are changes in the physical-chemical properties of milk, i.e., somatic cell count – SCC (predominantly leucocytes and epithelial cells) increases, and the pH value and concentration of certain ions vary. In the healthy lactating mammary gland, a cell count is often <100,000 cells/ml and in the subclinical mastitis increases to >1,000,000 cells/ml (Guidry, 2007; Jones and Bailey, 2009).

However, the clinical form of mastitis can be quickly recognized (diagnosed) in a herd by visible changes in an appearance of the mammary gland as well as milk composition and its physical properties. The udder is warm, red, hardened, and sore as well as sensitive with visible swelling. Floccus and changes of color and flavor appear in the milk. Clinical mastitis can be mild, causing small modification in milk, or heavy, with visible changes. Furthermore, in affected animals a fever and loss of appetite are observed (Bansal et al., 2005; Nyman et al., 2009). Therefore, the three types of clinical mastitis are distinguished into the following classes: pre-acute, acute and sub-acute. However, Cha et al. (2010) classified clinical mastitis in other three categories: 1) caused by Gram-positive bacteria, 2) caused by Gram-negative bacteria, and 3) induced by other microorganisms.

Incidence of Mastitis

Several works detail the frequency of udder inflammation, mostly in cows but in other species as well (Bansal et al., 2005; Nyman et al., 2009; van den Borne et al., 2010). According to Sharma et al. (2011), the prevalence of mastitis ranges from 29.34% to 78.54% in cows. Cases of environmental mastitis rarely exceed 10% of the total mastitis cases in the herd, which indicates a much greater incidence of contagious mastitis (Awale et al., 2012). Shearer and Harris (2003) pointed out that subclinical mastitis can be from 15 to 40-times more common than the clinical forms. However, Bansal et al.

(2005) suggested that subclinical mastitis can occur up to 50-times more than its clinical form in lactating cows. Van den Borne et al. (2010) showed that the average frequency of subclinical mastitis occurrence in dairy herds kept in Denmark is 12.8% in primiparous cows and 27.1% in multiparous. Furthermore, De Vliegher et al. (2004) and Steeneveld et al. (2008) detailed that subclinical mastitis diagnosed in primiparous cows in the initial stage of lactation was strongly correlated with a higher somatic cell count in the successive stages of lactation. Generally, this results in a loss of productivity and is also associated with a higher probability of clinical mastitis, and is culled as a consequence. However, clinical mastitis affects between 15 and 20% of cows each year (Osman et al., 2009). It is estimated that in Denmark mastitis is the cause of 30 to 40% of veterinary interventions undertaken, while in Canada and the U.S. about 50% of the cows one or more quarters are infected (Osman et al., 2009). Van den Borne et al. (2010) showed that the average frequency of clinical mastitis occurrence in dairy herds kept in Denmark is 20.2% in primiparous cows and 39.6% in multiparous. In the opinion of many authors (De Vliegher et al., 2004; Nyman et al., 2009; olde Riekerink et al., 2008), the number of clinical mastitis cases is generally high in multiparous cows. However, in the case of primiparous cows especially being in the early stage of lactation, the frequency of occurrence of this type of mastitis is even higher. The problem of mastitis in heifers with a calf and primiparous cows is also discussed by Malinowski and Smulski (2007). In multiparous cows, the risk of clinical mastitis developing increases with a subsequent lactation (Steeneveld et al., 2008), with the exception of very early stages of lactation where this relationship is reversed. Harmon (1994) reported that in older cows the probability of clinical mastitis increases with a rise in milk SCC.

Globally, there is a small number of publications dealing with cases and the incidence of the mammary gland inflammation in goats and sheep, as well as buffaloes, camels and horses (Contreras et al., 2007; Wernery et al., 2008; Monecke et al., 2011). It is estimated that the number of clinical mastitis cases occurring in small ruminants (goats and sheep) is typically lower than 5% but it can grow spontaneously. The incidence of the subclinical form of mastitis is estimated to be 5-30% and greater (Bergonier et al., 2003; Contreras et al., 2007). It has been assessed that 5-50% of the udders in dairy herds of cows, goats and sheep are subclinically infected with bacteria (Leitner et al., 2012). According to Leitner et al. (2004), subclinical mastitis can touch even 70% of the udder halves of goats. Both clinical as well as subclinical cases increase the cost of veterinary care, deteriorate milk yield and the quality of milk produced, as well as reduce cheese yield (Haenlein, 2002). In Poland, this problem occurs in more than 62% of herds (Bagnicka, 2007). Menzies and Ramanoon (2001), however, indicated the prevalence of mastitis in sheep. Its clinical type was the cause of 13 to 50% of the slaughters of sheep maintained in England. This percentage ranged from 1 to 3% in herds kept in the U.S. Moreover, the prevalence of mastitis ranges from 66.00%-70.32% in buffaloes maintained in India (Sharma et al., 2007). In buffalo herds maintained in Brazil (São Paulo state), the incidence of clinical and subclinical mastitis in buffaloes during lactation was 1.50 and 18.77%, respectively. Inflammation lead to the decline in productivity and quality of milk, which significantly affected the production of the original mozzarella cheese from the buffalo milk (Costa et al., 2000). A higher incidence of subclinical mastitis (5-20%), than clinical (1-10%), was also noted in buffalo herds in India (Awale et al., 2012).

Economic Losses Due to Mastitis

Mastitis is the most costly and difficult to control of the dairy animal's diseases, especially with traditional methods of treatment. Moreover, it is the most frequently cited reason for culling and use of antibiotics in lactating dairy cattle (Norberg, 2005). Mastitis causes huge losses in the economy, especially in the dairy industry, and is a serious threat to the stability of livestock population. According to Osman et al. (2009), mastitis was responsible in approximately 70% for avoidable economic losses beared by commercial dairy farmers. Depending on the species of animals, in various countries these costs vary but are always a large financial burden for dairy farms. It should also be emphasized that the type of inflammation is very crucial. Subclinical mastitis usually precedes the clinical type; however, because of the duration and difficulties in detecting its occurrence detecting, it is associated with high economic losses. According to Gröhn et al. (2005), mastitis reduces the profitability of dairy farms, and the losses are not only due to the decrease in milk production but also the costs of treatment and culling of animals. In addition, this disease increases the risk of new cases of mastitis (Nyman, 2007).

Losses associated with the inflammation are related to: 1) the unwanted changes in the chemical milk composition, 2) a deterioration of the technological quality of milk, 3) a poorer microbial quality, 4) diseases affecting calves fed milk from an unhealthy udder, 5) the need to stop the supplying of milk taken from the treated animals (the grace period), or 6) a risk of permanent damage or inactivation of some part or the whole of the mammary gland. According to Bar et al. (2008) and Huijps et al. (2008), the cost of mastitis treatment is about 70 EUR/cow/year, i.e., 65 EUR/cow/year in the Netherlands and 71 EUR/cow/year in the U.S., whereas the cost of the total treatment is much higher, approximately 180 EUR/cow/year. Nevertheless, according to Nielsen (2009), the cost of subclinical mastitis treatment in Sweden was much lower (60 EUR/cow/year) than its clinical form (275 EUR/cow/year). The author also pointed to much lower cost of prevention (50 EUR/cow/year) in relation to the expense incurred for the treatment of mammary gland inflammation. According to OTT (Petrovski et al., 2011), in the U.S. losses due to a production decrease resulting from an incidence of mastitis were 108 USD/cow in herds with an average SCC in milk in the range of 200,000-400,000/ml, and 295 USD in the herds with SCC above 400,000/ml. This loss in the dairy industry in the U.S. were estimated at approximately USD 1 billion, only from the occurrence of subclinical inflammation.

Effect of Mastitis on Milk Quality

Mastitis causes reduced milk production, not only at the initial occurrence but also throughout the rest of the lactation (Gröhn et al., 2004; Hagnestam et al., 2007). The research of Khan and Khan (2006) and Litwińczuk et al. (2011) indicate that the highly productive cow breeds are more susceptible to infection, which results in higher losses in milk production in such herds. Decreased synthetic activity of infected mammary gland are also revealed in the changes in individual milk component content and in the ratios between them. As a consequence, milk nutritional value and suitability for processing is reduced as shown in Figure 1. Inflammations cause changes in the distribution of proteins (i.e., the whey protein proportion increases at the expense of casein share) and lead to a decrease in fat and lactose content and changes in the concentration of minerals, mainly a calcium reduction. It is worth mentioning the increased concentration of blood serum components in mastitic milk, such as albumins, globulins, chlorine and sodium (Nudda et al., 2001; Stanek et al., 2004; Litwińczuk et al., 2006; Jones and Bailey, 2009; Barłowska et al., 2009; Król et al., 2010b; Litwińczuk et al., 2011; Petrovski et al., 2011; Olechnowicz and Jaśkowski, 2012).

Component	Direction of change	References	Reason for change
SCC	↑	Liebe et al., 1998; Leitner et al., 2004; Piccinini et al., 2006; Stelwagen et al., 2012	Leakage from blood
Whey protein			
Serum albumin	↑	Leitner et al., 2004; Piccinini et al., 2006; Jones and Bailey, 2009; Litwińczuk et al., 2011	Leakage from blood
Immunoglobulins	↑	Guliński et al., 2006; Jones and Bailey, 2009; Liu et al., 2009; Park et al., 2007; Boudry et al., 2008; Król et al., 2012	Leakage from blood
β-lactoglobulin	↓	Piccinini et al., 2006; Litwińczuk et al., 2011	Reduced synthesis
α-lactalbumin	↓	Piccinini et al., 2006; Litwińczuk et al., 2011	Reduced synthesis
Lactoferrin	↑	Lindmark-Månsson et al., 2000; Hagiwara et al., 2001; Leitner et al., 2004; Lindmark-Månsson et al., 2006; Piccinini et al., 2006; Jones and Bailey, 2009; Litwińczuk et al., 2011; Król et al., 2012; Soyeurt et al., 2012; Giacinti et al., 2013	Increased synthesis
Lysozyme	↑	Litwińczuk et al., 2011; Król et al., 2012	Increased synthesis
Lactoperoxidase	↑	Weiss et al., 1990; Dael et al., 1991; Fonteh et al., 2002; Seifu et al., 2007; O'Rourke, 2009	Increased synthesis
Basic milk components			
Cl	↑	Jones and Bailey, 2009	Increased synthesis
K	↓	Jones and Bailey, 2009	Reduced synthesis
Na	↑	Jones and Bailey, 2009	Increased synthesis
Lactose	↓	Harmon, 1994; Ikonen et al., 2004; Leitner et al., 2004; Lindmark-Månsson et al., 2006; Barłowska et al., 2009; Bleck et al., 2009; Król et al., 2010a;	Reduced synthesis
Casein	↓	Barłowska et al., 2009; Król et al., 2010a; Litwińczuk et al., 2011	Reduced synthesis
Fat	↓	Lindmark-Månsson et al., 2006; Barłowska et al., 2009; Król et al., 2010a	Reduced synthesis

Figure 1. Changes in selected milk constituents caused by mastitis.

In Pakistan, mastitis reduced a useful life (i.e., lactation) in buffaloes by 57 days averagely and caused the decrease of 438 kg in milk production per lactation (Cady et al., 1983). In addition, this disease deteriorates the quality of milk and dairy products (Khan and Khan, 2006). It should be noted that the bacterial contamination of milk from affected cows renders it unfit for human consumption and provides a mechanism of spread of diseases like tuberculosis, sore-throat, Q-fever, brucellosis or leptospirosis and has zoonotic importance (Sharif et al., 2009).

Despite the intensive research and implementation of many strategies of control and prevention, the problem of mastitis has not disappeared in recent decades. It is a challenge not only for farmers but especially for veterinarians. Although, the reduction in the incidence of subclinical mastitis has been obtained, no significant progress has been made on reducing the incidence of the clinical forms of mastitis (Petrovski et al., 2011). For an early diagnosis of subclinical inflammation of the mammary gland, dairy animal breeders need a cheap, quick and easy diagnostic indicator.

Indicators of Mammary Gland Health Status

Reference indicators of the inflammatory state used in routine diagnoses not only include a somatic cell count, but also serum albumin (SA) levels, activity of an enzyme destroying cell membranes of bacteria (N-acetyl-β-D-glucosaminidase – NAGase), or lactate dehydrogenase (LDH) (Oliszewski et al., 2002; Pyörälä, 2003; Leitner et al., 2004). Nevertheless, the most useful indicators of subclinical udder inflammation can be the lactose level, electrical conductivity, or a count of polymorphonuclear leukocytes (PMN).

Somatic Cell Count (SCC)

Research on the relationship between the level of somatic cells in milk and mammary gland health status began Prescott and Breed in 1910, but only at the end of 1960 were the somatic cells widely recognized as a diagnostic indicator of mammary gland health status (Harmon, 2001). Somatic cells (SC) are naturally present in breast milk obtained from healthy animals. The milk somatic cells from healthy animals include mainly the cells derived from blood (50-100%), including especially leukocytes, i.e., neutrophils, macrophages and lymphocytes, and exfoliated epithelial cells (0-50%). In milk from the healthy udder, leucocytes consist of 0-11% neutrophils (polymorphonuclear granulocytes or polymorphonuclear leukocytes – PMNs), 10-27% lymphocytes and 30-74% macrophages. It should be mentioned that the percentage of particular types of cells varies depending on the udder health status, age, stage of lactation, production season, farm size, body condition score (BCS) and metabolic or physiological "stress" (Burvenich et al., 2000; Aniulis et al., 2003; Sender et al., 2003; Litwińczuk et al., 2011; Sharma et al., 2011; Leitner et al., 2012; Olechnowicz and Jaśkowski, 2012). The somatic cell count is a commonly recognized indicator of bovine udder health, milk quality and its technological usability. Therefore, each cow has a defined milk somatic cell count (MSCC) which is the basis for abnormal milk control programs. Moreover, SCC in bulk tank milk (BTSCC) is also one of the admission criteria in the purchasing of cow milk. It is also used to monitor the spread of mastitis in a herd. BTSCC is a quality indicator of raw material taken to the dairy plant and generally indicates the hygienic conditions of milk production on a farm (Norberg, 2005; Contreras et al., 2007; van der Borne et al., 2010; Højsgaard and Friggens, 2010; Leitner et al., 2012; Olechnowicz and Jaśkowski, 2012).

In numerous studies it has been shown that milk somatic cell count is a good indicator of mammary gland health status. Furthermore, commonly occurring subclinical and clinical inflammations are associated with a significant increase in their count in milk. This is confirmed by generally high positive correlation coefficients between SCC and udder inflammation (at the level of 0.30-0.97) shown in Figure 2 (Lund et al., 1994; Kelly et al., 2000; Carlen et al., 2004; Rainard and Riollet, 2006; Bloemhof et al., 2009).

Correlation coefficient	References
0.97 (for SCC)	Lund et al., 1994
0.30-0.97 (for SCS)	Pösö and Mäntysaari, 1996; Rupp and Boichard, 1999; Carlen et al., 2004; Bloemhof et al., 2009
0.30-0.70 (for SCS)	Mrode et al., 1998
0.50-0.70 (for SCS)	Koivula et al., 2005

Figure 2. Genetic correlation coefficients (r_g) between SCC or SCS and mastitis.

It should be noted that the greatest changes in SCC are observed in the presence or absence of bacterial infection of the mammary gland (intramammary infection – IMI). An increase in the milk somatic cell count is the first informative sign about changes in the health status of mammary gland. The leukocyte percentage of neutrophils increases in milk not only in the case of bacterial infection, but also during tissue damage, stress, or late stage of lactation. Leukocytes are transported directly from the blood to the mammary gland in response to mediators released during inflammation. Macrophages and neutrophils (PMNs) are phagocytic cells which engulf and kill bacteria. However, in bovines, the phagocytic ability of milk PMNs can consume milk fat globules and casein, leading to putrefaction of milk. Lymphocytes are the only cells of the immune system that recognize a variety of antigenic structures through membrane receptors, which define their specificity, diversity and memory characteristics. Lymphocytes include both B-cells and T-cells, which play key roles in the specific immune reactions that may follow the initial response to an infection. With increasing levels of PMNs, a reduction in the share of lymphocytes and macrophages was observed. In milk from an infected udder, the leucocytes consisted of 40-90% neutrophils (PMNs), 27-45% lymphocytes and 12-16% macrophages. The epithelial cells of the glands are normally shed and get renewed; however, during infection their number increases, and the white blood cells serve as a defense mechanism to fight infection and assist in the repair of damaged tissue. The mammary epithelial cells play a protective role in the prevention of infection via ingestion and possible digestion of phagocytized microbes. They are able to produce a variety of inflammatory mediators such as cytokines, chemokines, host defense peptides and arachidonic acid metabolites (Aniulis et al., 2003; Sharma et al., 2011; Leitner et al., 2012). A change of defense cell activity is negatively correlated with the energy and metabolism balance, which affects the function of neutrophils and increases the risk of mastitis (Hoeben et al., 2000). According to Tripaldi et al. (1998), the share of PMNs was 38% of the somatic cell count which amounted to 100,000/ml and rose to 64% when the SCC reached a level higher than 200,000/ml. The authors noted, however, the positive correlation between the content of lymphocytes and SCC. The leukocytes were even up to 80% of the somatic cell population at a SCC above 5,000,000/ml.

During lactation, after the colostrum period, SCC in milk obtained from the uninfected bovine glands typically range from 10,000 to 100,000/ml. According to Bartocci et al. (2002), in the uninfected and non-inflammatory quarters of mammary gland, SCC was lower than 150,000/ml, with a simultaneously low neutrophil count (5-25% of the total SCC). It is assumed that the somatic cell count in cow milk exceeding 150,000/ml is one of the first signs of mammary gland infection. During the inflammation, an elevation in milk SCC is mainly due to an increase of the polymorphonuclear cell percentage by 99-100% (Schukken et al., 2003; Leitner et al., 2012). As the SCC limit, Harmon (1994) accepted only 50,000/ml. Hamann (2002) defined "the gold standard" for SCC at the level of 100,000/ml. In his opinion, a higher somatic cell count testified to a dysfunctional milk secretion, what leaded to reduction in daily milk production, changes in milk chemical composition and deterioration of its technological properties. However, Griffin et al. (1987) indicated the lower SCC limit of subclinical mastitis at a level of 125,000/ml and an upper limit of 250,000/ml. Moreover, Scheppers et al. (1997) established the so-called "physiological threshold level", i.e., a SCC limit of 200,000/ml, to differentiate between the healthy and infected quarter. Furthermore, they stated that each doubling of SCC above 50,000/ml results in loss of milk production. However, the number of somatic cells in the milk of bacteria free goats' and sheep' glands is typically higher than of cows, amounting to 500,000/ml, which results from species differences or udder build (Silanikove et al., 2010; Leitner et al., 2012). In Europe, in accordance to the Commission Regulation (EC) No 1662/2006 of 6 November 2006, modifying the Regulation (EC) No 853/2004 of the European Parliament and of the Council of 29 April 2004, milk intended for human consumption should not contain more than 400,000 of somatic cells in 1 ml of milk. The identical limits are applied in Canada and New Zealand as well. Furthermore, in the U.S. to 2011 the official standard was up to 750,000/ml. However, in order to allow the American producers to export dairy products to the European markets, a gradual reduction of the SCC limit to the requirements of the European Union is planned (NMC, 2011). Nevertheless, the widely used diagnostic indicator of bovine mastitis, which is the somatic cell count in 1 ml of milk, is not reliable in goats. It is difficult to determine the physiological limit for this parameter in the milk of other dairy animals. According to the legislation adopted in the European Union, in fresh goat milk somatic cell count shall not exceed 1,500,000/ml (EU Council Directive No 92/46 EEC of 16 June 1992). In practice, however, the clinically healthy animals in which milk the SCC is over 2,000,000/ml are often observed (Bagnicka et al., 2007; Pazzola et al., 2012). In the opinion of the Scientific Panel on Biological Hazards of the European Food Safety Authority, high SCC in milk cannot be used as a marker of udder infection in goats (EFSA, 2005). On the contrary, in the U.S. the legal MSCC limit established by the Food and Drug Administration for goats and sheep is 1,000,000/ml but many goat breeders are not able to meet this requirement because milk is very often not suitable for sale even if it is taken from the healthy mammary gland (Paape et al., 2007). However, in buffalos the SCC is accepted as the appropriate indicator of mastitis and its limit is 200,000/ml (Tripaldi et al., 2010).

Polymorphonuclear Leukocytes (PMNs)

A more specific marker of milk quality than the SCC is a count of polymorphonuclear neutrophils (PMNs or PMLs, i.e., polymorphonuclear leukocytes) – PMNC, the growth of which is the first sign informing about the changes in the health status of mammary gland. PMNs act by engulfing and destroying the invading bacteria via oxygen-dependent and oxygen-independent systems. They contain intracellular granules that store bactericidal proteins, peptides, enzymes (e.g., myeloperoxidase) as well as neutral and acidic proteases (e.g., cathepsin G, cathepsin B, cathepsin D and elastase). During the infection, PMNs migrate across the blood-milk barrier (Figure 3) and serve as the first line of cellular defense against bacteria. The released oxidants and proteases destroy the bacteria and some of the epithelial cells, resulting in a decrease in milk production and the release of enzymes, including N-acetyl-β-D-glucosaminidase (NAGase) and lactate dehydrogenase (LDH). Unfortunately, due to apoptosis most of the PMNs are eliminated. Subsequently, macrophages engulf and ingest the remaining PMNs. The dead and sloughed off epithelial cells and dead leukocytes are secreted into the milk, resulting in an SCC increase (Kelly et al., 2000; Paape et al., 2003 and 2007; Leitner et al., 2004; Jones and Bailey 2009; Awale et al., 2012). It should be noted that the PMNs may cause a direct adverse effect on milk quality, such as an increased proteolysis and lipolysis, potentially shortening the shelf life of liquid milk and reducing a curd cheese yield. Because of the negative effect of PMNs on milk components, PMNC is suggested as an alternative indicator of milk quality, including the bulk tank milk, and as the index of health in dairy herds (Kelly et al., 2000; Olechnowicz and Jaśkowski, 2012). O'Sullivan et al. (1994) obtained a high positive correlation coefficient ($r=0.94$) between PMN antigen and SCC in milk obtained from individual cows. Kelly et al. (2000) showed a significant rise in both SCC and PMN levels at the end of lactation (at $P<0.01$) in milk obtained from uninfected udders. It should be noted that that increase in SCC was at least partly due to an influx of PMNs. The somatic cell count also rose with the following lactations ($P<0.05$). Analyzing an effect of leukotoxic actions of *S. aureus* on polymorphonuclear leukocytes, Rainard et al. (2003) found that PMNs of small ruminants were more resistant to those leukotoxic actions than bovine PMNs.

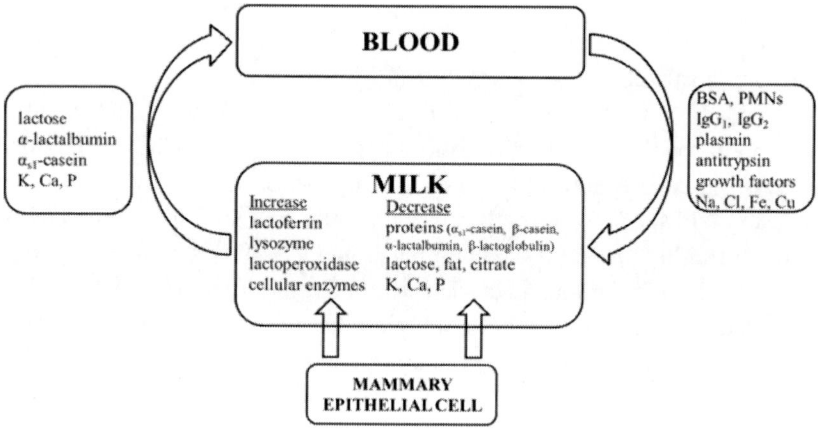

Figure 3. Movement of the components through the blood-milk barrier.

Protein	Correlation coefficient	References
BSA	0.310	Poutrel et al., 1983
	0.530	Lindmark-Månsson et al., 2000
	0.204	Nudda et al., 2001
	0.590	Litwińczuk et al., 2011
Lactoferrin	0.455	Lindmark-Månsson et al., 2000
	0.390	Nudda et al., 2001
	0.918	Lindmark-Månsson et al., 2006
	0.375*	Cheng et al., 2008
	0.650	Litwińczuk et al., 2011
	0.210*	Giacinti et al., 2013
Lizozym	0.630	Litwińczuk et al., 2011
IgG	0.252 (IgG1), 0.666 (IgG2)	Lindmark-Månsson et al., 2000
	0.350	Nudda et al., 2001
	0.540	Claus et al., 2006
	0.217*	Liu et al., 2009
	0.303*	Zhao et al., 2010

Figure 4. Genetic correlation coefficients (r_g) between protein content and SCC (as logSCC) or SCS (*).

Blood Serum Albumin (BSA)

Milk proteins consist of approximately 6-7% BSA. Serum albumin in milk is physically and immunologically identical to that of blood serum albumin, as it is not synthesized in the mammary secretory cells but derives from the so-called non-specific "leakage" from the blood to the milk. The influx of blood cells is mainly due to the weakening of the milk-blood barrier. The BSA concentration in milk is an indicator of the permeability of the blood-milk barrier in the mammary gland (Poutrel et al., 1983; Lieske et al., 2005; Litwińczuk et al., 2011).

The main factors increasing the permeability of cell membranes of mammary gland are udder inflammations. There is a positive relationship between level of somatic cells and milk serum albumin content as shown in Figure 4 (Urech et al., 1999; Lindmark-Månsson et al., 2000; Batavani et al., 2007; Litwińczuk et al., 2011). Milk of a healthy cow contains approximately 0.1-0.4 g/l of albumin, which comprises between 0.3 and 1.0% of the total nitrogen (Lieske et al., 2005; Park et al., 2007). In milk with higher SCC (above 400,000/ml), the SA level increased from 0.11 g/l to 0.21 g/l (Urech et al., 1999).

In the studies of Litwińczuk et al. (2011), cow milk with the highest somatic cell count (500,000-1,000,000/ml), compared to milk with SCC below 100,000/ml, had a higher BSA average by 64.7%. The authors obtained the significant interactions ($P \leq 0.01$) between breed and SCC for BSA content in milk, which indicated a various sensitivity of the analyzed breeds of cows (Holstein-Friesian, Simmental and Jersey) on increasing somatic cell count. In a certain sense, that hypothesis was confirmed by the different values of correlation coefficients calculated between BSA content and SCC in milk of different breeds of cows. The highest relationship ($r=0.711$) was obtained for Holstein-Friesian cows, while a noticeably lower dependence was found for Simmental ($r=0.577$) and Jersey cows ($r=0.472$). Therefore, it can be assumed that in Simmental and Jersey cows the SCC growth was not followed by such intensive permeation of bovine serum albumin from blood to milk, as it was observed in Holstein-Friesian cows. That would indicate a higher resistance of Simmental and Jersey cows to mammary gland infections. However, an excessively high protein fraction content interferes with IgG absorption by the intestinal epithelium of calves (Garry et al., 1996).

NAGase (N-Acetyl-β-D-Glucosaminidase)

A promising parameter, indicating damage to the udder epithelial cells and an occurrence of subclinical inflammations in cows, proved to be NAGase activity – an enzyme destroying of cell membranes of bacteria present in milk (Urech et al., 1999; Pyörälä, 2003). That was also confirmed in the research of goat milk. Oliszewski et al. (2002) and Leitner et al. (2004) showed significantly greater activity of NAGase in milk derived from the infected halves of goat's udder. Urech et al. (1999) found that the activity of N-acetyl-β-D-glucosaminidase was more appropriate indicator of subclinical mastitis and correlated better with protein degradation than did SCC. Bansal et al. (2005) obtained the correlation coefficients between NAGase and SCC for cow milk in the range of 0.44 to 0.50, depending on a phase of milking. Positive correlation between NAGase and SCC may indicate an increase in NAGase concentration both at the beginning and in the advanced (i.e., intensive) stage of mastitis (Malinowski et al., 2008). The activity of this marker is mainly used in scientific research and is not yet widely used in the mastitis diagnosis.

L-Lactate Dehydrogenase (LDH)

Besides NAGase, one of the biomarkers associated with the onset of the udder inflammation is lactate dehydrogenase. Indigenous L-lactate dehydrogenase in milk originates mainly from somatic cells, leucocytes and invading microorganisms. Milk LDH activity has potential as an indicator of clinical and subclinical mastitis not only in the herds of dairy cows, but also in other dairy animals. LDH is used today to detect mastitis in cows in commercial farms (Larsen, 2005; Mohammadian, 2011). Mohammadian (2011) stated that the mean LDH activity was significantly higher in milk from inflamed SCM quarters than in normal milk. The results obtained by De Ying et al. (2009) showed that compared to the healthy Holstein cows, LDH activity in the milk of subclinical mastitis cows increased significantly. There was a positive correlation between SCC and LDH activity (r^2=0.93). It should be noted that the LDH activity higher than 100 IU/l is considered to be the threshold to diagnose of subclinical mastitis.

Lactose Level

The most sensitive milk component to mammary gland inflammation is lactose. It is responsible, along with some elements (primarily Na and Cl), for regulating the osmotic pressure in udder, which must be in balance with the osmotic pressure of blood (Bleck et al., 2009). Increased SCC effects a decline in lactose concentration, as a result of reduced synthetic activity of mammary gland as shown in Figure 1 (Harmon, 1994; Bleck et al., 2009; Ikonen et al., 2004). This leads to flow of higher quantity of Cl^- and Na^+ from blood to milk and K^+ into the blood to compensate for the osmotic pressure in the mammary gland (Bansal et al., 2005). Forsbäck et al. (2009) indicated that at the SCC level ≤100,000/ml (healthy udder) lactose content was 4.66 g/100 ml and at the SCC>200,000/ml (threshold physiological limit) was 4.51 g/100 ml. Ogola et al. (2007) showed a reduction in lactose content from 48.8 g/l at a SCC level <250,000/ml to 43.8 g/l at SCC>750,000/ml. A significant decrease in lactose content with increasing SCC was also noted by others (Barłowska et al., 2009; Król et al., 2010; Litwińczuk et al., 2011). A relatively high negative correlation coefficients between SCC in milk and lactose concentration (from r=-0.250 to r=-0.774) (Zumbo et al., 2004; Bansal et al., 2005; Sawa et al., 2007; Bleck et al., 2009; Pazzola et al., 2012) confirm this relationship depicted in Figure 5.

Correlation coefficient	References
-0.448	Zumbo et al., 2004
-0.250	Bansal et al., 2005
-0.774	Lindmark-Månsson et al., 2006
-0.380	Sawa et al., 2007
-0.485 – herd I -0.501 – herd II	Bleck et al., 2009
-0.448 (for logSCC)	Pazzola et al., 2012

Figure 5. Genetic correlation coefficients (r_g) between lactose content and SCC.

Juozaitiene et al. (2004) indicated that the values of this coefficient oscillated from -0.38 in lactation I to -0.44 in lactation III ($P \leq 0.01$). However, Lindmark-Månsson et al. (2000) and others reported a totally different relationship between $\log_{10}$SCC and lactose percentage (0.073). A reduction of lactose content is also observed in milk from endotoxin-infused mammary glands in both cows and goats. This is due to a reduced secretory activity of the udder epithelial cells and movement of lactose from the milk to the blood (Oliver and Calvinho, 1995). It is suggested that the etiology of mastitis is associated with oxidative stress, which may be expressed either by the FRAP (ferric ion reducing antioxidant power) indicator in blood plasma or by the milk production and content of lactose. Both the FRAP indicator and the content of lactose in milk indicate the significance of antioxidants in retaining the health status of the cow mammary gland (Bansal et al., 2005; Jóźwik et al., 2012).

Electrical Conductivity (EC)

Electrical conductivity measures the ability of a solution to conduct an electric current between two electrodes. A unit of this parameter is milliSiemens (mS). EC of milk is conditioned by the concentration of anions and cations, especially Na^+, K^+ and Cl^-. In the healthy mammary gland, Na^+ and K^+ ions are transported passively between the secretory cells and the milk across the apical membrane. Na^+ and Cl^- are moving into the milk, while K^+ and lactose into the extracellular fluid (Peaker, 1983). It was showed that during intramammary infection, EC of the milk increases. This occurs as a result of an increased concentration of Na^+ and Cl^- moving from blood to the milk. Simultaneously, the potassium and lactose content decreases in milk and its pH value raises. Measurement of the milk electrical conductivity enables the detection of subclinical and clinical mastitis before the onset of visible changes in udder tissue or milk obtained. An electric current flows easier through inflammatory secretion than through the milk from a healthy udder. EC for normal milk from an uninfected udder, measured at a milk temperature of 25 °C, is 4-5 mS for cows, 5-6 mS for goats, and 4-6 mS for sheep. In the case when it is measured in-line (AMS) in cow herds, the milk temperature is higher (38 °C) which results in higher EC values of for normal milk. As it was mentioned, milk taken from the udder affected by mastitis, both clinically and subclinically, has higher conductivity than from healthy, uninfected one. Norberg et al. (2004a) found that the mean EC for healthy, subclinically infected and clinically infected cows was 5.3±0.03 mS, 5.75±0.04 mS and 6.73±0.06 mS, respectively. Ying et al. (2004) found that mastitis in a Saanen goat breed produces an increase of 0.2 mS/cm (from 5.6 to 5.8 mS/cm), while in Alpina breed the effect was a higher decrease of EC (from 6.1 to 5.4 mS/cm). However, Romero et al. (2012) obtained the values for Murciano-Granadina goats, local Spanish breed, varies between 4.75 and 6.60 mS/cm; however, according to Díaz et al., (2012), these values could be elevated by the presence of mastitis. The idea of using EC as an indicator trait in a breeding program was first suggested by Schukken et al. (1997). Over the last twenty years, electrical conductivity has been used to current monitor mastitis in dairy herds (Norberg, 2005; Jones and Bailey, 2009; Højsgaard and Friggens, 2010). Moderate to high genetic correlation coefficients between the lactation means of EC and clinical mastitis, which have been obtained by Rogers (2002) and Norberg et al. (2004b), support the use of EC as the indicator of udder inflammation as shown in Figure 6. However, Bansal et al. (2005) obtained the correlation coefficients between EC and SCC in cow milk from 0.41 to 0.58, depending on a phase of milking.

At the time of the inflammatory process initiation, an increase of antimicrobial activity of a number of milk components, such as lactoferrin, lysozyme and lactoperoxidase, occurs. According to many authors, these compounds can also be used as the indicators of udder health status (Rupp and Boichard, 1999; Wojdak-Maksymiec et al., 2006; Soyeurt et al., 2012).

Correlation coefficient	References
0.65 (for primiparous cows) 0.80 (for cows in 2nd lactation)	Rogers, 2002
0.75 (for primiparous cows)	Norberg et al., 2004b

Figure 6. Genetic correlation coefficients (r_g) between lactation means of EC and clinical mastitis.

Lactoferrin (Lf)

Lactoferrin is a glycoprotein with a molecular weight of about 80 kDa. It occurs as a single polypeptide chain which consists of about 690 amino acids.

Lf belongs to the transferrin family and has a specific ability to bind iron (Baker and Barker, 2005; Małaczewska and Rotkiewicz, 2007; Park et al., 2007; Legrant et al., 2008). Its presence has been noted also in other secretions such as saliva, tears, semen, bronchial mucous secretion, digestive and genital tract. Lactoferrin is a component of the secondary granules of neutrophils, from which it is released into the blood in the case of an injury, infection or inflammation (Baker and Barker, 2005; Małaczewska and Rotkiewicz, 2007; Artym, 2010; Garcia-Mantoya, 2011). It should be emphasized that this protein is an essential component of non-specific innate immunity of humans and other mammals (Kruzel et al., 2007; Legrant et al., 2008). By binding and sequestrating iron, Lf exhibits the antibacterial properties against Gram-positive and Gram-negative bacteria, non-capsular and capsular viruses as well as against various types of fungi and parasites (Steijns and Hooijdonk, 2000; Orsi, 2004; Wakabayashi et al., 2006; Małaczewska and Rotkiewicz, 2007). Lactoferrin exhibits non-specific immunological actions through activity as both bacteriostatic and bactericidal on a growth of numerous microorganisms (e.g., *Escherichia coli, Salmonella typhimurium, Shigella dysenteria, Listeria monocytogenes, Streptococcus mutans* and *Bacillus subtilis*). The bacteriostatic effect of Lf results partially from the high affinity of this protein to chelate iron (Fe^{3+} ions) and subsequently removing this element from the environment of microbial growth. An additional advantage of Lf in the fight against bacterial infections is the possibility of increasing a bacteria sensitivity to certain antibiotics (e.g., vancomycin and penicillin) and lowering their effective doses. The combination of penicillin with lactoferrin doubles as an inhibitory activity of antibiotic against *Staphylococcus aureus* (Diarra et al., 2002). An important function of lactoferrin is also protecting the immune cells from free radicals produced by the body during inflammation and infection (Lönnerdal et al., 1995). In milk originating from a healthy cow, lactoferrin levels are 0.25-0.40 g/l, and increases during a course of lactation (Hagiwara et al., 2003; Król et al., 2010b). The increase in concentration of this protein is also noted in inflammations or injuries (Baker and Barker, 2005; Małaczewska and Rotkiewicz, 2007; Artym, 2010; Garcia-Mantoya, 2011). Lactoferrin level reaches a value of 0.50 g/l in subclinical mastitis and 0.75 g/l in the clinical stages (Kawai et al., 1999; Hagiwara et al., 2003). In several studies, a positive correlation coefficients between SCC and lactoferrin content in milk were shown (Lindmark-Månsson et al., 2000; Lindmark-Månsson et al., 2006; Litwińczuk i wsp. 2011). According to Lindmark-Månsson et al. (2000 and 2006), SCC of over 5,000/ml increases Lf content in milk, and a close relationship between this component and udder health status was confirmed by very high correlation coefficients between milk lactoferrin concentration and SCC (r=0.962 and r=0.918) obtained from two independent studies. A significant rise in lactoferrin content with a concurrent progression of mammary gland disease was also noted in goat and buffalo milk (Leitner et al., 2004; Piccinini et al., 2006; Giacinti et al., 2013). Therefore, research indicates the large scale potential use of lactoferrin in animal breeding programs to increase the selection accuracy for mastitis resistance in dairy cows. In addition, a naturally increasing content of lactoferrin in milk, as a result of natural genetic selection, may also have a beneficial effect on human health.

Lysozyme (Lz)

Lysozyme (N-acetylmuramide glycanhydrolase, E.C.3.2.1.17) is a low molecular weight (14.4 kDa) enzymatic protein from the hydrolase group. Lz is widely distributed in nature, occurring in many body fluids and tissues of living organisms (Fox and Kelly, 2005). Lysozyme is a natural defense mechanism of an organism. An antibacterial activity of Lz bases on the hydrolysis of β-glycosidic bonds between N-acetylglucosamine and N-acetylmuramic acid in the polysaccharides which are present in the cell walls of Gram-positive bacteria. Resistance of Gram-negative bacteria to lysozyme can be reduced by the use of detergents in the lipid components of cell wall. It was shown that the coupling of Lz with dextran gave an active product against these bacteria (Masschalck and Michiels, 2003; Séverin and Wenshui, 2005; Leśnierowski, 2009). Under natural conditions, the antibacterial activity of monomeric lysozyme is limited to Gram-positive bacteria. Only after modification, which reduces its hydrolytic activity, does its bactericidal activity extends Gram-negative bacteria including many pathogenic bacteria (Masschalck et al., 2001; Chang and Li, 2002; Benkerroum, 2008; Leśnierowski, 2009). Besides lactoferrin, lysozyme also occurs to be one of the most crucial component of the non-specific humoral immune response (Montagne et al., 2001; Benkerroum, 2008). Concentration of the protein varies according to an udder health. It is in much higher levels in colostrum and mastitis milk of cows than in normal milk, so it has utility in the mastitis diagnosis as shown in Figure 1. There was also a noticed synergistic effect of the enzyme with immunoglobulins and lactoferrin against *Escherichia coli* and *Micrococcus luteus* (Séverin and Wenshui, 2005; Moatsou, 2010). Lysozyme content in milk is at the level of 0.073 μg/ml, while in colostrum is much higher, i.e., 0.401 μg/ml (Boudry et al., 2008). Lysozyme activity decreases with a rise in SCC in mammary gland secretions (Person et al., 2000).

Lactoperoxidase (Lp)

Lactoperoxidase (EC 1.11.1.7) is a 78 kDa protein that has the enzymatic properties of the oxidoreductases (Boudry et al., 2008). Lactoperoxidase is synthetized mainly by the polymorphonuclear leukocytes. Its concentration in bovine milk is approximately 30 mg/l. It catalyzes the oxidation of thiocyanate (SCN^-) in the presence of hydrogen peroxide (H_2O_2) in the volatile, toxic compounds which inhibit the metabolism of many microorganisms, i.e., lactoperoxidase-thiocyanate-hydrogen peroxide system (Boots and Floris, 2006). Found in both the mammary gland and the gastrointestinal tract of newborns, Lp is a component of non-specific cellular immunity. It is a natural bacteriostatic and bactericidal factor present in milk and other body fluids. Lactoperoxidase effects bactericidally not only on Gram-negative bacteria (e.g., *E. coli*, *Salmonella spp.*, *Pseudomonas spp.* and *Campylobacter spp.*) but also Gram-positive ones (e.g., *Listeria spp.*, *Staphylococcus spp.* and *Streptococcus spp.*) (Zimecki and Artym, 2005). Together with lysozyme, lactoperoxidase requires interaction with lactoferrin to fight infection (Zimecki and Artym, 2005; Boudry et al., 2008; Struff and Sprotte, 2008). It is also used as an index of pasteurization efficiency in milk. Along with the other ingredients contained in colostrum, including properidne, conglutinin, ubiquitin and the components of complement system, Lp actively participates in the defense mechanism against infection as an inhibitor. The mean lactoperoxidase activity in cows ranged from 1.5 to 2.7 U/ml with an overall mean of 2.3 U/ml, which corresponds to a content of 20 mg/l (Fonteh et al., 2002). The minimum amount of Lp in milk required to activate the lactoperoxidase system is 0.02 U/ml. However, Lp content and activity in milk increases with the rise in SCC; therefore, it has been stated that this enzyme can be used to detect mastitis, particularly in cows. The confirmation of this is a negative relationship between lactoperoxidase level in milk and mastitis causing pathogens (e.g., *Streptylococus agalacte* and *Staphylococcus aureus*) (Weiss et al., 1990; O'Rourke, 2009). Seifu et al. (2007), obtaining a significantly ($P<0.01$) positive correlation between Lp activity and SCC in milk of South African Indigenous ($r=0.91$) and Saanen ($r=0.95$) clinically healthy goats, pointed to the possibility of using of this enzyme activity measurement to detect mastitis in dairy goats.

Immunoglobulins (Ig)

Immunoglobulins are high molecular globulins that occur in plasma and body fluids. Depending on the physical-chemical structure and biological activity, three major classes of immunoglobulins include IgG, IgM and IgA. IgG predominates (approximately 80%) in the milk of ruminants, while in other mammalian milk, including human, IgA does (approximately 90%). They determine the specific humoral immunity of a body (El-loly and Farrag, 2007; Boudry et al., 2008). During the process of antigen binding and phagocytosis or complement activation, these proteins are involved in the destruction of pathogenic microorganisms, e.g., *Escherichia coli*, *Shigella flexneri*, *Clostridium difficile*, *Candida albicans*, *Streptococcus mutans* and *Helicobacter pylori* (Korhonen, 2004; Gapper et al., 2007). Nevertheless, a positive relationship exists between the level of immunoglobulins in the blood serum of cows and their level in the mammary gland secretion (Guliński et al., 2006; Boudry et al., 2008). Immunoglobulins are selectively transported from the plasma to the mammary gland. The average level of IgG, IgM and IgA in the colostrum of healthy dairy cows is 47.6, 4.2 and 3.9 mg/ml, respectively. Their content in milk decreases rapidly and remains at a level many times lower (IgG is 590 μg/ml, IgM is 50 μg/ml and IgA is 140 μg/ml) (Park et al., 2007; Boudry et al., 2008). Research suggests that inflammation contributes to a colostrum and milk value reduction, negatively affecting the degree of utilization of immunoglobulins by calves (Ontsouka et al., 2003; Błaszkowska and Twardoń, 2006).

α-Lactalbumin (α-LA)

A potential indicator of a milk quality evaluation can be also α-lactalbumin, which contributes actively in the control of lactation and milk secretion, and is an indispensable component of lactose synthetase. It plays a crucial role in regulating lactose content and directly affects milk yield. α-LA also shows anti-carcinogenic, anti-bacterial (against Gram-positive) and antiviral activity, and functions as an immunological factor to increase a neonatal immunity. α-lactalbumin is a low molecular weight protein (approximately 14.2 kDa). A single polypeptide chain of this protein is composed of 123 amino acid residues. Bovine milk contains an average of 1.0-1.5 g/l of α-LA, which represents approximately 20% of the total whey protein content (Chatterton et al., 2006; Kanwar et al., 2009; Litwińczuk et al., 2011).

During a typical lactation, a decline in α-LA concentration is correlated with the decrease of lactose content in milk. Lowering the amount of the protein, with a simultaneous reduction of lactose level, is also observed in cows with udder inflammation. α-LA is suggested to be a negative acute phase protein (APP) in bovine milk because its concentration decreases, potentially as a consequence of the onset of the acute phase response (Oliver and Calvinho, 1995; Bleck et al., 2009). According to Ushida et al. (2007), the decline in α-LA level during udder inflammation is unfavorable because this protein shields the gastric mucosa and protects it against the development of ulcers. Harmon et al. (1976) stated that in mammary gland returning to a normal healthy state, the production of α-lactoalbumin returned to a preinfection level which was accompanied by a reduction in lactoferrin production.

Cytokines

Cytokines are small proteins (less than 50 kDa) that act as intercellular communication signals in hematopoiesis, stress, inflammation, immunity and tissue repair. The identification of a large number of cytokines and disclosure of their pathophysiological mechanisms has opened innovative frontiers into diagnosis and therapy. In the healthy mammary gland, numerous cytokines have been detected. These cytokines have been used in the attempt to raise a resistance or potentiate the immune system of bovine mammary gland infected with *Escherichia coli* or *Staphylococcus aureus*. Once inside the teat, bacteria must elude the cellular and humoral defense mechanisms of the udder. If bacteria are not eliminated, they start multiplying in the teat. They produce toxins and induce leukocytes and epithelial cells to release chemoattractants, including cytokines such as tumour necrosis factor-α (TNF-α), interleukins IL-1 and IL-8, eicosanoids (e.g., prostaglandin $F_{2\alpha}$), oxygen radicals and acute phase proteins (APPs) such as haptoglobin (HP) and serum amyloid A (SAA). This attracts circulating immune effector cells, mainly polymorphonuclear neutrophils, to the site of infection (Paape et al., 2003; Alluwaimi, 2004; Awale et al., 2012). Changes in the activity of various cytokines indicate a role of the immune system in the initiation and ending of inflammatory process. During the inflammation an increase in the activity of pro-inflammatory cytokines (i.e., TNF-α, IL-1β, IL-6, IL-8, IL-12 and GM-CSF) secreted by somatic cells, primarily by macrophages, was always observed. However, in the case of INF-γ no growth or decrease was noticed (Alluwaimi, 2004; Malinowski et al., 2008).

Growth Factors

Growth factors include IGF I and II (IGF, insulin-like growth factor), TGF-α and TGF-β (TGF, transforming growth factor) as well as EGF (epidermal growth factor) (Tripathi and Vashishtha, 2006; Boudry et al., 2008; Penchev, 2008). IGF-I and II are polypeptide chains with molecular weights of approximately 7.6 and 7.5 kDa, respectively (Boudry et al., 2008).

In cattle, pigs and humans they have identical sequences. IGF-I and II move from the blood to the colostrum and milk. They are also synthesized locally in the mammary gland. IGF I and II are responsible for hormonal balance and glucose metabolism. Moreover, they stimulate DNA and RNA synthesis (Rauprich et al., 2000; Penchev, 2008). IGF-I has a higher biological activity than IGF-II. IGF-I content in colostrum is around 100-2000 μg/l and IGF-II about 200-600 μg/l.

The concentration of these two milk fractions decreases rapidly in milk (<25 μg/l and <10 μg/l, respectively) (Boudry et al., 2008). Moreover, transforming growth factors, mainly responsible for the differentiation of intestinal epithelial cells of calves, are characterized by higher level in colostrum (20-40 mg/l) than in milk (1-2 mg/l) (Boudry et al., 2008; Penchev, 2008).

Like other growth factors, they are polypeptides with molecular weights of 6 kDa (TGF-α) and 25 kDa (TGF-β). TGF-β plays a crucial role in embryogenesis, tissue repair, formation of bone cartilage and in control of the immune system (Tripathi and Vashishtha, 2006; Boudry et al., 2008; Penchev, 2008).

During injury, TGF-β plays an important role in embryogenesis, tissue repair, bone and cartilage formation in the regulation of the immune system (Tripathi and Vashishtha, 2006; Boudry et al., 2008; Penchev, 2008). However, EGF is a 6 kDa polypeptide which is composed of 53 amino acids. The peptide is highly homologous among species and elicits similar effects across species. EGF prevents bacterial translocation thus limiting the migration of bacteria through the gastrointestinal tract wall to reduce the probability of organism infection (Rauprich et al., 2000; Tripathi and Vashishtha, 2006). Its level in milk is approximately 2 μg/l (Boudry et al., 2008).

Genetic Markers in the Fight Against Mastitis

Genetic markers revealing a susceptibility or resistance to mastitis (so-called MAS – marker assisted selection) are also being identified (Sender et al., 2003; Żukiewicz et al., 2012). MAS uses genetic markers to identify the specific regions of chromosomes where the genes affecting on various quantitative traits, so-called quantitative trait loci (QTL) are located. This is used to predict the genetic value of animals, including the selection of individuals which are less susceptible to mastitis. A potential for use of class II BoLA genes and lactoferrin in the selection of cows resistant to mastitis exists. The lactoferrin gene is located on the 22nd chromosome in cattle and is composed of 17 exons.

A large variability of single-nucleotide polymorphism (SNPs), more than 140 in the lactoferrin gene, indicates that there is a high probability for a mastitis-resistance marker or a marker of milk yield (Wojdak-Maksymiec et al., 2006; Żukiewicz et al., 2012). It should be emphasized that lactoferrin genotype is associated with SCC. According to Sender et al. (2012), the BB genotype of lactoferrin was the most preferred in a reducing of mastitis incidence because the lowest SCC was observed in the group of cows with a BB genotype.

Unfortunately, it should be noted that the BB genotyped cows are of a low frequency in the cattle population. Nevertheless, in the studies of Wojdak-Maksymiec et al. (2006), the animals with an AA lactoferrin genotype were characterized by the lowest SCC. However, Kamiński et al. (2006) suggested that the G allele reduced an expression of lactoferrin which in turn was manifested by a lower somatic cell count.

On the other hand, a C allele enhanced the expression of lactoferrin, resulting in a strengthening of the immune response and an increase in SCC in milk. Moreover, the relationship between class II BoLA allele and the occurrence of mastitis in cows was also shown. In this respect, the most promising seems to be the BoLA DRB3.2*16 allele (Sharif et al., 2000; Sender et al., 2005).

This gene appears on the 23rd chromosome in cattle. The studies indicate a significant relationship of this allele with the occurrence of mastitis. A significant decrease in SCC was observed in the group of cows carrying this allele.

Conclusion

For early diagnosis of udder subclinical inflammations, a cheap and easy diagnosis indicator is needed. The commonly used diagnostic indicator of the mammary gland health, especially in cattle, is somatic cell count. However, SCC is not a reliable indicator in other species because it is difficult to determine the physiological norm for this parameter. The existence of other more credible physiological indicators can allow for the diagnosis of the mammary gland mastitis cases. These indicators are becoming increasingly used in the routine diagnosis of udder inflammations. It should be emphasized that early detection of mastitis allows for the reduction of economic losses, prolong the use of animals, as well as contribute to a significant improvement in the quantity and quality of milk obtained that is suitable for processing.

References

Alluwaimi A.M. (2004) The cytokines of bovine mammary gland: prospects for diagnosis and therapy. *Research in Veterinary Science*, 7, 211-222.

Aniulis E., Japertas S., Klimaite J., Aniuliene A. (2003) Prevalence and treatment of subclinical mastitis in cows. *Medycyna Weterynaryjna* 59, 10, 872-875.

Artym J. (2010) Udział laktoferyny w gospodarce żelazem w organizmie. Część II. Działanie przeciwmikrobiologiczne i przeciwzapalne poprzez sekwestrację żelaza. *Postępy Higieny i Medycyny Doświadczalnej*, 64, 604-616. (in Polish)

Awale M.M., Dudhatra G.B., Avinash K., Chauhan B.N., Kamani D.R., Modi C.M., Patel H.B., Mody S.K. (2012) *Bovine Mastitis: A threat to economy. Open Access Scientific Reports,* 1:295. doi:10.4172/scientificreports.295.

Bagnicka E., Strzałkowska N., Jóźwik A., Kaba J., Krzyżewski J. (2007) Czy liczba komórek somatycznych w mleku kóz jest wiarygodnym wskaźnikiem stanu zdrowotnego wymienia? *Wiadomości Zootechniczne*, 1-2, 35-41. (in Polish)

Baker E.N., Baker H.M. (2005) Molecular structure, binding properties and dynamics of lactoferrin. *Cellular and Molecular Life Sciences*, 62, 2531-2539.

Bansal B.K., Hamann J., Grabowski N.T., Singh K.B. (2005) Variation In The Composition Of Selected Milk Fraction Samples From Healthy And

Mastitis Quarters, And Its Significance For Mastitis Diagnosis. *Journal Of Dairy Research,* 72, 144-152.

Bar D., Tauer L.W., Bennett G., Gonza´lez R.N., Hertl J.A., Schukken Y. H., Schulte H.F., Welcome F.L., Grohn Y.T. (2008) The cost of generic clinical mastitis in dairy cows as estimated by using dynamic programming. *Journal of Dairy Science,* 91, 2205–2214.

Barłowska J., Litwińczuk Z., Wolanciuk A., Brodziak A. (2009) Relationship of somatic cell count to daily yield and technological usefulness of milk from different breeds of cows. *Polish Journal of Veterinary Sciences* 12, 1, 75-79.

Bartocci S., Tripaldi C., Terramoccia S. (2002) Characteristics of foodstuffs and diets, and the quanti-qualitative milk parameters of Mediterranean buffaloes bred in Italy using the intensive system an estimate of the nutritional requirements of buffalo herds lactating or dry. *Livestock Production Science,* 77, 45-58.

Batavani R.A., Asri S., Naebzadeh H. (2007) The effect of subclinical mastitis on milk composition in dairy cows. *Iranian Journal of Veterinary Research*, 8, 20, 205-211.

Benkerroum N. (2008) Antimicrobial activity of lysozyme with special relevance to milk. *African Journal of Biotechnology*, 7, 25, 4856-4867.

Bergonier D., de Cremoux R., Rupp R., Lagriffoul G., Berthelot X. (2003) Mastitis of dairy small ruminants. *Veterinary Research*. 34, 5, 689-716.

Błaszkowska M., Twardoń J. (2006) Wpływ koncentracji immunoglobulin całkowitych w siarze i surowicy krów na poziom odporności biernej u potomstwa. *Medycyna Weterynaryjna*, 2, 185-188. (in Polish)

Bleck G.T., Wheeler M.B., Hansen L.B., Chester-Jones H., Miller D.J. (2009) Lactose synthesis components in milk: concentrations of alpha lactalbumin and beta 1,2-galactosyltransferase in milk of cows from several breeds at various stages of lactation. *Reproduction of Domestic Animals*, 44, 241-247.

Bloemhof S., de Jong G., de Haas Y. (2009) Genetic parameters for clinical mastitis in the first three lactations of Dutch Holstein cattle. *Veterinary Microbiology,* 134, 165-171.

Boots J.W., Floris R. (2006) Lactoperoxidase: From catalytic mechanism to practical applications. *International Dairy Journal* 16, 11, 1272-1276.

Boudry C., Dehoux J., Portetelle D., Buldgen A. (2008) Bovine colostrum as a natural growth promotor for newly weaned piglets: a review. *Biotechnolgy Agronomy, Society and Environment,* 12, 2, 157-170.

Burvenich C., Detilleux J., Paape M.J., Massart-Leen A.M. (2000). Physiological and genetic factors that influence the cows' resistance to mastitis, especially during early lactation. [In:] *Proc. IDF Symp. on Immunology of Ruminant Mammary Gland*. Stresa, Italy, pp. 9-20.

Cady R.A., Shah S.K., Schermerhorn E.C., McDowell R.E. (1983) Factors affecting performance of Nili Ravi buffaloes in Pakistan. *Journal of Dairy Science*, 66, 578-586.

Carlen E., Strandberg E., Roth A. (2004) Genetic parameters for clinical mastitis, somatic cell score, and production in the first three lactations of Swedish Holstein cows. *Journal of Dairy Science,* 87, 3062-3070.

Cha E., Hertl J.A., Bar D. Gröhn Y.T. (2010) The cost of different types of lameness in dairy cows calculated by dynamic programming. *Preventive Veterinary Medicine*, 97, 1-8.

Chang J.Y., Li L. (2002) The unfolding mechanism and disulfide structures of denatured lysozyme. *FEBS Letters,* 511, 73-78.

Chatterton D.E.W., Smithers G., Roupas P., Brodkorb A. (2006) Bioactivity of α-lactoglobulin and β-lactalbumin – technological implications for processing. *International Dairy Journal*, 16, 1229-1240.

Cheng J.B., Wang J.Q., Bu D.P., Liu G.L., Zhang C.G., Wei H.Y., Zhou L.Y., Wang J.Z. (2008) Factors affecting the lactoferrin concentration in bovine milk. *Journal of Dairy Science*, 91, 3, 970-976.

Claus M.A., Levy J.K., MacDonald K., Tucker S.J., Crawford P.C. (2006) Immunoglobulin concentrations in feline colostrum and milk, and the requirement of colostrum for passive transfer of immunity to neonatal kittens. *Journal of Feline Medicine and Surgery*, 8, 184-191.

Contreras A., Sierra D., Sanchez A., Corrales J.C., Marco J.C., Paape M.J., Gonzalo C. (2007) *Mastitis in small ruminants. Small Ruminant Diseases and Resources,* 68, 145-153.

Costa E.O., Garino F.G., Melville P.A., Ribeiro A.R., Silva J.A., Watanabe E.T., Valle C. R. (2000) Estudo da etiologia das mastites bovinas nas sete principais bacias leiteiras do Estado de São Paulo. *Napgama*, 4, 6-13.

De Vliegher S., Barkema H.W., Stryhn H., Opsomer G., de Kruif A. (2004) Impact in dairy heifers of early lactation somatic cell count on somatic cell counts during the first lactation. *Journal of Dairy Science*, 87, 3672-3682.

De Ying Y., Zhong C.S., Min Y.S., Ping Y.X., Song L.C., Xin D.L. (2009) Research on lactate dehydrogenase activity in cow's milk as an indicator of subclinical mastitis. *Chinese Journal of Veterinary Science*, 29, 6, 761-764.

Diarra M.S., Petitelere D., Lacasse P. (2002) Effect of lactoferrin in combination with penicillin on the morphology and the physiology of *Staphylococcus aureus* isolated from bovine mastitis. *Journal of Dairy Science*, 85, 1141-1149.

Díaz J.R., Romero G., Muelas R., Alejandro M., Peris C. (2012) Effect of intramammary infection on milk electrical conductivity in Murciano-Granadina goats. *Journal of Dairy Science*, 95, 2, 718-726.

EFSA (2005) Opinion on the usefulness on somatic cell counts for safety on milk and milk derived products from goats. EFSA J. 305, 1-19. doi: *http://www.efsa.europa.eu.*

El-Loly M.M., Farrag A.F. (2007) Isolation of immunoglobulin-rich fractions from whey. *Milchwissenschaft* 62, 2, 199-202.

Fonteh F.A, Grandison A.S., Lewis M.J. (2002) Variations of lactoperoxidase activity and thiocyanate content in cows' and goats' milk throughout lactation. *Journal of Dairy Research*, 69, 3, 401-409.

Forsbäck L., Lindmark-Månsson H., Andren A., Akerstedt M., Svennersten-Sjaunja K. (2009) Udder quarter milk composition at different levels of somatic cell count in cow composite milk. *Animal* 3, 5, 710-717.

Fox P.F., Kelly A.L. (2005) Indigenous enzymes in milk: Overview and historical aspects – Part 2. *International Dairy Journal*, 16, 517-532.

Gapper L.W., David E.J., Copestake D.E.J., Otter D.E., Indyk H.E. (2007) Analysis of bovine immunoglobulin G in milk, colostrum and dietary supplements: a review. *Analytical of Bioanalytical Chemistry*, 389, 93-109.

Garcia-Mantoya I.A., Cendon T.S., Arevalo-Gallegos S., Rascon-Cruz Q. (2011) Lactoferrin a multiple bioactive protein: An overview. *Biochemica et Biophysica Acta*, doi:10.1016/j.bbagen.2011.06.018, 1-11.

Garry F. B., Adams R., Cattell M.B., Dinsmore R.P. (1996) Comparison of passive immunoglobulin transfer to dairy calves fed colostrum or commercially available colostral-supplement products. *Journal of the American Veterinary Medical Association,* 208, 107-110.

Giacinti G., Basirico L., Ronchi B., Bernabucci U. (2013) Lactoferrin concentration in buffalo milk. *Italian Journal Animal Science*, 12, 23, 139-143.

Griffin T.K., Morant S.V., Dodd F.H. (1987) Bovine mastitis: initiation and guidelines for diagnosis. *Bulletin of the International Dairy Federation*, 211, 72, 1900-1906.

Gröhn Y.T., Wilson D.J., Gonzalez R.N., Hertl J.A., Schulte H., Bennett G., et al. (2004) Effect of pathogen-specific clinical mastitis on milk yield in dairy cows. *Journal of Dairy Science*, 87, 3358-3374.

Gröhn Y.T., González R.N., Wilson D.J., Hertl J.A., Bennett G., Schulte H., Schukken Y.H. (2005) Effect of pathogen-specific clinical mastitis on herd life in two New York State dairy herds. *Preventive Veterinary Medicine*, 71, 105-125.

Guidry A.J. (2007) Mastitis and the immune system of the mammary gland. [In:] *Lactation*. Larson, B.L. (eds). The Iowa State University Press, Ames, Iowa, USA. pp. 229-262.

Guliński P., Młynek K., Giersz B. (2006) Wpływ długości okresu po wycieleniu i wieku krów na poziom immunoglobulin w siarze. *Roczniki Naukowe Zootechniki*, 33, 2, 193-200. (in Polish)

Haenlein G.F.W. (2002) Relationship of somatic cell count in goat milk to mastitis productivity. *Small Ruminant Diseases and Resources*, 45, 163-178.

Hagiwara S., Kawai K., Anri A., Nagahata H. (2003) Lactoferrin concentrations in milk from normal and subclinical mastitis cows. *The Journal of Veterinary Medical Science*, 65, 3, 319-323.

Hagnestam C., Emanuelson U., Berglund B. (2007) Yield losses associated with clinical mastitis occurring in different weeks of lactation. *Journal Dairy Science*, 90, 2260-2270.

Hamann J. (2002) Relationship between somatic cell count and milk composition. *Bulletin FIL-IDF*, 372, 56-59.

Harmon R.J. (1994) Physiology of mastitis and factors affecting somatic cell counts. *Journal Dairy Science*, 77, 2103-2112.

Harmon R.J. (2001) Somatic cell counts: A primer. *Madison to Reno, National Mastitis Council Annual Meeting Proceedings*, pp. 3-9.

Harmon R.J., Schanbacher F.L., Ferguson L.C., Smith K.L. (1976) Changes in lactoferrin, immunoglobulin G, bovine serum albumin, and alpha-lactalbumin during acute experimental and natural coliform mastitis in cows. *Infection Immunity*, 13, 2, 533-542.

Hoeben D., Burvenich C., Trevisi E., Bertoni G., Hamann J., Bruckmaier R.M., Blum J.W. (2000) Role of endotoxin and TNF-alpha in the pathogenesis of experimentally induced coliform mastitis in periparturient cows. *Journal of Dairy Research*, 67, 503-514.

Højsgaard S., Friggens N.C. (2010) Quantifying degree of mastitis from common trends in a panel of indicators for mastitis in dairy cows. *Journal of Dairy Science*, 93, 582-592.

Huijps K., Lam T.J.G.M., Hogeveen H. (2008) Costs Of Mastitis: Facts And Perception. *Journal of Dairy Research*, 75, 113-120.

Ikonen T., Morri S., Tyrisevä A.M., Ruottinen O., Ojala M. (2004) Genetic and phenotypic correlations between milk coagulation properties, milk production traits, somatic cell count, casein content, and pH of milk. *Journal of Dairy Science*, 87, 458-467.

Jones G.M., Bailey T.L. (2009) Understanding the Basics of Mastitis. Virginia Cooperative Extension, Publication 404-233. Virginia Tech, USA, pp. 1-5. doi: *http://pubs.ext.vt.edu/404/404-233/404-233.*

Jóźwik A., Krzyżewski J., Strzałkowska N., Poławska E., Bagnicka E., Wierzbicka A., Niemczuk K., Lipińska P., Horbańczuk J. (2012) Relations between the oxidative status, mastitis, milk quality and disorders of reproductive functions in dairy cows – a review. *Animal Science Papers and Reports*, 30, 4, 297-307.

Juozaitiene V., Zakas A., Juozaitis A. (2004) Relationship of somatic cell count with milk yield and composition in the herds of Black-and-White cattle. *Medycyna Weterynaryjna*, 60, 7, 701-704.

Kamiński S., Oleński K., Brym P., Malewski T., Sazanov A.A. (2006) Single nucleotide polymorphism In the promotor region of the lactoferrin gene and its associations with milk performance traits in Polish Holstein cows. *Russian Journal Genetic,* 42, 8, 924-927.

Kanwar J.R., Kanwar R.K., Sun X., Punj V., Matta H., Morley S.M., Parratt A., Puri M., Sehgal R. (2009) Molecular and Biotechnological Advances in Milk Proteins in Relation to Human Health. *Current Protein and Peptide Science,* 10, 4, 308-338.

Kawai K., Hagiwara S., Anri A., Nagahata H. (1999) Lactoferrin concentration in milk of bovine clinical mastitis. *Veterinary Research Communications*, 23, 7, 391-398.

Kelly A.L., Tiernan D., O'Sullivan C., Joyce P. (2000) Correlation between bovine milk somatic cell count and polymorphonuclear leukocyte level for samples of bulk milk and milk from individual cows. *Journal of Dairy Science*, 83, 300-304.

Khan M.Z., Khan A. (2006) Basic facts of mastitis in dairy animals: A review. *Pakistan Veterinary Journal*, 26, 4, 204-208.

Koivula M., Mantysaari E.A., Negussie E., Serenius T. (2005) Genetic and phenotypic relationships among milk yield and somatic cell count before and after mastitis. *Journal of Dairy Science*, 88, 827-833.

Korhonen H. (2004) Isolation of immunoglobulins from colostrums. *Bulletin of the IDF*, 389, 78-84.

Król J., Brodziak A., Florek M., Litwińczuk Z. (2010a) Effect of somatic cell counts in milk on its quality subject to cow breed and season. *Annales UMCS*, Sec. EE, XXVIII, 3, 9-17.

Król J., Litwińczuk Z., Brodziak A., Barłowska J. (2010b) Lactoferrin, lysozyme and immunoglobulin G content in milk of four breeds of cows manager under intensive production system. *Polish Journal of Veterinary Science*, 13, 2, 357-361.

Król J., Brodziak A., Litwińczuk Z., Barłowska J. (2012) Selected factors determining the content of lactoferrin, lysozyme and immunoglobulin G in bovine milk [In:] *A Search for Antibacterial Agents*. Ed. Varaprasad Bobbarala, InTech - Open Access Publisher, Chapter 7, 107-125, ISBN 978-953-51-0724-8.

Kruzel M.L., Actor J.K., Boldogh I., Zimecki M. (2007) Lactoferrin in health and disease. *Postępy Higieny i Medycyny Doświadczalnej*, 61, 261-267.

Larsen T. (2005) Determination of lactate dehydrogenase (LDH) activity in milk by a fluorometric assay. *Journal of Dairy Research*, 72, 2, 209-216.

Legrand D., Pierce E., Carpentier M., Mariller C., Mazurier J. (2008) Structure and function lactoferrin. *Advances in Experimental Medicine and Biology*, 606, 94, 163.

Leitner G., Merin U., Silanikove N. (2004) Changes in milk composition as affected by subclinical mastitis in goats. *Journal of Dairy Science*, 87, 1719-1726.

Leitner G., Merin U., Krifucks O., Blum S., Rivas A.L., Silanikove N. (2012) Effects of intra-mammary bacterial infection with coagulase negative staphylococci and stage of lactation on shedding of epithelial cells and infiltration of leukocytes into milk: comparison among cows, goats and sheep. *Veterinary Immunology and Immunopathology*, 147, 202-210.

Leśnierowski G. (2009) Nowe sposoby fizykochemicznej modyfikacji lizozymu. *Nauka Przyroda Technologie*, 3, 4, 1-18. (in Polish)

Lieske B., Jantz., Finke B. (2005) An improved analytical approach for the determination of bovine serum albumin in mil. *Dairy Science and Technology*, 85, 237-248.

Lindmark-Månsson H., Sensson U., Paulsson M., Alden G., Frank B., Johnsson G. (2000) Influence of milk components, somatic cells and supplemental zinc on milk processability. *International Dairy Journal*, 10, 423-433.

Lindmark-Månsson H., Brånning C., Alden G., Paullsson M. (2006) Relationship between somatic cell count, individual leukocyte populations and milk components in bovine udder quarter milk. *International Dairy Journal*, 16, 717-727.

Litwińczuk Z., Teter U., Teter W., Stanek P., Chabuz W. (2006) Ocena wpływu niektórych czynników na wydajność i jakość mleka krów utrzymywanych w gospodarstwach farmerskich. *Roczniki Naukowe Polskiego Towarzystwa Zootechnicznego*, 2, 1, 133-140. (in Polish)

Litwińczuk Z., Król J., Brodziak A., Barłowska J. (2011) Changes of protein content and its fractions in bovine milk from different cow breeds subject to somatic cell count. *Journal of Dairy Science*, 94, 684-691.

Liu G.L., Wang J.Q., Bu D.P., Cheng J.B., Zhang C.G., Wei H.Y., Zhou L.Y., Zhou Z.F., Hu H., Dong X.L. (2009) Factors affecting the transfer of immunoglobulin G1 into the milk of Holstein cows. *The Veterinary Journal,* 182, 79-85.

Lönnerdal B., Iyer S. (1995) Lactoferrin: molecular structure and biological function. *Annual Review of Nutrition*, 15, 93-110.

Lund T., Miglior F., Dekkers J.C.M., Burnside E.B. (1994) Genetic relationships between clinical mastitis, somatic cell count and udder conformation in Danish Holsteins. *Livestock Production Science*, 39, 243-251.

Małaczewska J., Rotkiewicz Z. (2007) Laktoferyna – białko multipotencjalne. *Medycyna Weterynaryjna*, 63, 2, 136-139. (in Polish)

Malinowski E., Kłossowska A., Smulski S. (2008) Zmiany stężeń biologicznie aktywnych składników mleka krowiego wskutek mastitis. *Medycyna Weterynaryjna*, 64, 1, 14-19.

Malinowski E., Smulski S. (2007) Występowanie i profilaktyka zakażeń i zapaleń gruczołu mlekowego u jałówek. *Życie Weterynaryjne,* 82, 6, 476-482. (in Polish)

Masschalack B., van Houdt R., van Haver E.G., Michiels C.W. (2001) Inactivation of gram-negative bacteria by lysozyme, denatured lysozyme, and lysozyme-derived peptides under high hydrostatic pressure. *Applied and Environmental Microbiology*, 67, 1, 339-344.

Masschalck B., Michiels C.W. (2003) Antimicrobial properties of lysozyme in relation to foodborne vegetative bacteria. *Critical Reviews in Microbiology,* 29, 3, 191-214.

Menzies P.I., Ramanoon S.Z. (2001) Mastitis of sheep and goats. *Veterinary Clinics of North America: Food Animal Practice*, 17, 2, 333-358, vii.

Moatsou G. (2010) Indigenous enzymatic activities in ovine and caprine milks. *International Journal of Dairy Technology*, 63, 1, 16-31.

Mohammadian B. (2011) The effect of subclinical mastitis on lactate dehydrogenase in dairy cows. *International Journal of Animal and Veterinary Advances*, 3, 161-163.

Monecke S., Ehricht R., Slickers P., Wernery R., Johnson B., Jose S., Wernery U. (2011) Microarray-based genotyping of *Staphylococcus aureus* isolates from camels. *Veterinary Microbiology*, 150, 309-314.

Montagne P., Cuillière ML., Molé C., Béné MC., Faure G. (2001) Changes in lactoferrin and lysozyme levels in human milk during the first twelve weeks of lactation. *Advances in Experimental Medicine and Biology*, 501, 241-247.

Mrode R.A., Swanson G.J.T., Winters M.S. (1998) Genetic parameters and evaluations for somatic cell counts and its relationship with production and type traits in some dairy breeds in the United Kingdom. Animal. *Science*, 66, 569-576.

Nielsen C. (2009) Economic impact of mastitis in dairy cows. Doctoral Thesis, Swedish University of Agricultural Sciences, Uppsala. *Acta Universitatis Agriculturae Sueciae,* 29. ISBN 978-91-86195-76-2.

NMC (2011) *National Mastitis Council, the 50th Annual Meeting Proceedings,* Arlington, Virginia.

Norberg E. (2005) Electrical conductivity of milk as a phenotypic and genetic indicator of bovine mastitis: A review. *Livestock Production Science*, 96, 129-139.

Norberg E., Hogeveen H., Korsgaard I.R., Friggens N.C., Lbvendahl P. (2004a) Electrical conductivity of milk-ability to predict mastitis status. *Journal of Dairy Science,* 87, 1099-1107.

Norberg E., Rogers G.W., Madsen P. (2004b) Genetic parameters for electrical conductivity of milk. *Proceeding 55th Annual EAAP Meeting, Bled.*

Nudda A., Feligini M., Battacone G., Murgia P., Pulina G. (2001) Relationship between somatic cells count, whey protein and coagulation properties in sheep milk. *Proceedings of the ASPA XIV Congress, Firenze, Italy*, 511-513.

Nyman A.K., Ekman T., Emanuelson U., Gustafsson A.H., Holtenius K., Waller P.K., Sandgren C.H. (2007) Risk factors associated with the incidence of veterinary-treated clinical mastitis in Swedish dairy herds with a high milk yield and a low prevalence of subclinical mastitis. *Preventive Veterinary Medicine*, 78, 142-160.

Nyman A.K., Emanuelson U., Gustafsson A.H., Waller P.K. (2009) Management practices associated with udder health of first-parity dairy cows in early lactation. *Preventive Veterinary Medicine*, 88, 138-149.

O'Rourke D. (2009) Nutrition and udder health in dairy cows: a review. *Irish Veterinary Journal,* 62, 15-20.

Ogola H., Shitandi A., Nanua J. (2007) Effect of mastitis on raw milk compositional quality. *Journal of Veterinary Science*, 8, 3, 237-242.

Olde Riekerink R.G.M., Barkema H.W., Kelton D.F., Scholl D.T. (2008) Incidence rate of clinical mastitis on Canadian dairy farms. *Journal of Dairy Science*, 91, 1366-1377.

Olechnowicz J., Jaśkowski J.M. (2012) Somatic cells count in cow's bulk tank milk. *Journal of Veterinary Medical Science*, 74, 681-686.

Oliszewski R., Nunez de Kairuz M.S., Elias de Gonzalez S.N., Oliver G. (2002) Assessment of beta-glucuronidase levels in goat's milk as an indicator of mastitis: comparison with other mastitis detection methods. *Journal of Food Protection,* 6, 864-866.

Oliver S.P., Calvinho L.F. (1995) Influence of inflammation on mammary gland metabolism and milk composition. *Journal of Animal Science*, 73 (Suppl. 2), 18-33.

Ontsouka C.E., Bruckmaier R.M., Blum J.W. (2003) Fractionized milk composition during removal of colostrum and mature milk. *Journal of Dairy Science*, 86, 2005-2011.

Orsi N. (2004) The antimicrobial activity of lactoferrin: current status and perspectives. *Biometals*, 17, 189-196.

Osman K.M., El-Enbaawy M.I., Ezzeldeen N.A., Hussein H.M.G. (2009) Mastitis in dairy buffalo and cattle in Egypt due to *Clostridium perfringens*: prevalence, incidence, risk factors and costs. *Revue scientifique et technique* (International Office of Epizootics), 28, 3, 975-986.

O'Sullivan C.A., Joyce P.J., Sloan T., Shattock A.G. (1992) Capture immunoassay for the diagnosis of bovine mastitis using a monoclonal antibody to polymorphonuclear granulocytes. *Journal of Dairy Research*, 59, 123-133.

Paape M.J., Bannerman D.D., Zhao X., Lee J.W. (2003) The bovine neutrophil: structure and function in blood and milk. *Veterinary Research,* 34, 597-627.

Paape M.J., Wiggans G.R., Bannerman D.D., Thomas D.L., Sanders A.H., Contreras A., Moroni P., Miller R.H. (2007) Monitoring goat and sheep milk somatic cell counts. *Small Ruminant Research*, 68, 114-125.

Park Y.W., Juarez M., Ramos M., Haenlein G.F.W. (2007) Physico-chemical characteristics of goat and sheep milk. *Small Ruminant Research*, 68, 88-113.

Pazzola M., Balia F., Carcangiu V., Dettori M.L., Piras G., Vacca G.M. (2012) Higher somatic cells counted by the electronic counter method do not influence renneting properties of goat milk. *Small Ruminant Research,* 102, 1, 32-36.

Peaker M. (1983) Secretion of ions and water. [In:] Mepham, T.B. (Ed.), *Biochemistry of Lactation*. Elsevier, Amsterdam, pp. 285-305.

Penchev G.I. (2008) Difference in chemical composition between cow colostrums and milk. *Bulgarian Journal of Veterinary Medicine*, 11, 1, 3-12.

Person M.D., Person C.N., Lester T.D., Rorie R.W. (2000) Effects of Milk Antimicrobial proteins on incidence of mastitis in dairy cattle. *Arkansas Animal Science Department Report,* 54-55.

Petrovski K.R., Williamson N.B., Lopez-Villalobos N., Parkinson T.J., Tucker I.G. (2011) Culture results from milk samples submitted to veterinary diagnostic laboratories from August 2003 to December 2006 in New Zealand. *New Zealand Veterinary Journal* 59, 6, 317-322.

Piccinini R., Mirelli M., Ferri B., Tripaldi C., Belotti M., Dapra V., Orlandini S., Zecconi A. (2006) Relationship between cellular and whey components in buffalo milk. *Journal of Dairy Research*, 73, 129-133.

Pösö J., Mäntysaari E.A. (1996) Relationships between clinical mastitis, somatic cell score, and production for the first three lactations of Finnish Ayrshire. *Journal of Dairy Science*, 79, 1284-1291.

Poutrel B., Caffin J., Rainard P. (1983) Physiological and pathological factors influencing bovine serum albumin content of milk. *Journal of Dairy Science,* 66, 535-541.

Pyörälä S. (2003) Indicators of inflammation in the diagnosis of mastitis. *Veterinary Research*, 34, 565-568.

Rainard P., Corrales J.C., Barrio M.B., Cochard T., Poutrel B. (2003) Leucotoxic activities of *Staphylococcus aureus* strains isolated from cows, ewes, and goats with mastitis: importance of LukM/LukF'-PV leukotoxin. *Clinical and Diagnostic Laboratory Immunology*, 10, 2, 272-277.

Rainard P., Riollet C. (2006) Innate immunity of the bovine mammary gland. *Veterinary Research*, 37, 369-400.

Rauprich A.B.H., Hammon J., Blum W. (2000) Influence of feeding different amounts of first colostrums on metabolic, endocrine, and health status and on growth performance in neonatal calves. *Journal of Animal Science,* 78, 896-908.

Rogers G.W. (2002) Aspects of milk composition, production life and type traits in relation to mastitis and other diseases in dairy cattle. *Proceeding*

7th World Congr. Gen. Appl. Livest. Prod., Montpellier, France, communication no 09-18.

Romero G., Díaz J.R., Sabater J.M., Perez C. (2012) Evaluation of commercial probes for on-line electrical conductivity measurements during goat gland milking process. *Sensors* (Basel), 12, 4, 4493-4513.

Rupp R., Boichard D. (1999) Genetic parameters for clinical mastitis, somatic cell score, production, udder type traits, and milking ease in first lactation Holsteins. *Journal of Dairy Science*, 82, 2198-2204.

Sawa A., Neja W., Bogucki M. (2007) Relationships between cytological quality and composition of milk and the effect of some environmental factors on the frequency of recurrent mastitis in cow. *Journal of Central European Agriculture*, 8, 3, 25-30.

Scheppers A.J., Lam T.J.G.M., Schukken Y.H., Wilmink J.B.M., Hanekamp W.B.A. (1997) Estimation of variance components for somatic cell counts to determine thresholds for uninfected quarters. *Journal of Dairy Science*, 80, 1833-1840.

Schukken Y.H., Lam T.J.G.M., Barkema H.M. (1997) Biological basis for selection on udder health traits. Proceedings, International Workshop on Genetic Improvement of Functional Traits in Cattle Health. Uppsala, Sweden, *Bulletin Interbull*, 15, 27-32.

Schukken Y.H., Wilson D.J., Welcome F., Garrison-Tikofsky L., Gonzalez R.N. (2003) Monitoring udder health and milk quality using somatic cell counts. *Veterinary Research*, 34, 579-596.

Seifu E., Donkin E.F., Buys E.M. (2007) Potential of lactoperoxidase to diagnose subclinical mastitis in goats. *Small Ruminant Research,* 69, 154-158.

Sender G., Korwin-Kosakowska A., Stępińska U. (2003) Wykorzystanie markerów genetycznych w programie zwalczania mastitis. *Medycyna Weterynaryjna,* 59, 10, 853-856. (in Polish)

Sender G., Korwin-Kossakowska A., Gralak B. (2005) Wpływ polimorfizmu genu BoLA-DRB3 na występowanie mastitis u krów. *Medycyna Weterynaryjna*, 61, 540-542. (in Polish)

Sender G., Oprządek J., Pawlik A., Urtnowski P., Kubasik D. (2012) Możliwości wykorzystania polimorfizmu genu laktoferyny w selekcji krów odpornych na zapalenie wymienia. *Roczniki Naukowe Zootechniki*, 8, 1, 9-16. (in Polish)

Séverin S., Wenshui X. (2005) Milk biologically active components as nutraceuticals: Review. *Critical Reviews in Food Science and Nutrition*, 45, 645-656.

Sharif S., Mallard B.A., Sargeant J.M. (2000) Presence of glutamine at position 74 of pocket 4 in the BoLA-DR antigen binding groove is associated with occurrence of clinical mastitis caused by *Staphylococcus* species. *Veterinary Immunology and Immunopathology*, 76, 231-238.

Sharif A., Umer M., Muhammad G. (2009) Mastitis control in dairy production. *Journal of Agriculture & Social Sciences*, 5, 102-105.

Sharma N., Gupta S.K., Sharma U., Hussai K. (2007) Treatment of clinical mastitis in buffalo-A case report. *Buffalo Bulletin*, 26, 2, 56-58.

Sharma N., Singh N.K., Bhadwa M.S. (2011) Relationship of somatic cell count and mastitis: An overview. Asian - *Australasian Journal of Animal Sciences,* 24, 3, 429-438.

Shearer J.K., Harris B. (2003) *Mastitis in dairy goats*. Anim. Sci. Dept. Florida Coop. Ext. Serv., Institute of Food and Agricultural Sciences, University of Florida, Gainesville, USA, pp. 1-6.

Silanikove N., Leitner G., Merin U., Prosser C.G. (2010) Recent advances in exploiting goat's milk: Quality safety and production aspects. *Small Ruminant Research*. doi: 101016/jsmallrumres200912033.

Smulski S., Malinowski E., Kaczmarowski M., Lassa H. (2011) Occurrence, forms and etiologic agents of mastitis in Poland depending on size of farm. *Medycyna Weterynaryjna*, 67, 90-193.

Soyeurt H., Bastin C., Colinet F.G., Arnould V. M.-R., Berry E. Wall D. P., Dehareng F., Nguyen H. N., Dardenne P., Schefers J., Vandenplas J., Weigel K., Coffey M., Théron L., Detilleux J., Reding E., Gengler N., McParland S. (2012) Mid-Infrared prediction of lactoferrin content in bovine milk: Potential indicator of mastitis. *Animal*, 6, 11, 1830-1838.

Stanek P., Litwińczuk Z., Teter U., Jankowski P. (2004) Skład chemiczny i jakość cytologiczna mleka krów czarno-białych utrzymywanych w gospodarstwach farmerskich Lubelszczyzny z uwzględnieniem pory roku i ich dziennej produkcyjności. *Zeszyty Naukowe Przeglądu Hodowlanego*, 72, 1, 153-159.

Steeneveld W., Hogeveen H., Barkema H.W., van den Broek J., Huirne R.B.M. (2008) The influence of cow factors on the incidence of clinical mastitis in dairy cows. *Journal of Dairy Science*, 91, 4, 1391-1402.

Steijns J.M., Hooijdonk A.C.M. (2000) Occurrence, structure, biochemical properties and technological characteristics of lactoferrin. *British Journal of Nutrition*, 84 (Suppl. 1), 11-17.

Struff W.G., Sprotte G. (2008) Bovine colostrum as a biologic in clinical medicine: a review – part II: clinical studies. *International Journal of Clinical Pharmacology and Therapeutics,* 46, 5, 211-225.

Sudhan N.A., Sharma N. (2010) Mastitis – An important production disease of dairy animals. *SMVS' Dairy Year Book*, pp. 72-88.

Tripaldi C., Martillotti F., Terramoccia S. (1998) Content of taurine and other free amino acids in milk of goats breed in Italy. *Small Ruminant Research,* 30, 127-136.

Tripaldi C., Palocci G, Miarelli M., Catta M., Orlandini S., Amatiste S., Di Bernardini R., Catillo G. (2010) Effects of Mastitis on Buffalo Milk Quality. *Asian-Australasian Journal of Animal Sciences*, 23, 10, 1319-1324.

Tripathi V., Vashishtha B. (2006) Bioactive compounds of bovine colostrums. *Food Reviews International*, 22, 225-244.

Urech E., Puha Z., Schallibaum M. (1999) Changes in milk protein fraction as affected by subclinical mastitis. *Journal of Dairy Science*, 82, 2402-2411.

Ushida Y., Shimokawa Y., Toida T., Matsui H., Takase M. (2007) Bovine alpha-lactoglobulin stimulates mucus metabolism in gastric mucosa. *Journal of Dairy Science,* 90, 541-546.

van den Borne B.H., van Schaik G., Lam T.J., Nielen M. (2010) Variation in herd level mastitis indicators between primi- and multiparae in Dutch dairy herds. *Preventive Veterinary Medicine*, 96, 1-2, 49-55.doi:10.1016/j.prevetmed.
2010.05.010.

Wakabayashi H., Yamauchi K., Takase M. (2006) Lactoferrin research, technology and applications. *International Dairy Journal*, 16, 1241-1251.

Weiss W.P., Hogan J.S., Smith K.L., Hoblet K.H. (1990) Relationships among selenium, vitamin e, and mammary gland health in commercial dairy herds. *Journal of Dairy Science*, 73, 381-390.

Wernery U., Johnson B., Jose S. (2008) The most important dromedary mastitis organisms. *Journal of Camel Practice and Research*, 15, 159-161.

Wojdak-Maksymiec K., Kmiec M., Ziemak J. (2006) Associations between bovine lactoferrin gene polymorphism and somatic cell count in milk. *Veterinary Medicine*, 51, 14-20.

Ying C., Yang C.B., Hsu J.T. (2004) Relationship of somatic cell count, physical, chemical and enzymatic properties to the bacterial standard plate count in different breeds of dairy goats. *Asian-Australasian Journal of Animal Sciences,* 17, 554-559.

Zhao S., Zhang C., Wang J., Liu G., Bu D., Cheng J., Zhou L. (2010) Variation of immunoglobulins in colostrum and immune milk as affected by antigen releasing devices. *Asian-Australasian Journal of Animal Sciences*, 23, 9, 1184-1189.

Zimecki M., Artym J. (2005) Właściwości terapeutyczne białek i peptydów z siary i mleka. *Postępy Higieny i Medycyny Doświadczalnej*, 59, 309-323. (in Polish)

Zumbo A., Chiofalo B., Liotta L., Rundo Sotera A., Chiofalo V. (2004) Quantitative and qualitative milk characteristics of Nebrodi goats. *South African Society for Animal Science*, 34 (Suppl. 1), 155-157.

Żukiewicz A., Grzesiak W., Szatkowska I., Błaszczyk P., Dybus A. (2012) Genetic Factors of Milk Yield in Dairy Cattle – Advances in the Quest for Universal Markers *Israel Journal of Veterinary Medicine*, 67, 2, 82-91.

In: Mammary Glands
Editor: Edmund B. Rucker

ISBN: 978-1-62948-853-0

Chapter IX

Effect of Lipopolysaccharide on Cell Populations in the Bovine Mammary Gland

***Petr Slama*[*,1], *Zdenek Havlicek*[1] and *Jiri Skladanka*[2]**
[1]Department of Animal Morphology, Physiology and Genetics, Mendel University in Brno, Czech Republic
[2]Department of Animal Nutrition and Forage Production, Mendel University in Brno, Czech Republic

Abstract

Lipopolysaccharide, a component of Gram-negative bacteria cell wall, has an ability to induce an inflammatory response in the bovine mammary gland. *Escherichia coli* is one of the most important pathogens causing bovine mastitis. In this respect, it is very important to study the effect of *E. coli* or lipopolysaccharide (LPS) on cell populations in the bovine mammary gland in order to improve our knowledge for the prevention and treatment of infections. Lipopolysaccharide can affect different cellular processes, for example, programmed cell death (e.g., apoptosis) and the expression of some cell receptors on leukocytes such

[*] Corresponding author: Department of Animal Morphology, Physiology and Genetics, Mendel University in Brno, Zemedelska 1, 613 00 Brno, Czech Republic. Tel: +420545133146. E-mail: petr.slama@mendelu.cz (P. Slama).

as neutrophils, lymphocytes and macrophages in the mammary gland. This mini-review summarizes information about the effects of lipopolysaccharide on leukocytes in the bovine mammary gland.

Keywords: Lipopolysaccharide, apoptosis, neutrophil, lymphocyte, macrophage, mammary gland, mastitis

Introduction

Escherichia coli is a Gram-negative bacterium which is commonly found in the small intestine. Most *E. coli* strains are harmless, but some of them can cause serious food poisoning in humans (Vogt and Dippold, 2005). This bacterium is also one of the most important pathogens that can cause inflammation of bovine mammary gland. This environmental bacterium produces lipopolysaccharides (LPSs). Bacterial LPSs are toxins released from the cell wall of Gram-negative bacteria. Application of LPS into the bovine mammary gland induces an inflammatory response that is a very good model for experimental studies of the immunological aspects of mammary gland inflammation (Sladek et al., 2002). Intramammary infusion of *E. coli* LPS induces an inflammatory response in the bovine mammary gland similar to other bacterial toxins and chemical such as muramyl dipeptide (Sladek and Rysanek, 2000b; Rysanek et al. 2001; Sladek et al., 2002; Langrova et al., 2008).

Inflammation of the mammary gland, or mastitis, is a very important disease found in lactating cows which decreases the quality and quantity of produced milk. Therefore, it is very important to study the processes found in the progression of this disease. Resident and infiltrating cells play an important role in the mammary gland defence system against invading pathogens. Lymphocytes and macrophages are the predominant resident cells in the healthy mammary gland. An intramammary infection induces the flux of leukocytes from the circulating blood into the infected mammary gland (Concha et al., 1986; Miller et al., 1991). Leukocytes accumulate at the site of inflammation and have the potential to damage the neighbouring cells and tissue through the release of inflammatory mediators or through their necrosis. Necrosis is a type of cell death that results in the release of toxic cellular contents (Weiss, 1989). Leukocytes in the mammary gland can undergo apoptosis and subsequent phagocytosis by macrophages (Sladek and Rysanek, 2000a; Sladek and Rysanek, 2000b; Sladek and Rysanek, 2001). In contrast to necrosis, apoptosis is a type programmed cell death that occurs without the release of cellular contents. This process is critical for the resolution of inflammation within the bovine mammary gland. Apoptosis of neutrophils reduces tissue destruction, decreases the influx of cells into the site of infection, and supports the termination of the innate immune response by limiting the pro-inflammatory capacity (Kobayashi et al., 2003).

Since mastitis is a multifactorial disease, it is very important to examine sources of contamination from the environment, such as the quality of feed for cattle. A prerequisite for high-quality fodder is a clean and healthy phytomass. Epiphyte flora of plants consist of a number of microorganisms, including undesirable microorganisms such as clostridia and fungi. The continued development of microscopic fungi may lead to the formation of mycotoxins. Mycotoxins are secondary metabolites produced by fungi, especially *Aspergillus*, *Penicillium* and *Fusarium*. The production of mycotoxins is caused by interactions and reactions of fungi based on changing environmental conditions. Mycotoxin production is associated with stress that can be caused by extreme weather conditions or damage caused by insects or animals. Mycotoxins have a natural negative impact on livestock. They can cause alterations in hormonal functions, poor feed utilization, lower weight gain, and sometimes death. Moreover, some mycotoxins may pass into the milk, which would affect those that consume the contaminated product (Skladanka et al., 2011; Skladanka et al., 2012).

In this mini-review, we briefly detail the effects of LPS on cell populations within the bovine mammary gland, especially those effects on apoptosis and the expression of cell receptors of leukocytes such as macrophages, neutrophils and lymphocytes.

Effect of LPS on Macrophages

Monocytes migrate from the blood into the mammary gland during an inflammatory reaction. These inflammatory macrophages are called 'non-vacuolized' macrophages (Jensen and Eberhart, 1975; Sladek and Rysanek, 2008). Structural changes arise during the maturation to a fully immune-competent cells. These cells increase in size and show an abundant cytoplasm which contains many granules (Wardley et al., 1976). These cells are called 'vacuolized' macrophages (Jensen and Eberhart, 1975; Sladek and Rysanek, 2008). These macrophages represent the dominant population of macrophages in the resolution of mammary gland inflammatory responses (Wardley et al., 1976; Sladek and Rysanek, 2008). Non-vacuolized macrophages in the mammary gland are migrant blood monocytes with their associated morphological features (Sladek et al., 2002). Functional maturation of macrophages is represented as the transition from monocytes to the activated cells. Bacteria and their products play an important role in the activation of macrophages. Peptidoglycan and muramyl dipeptide of Gram-positive bacteria cause an increase the expression of CD14 on monocytes (Wang et al., 2001; Takada et al., 2002). A higher proportion and number of $CD14^+$ non-vacuolized macrophages was found in the first phase of infection as a result of macrophage activation following their interaction with bacteria. A higher number of $CD14^+$ non-vacuolized macrophages was found 24 hours following infection with *S. uberis*. Contrary to that, infection with *S. uberis* down-regulates CD14 surface expression on vacuolized macrophages during the first phase of infection. Inflammation of bovine mammary gland caused by *S. uberis* induces a local immune response characterised by an increase predominantly in the number of $CD14^+$ neutrophils and $CD14^+$ macrophages. A resolution of inflammation is accompanied by an increase in the proportion of $CD14^+$ neutrophils, $CD14^+$ vacuolized macrophages and apoptotic neutrophils. This suggests the possibility of involving CD14 in the recognition of apoptotic neutrophils by macrophages (Sladek and Rysanek, 2006).

Macrophages play an important role in the defence of the mammary gland (Hill et al., 1994; Grant and Finch, 1996). Mononuclear phagocytes (e.g., monocytes and macrophages) are activated by LPS as reported by Chen et al. in 1992 (Sladek et al., 2002). The LPS-mediated activation of these cells involves two key proteins: 1) LPS-binding protein and 2) CD14 receptors (Ulevitch and Tobias, 1995; Sladek et al., 2002). Activated cells express CD14 on their surface which binds LPS in an aggregate with LPS-binding protein. This binding complex induces the production of inflammatory cytokines (e.g., tumor necrosis factor alpha, TNFα and interleukin 6, IL-6) in macrophages (Dentener et al., 1993; Sladek et al., 2002). LPS also initiates the production of other inflammatory cytokines in bovine mammary gland leukocytes such as interleukin 10 (IL-10) and transforming growth factor beta 1 (TGFβ1) (Slama et al., 2011b; Slama et al., 2012). CD14 also binds to other cell components of Gram-positive bacteria and fungi, which shows that CD14 is a polyspecific receptor that has a multiple recognition potential (van Miert, 1991; Otterlei et al., 1993; Sladek et al, 2002). Stimulation of mammary glands with LPS causes an increase in the total count and the proportion of $CD14^+$ non-vacuolized macrophages. This increase is probably caused by activation of newly migrated macrophages from the blood which is induced by bacterial components (Paape et al., 1996; Sladek et al., 2002; Sladek et al., 2010). LPS increases the expression of CD14 on macrophages through an increase in CD14 gene expression (Pure and Cuff, 2001). Landmann et al. (1991) and Chen et al. (1992) described this up-regulating effect of LPS on macrophages. Sladek et al. (2002) observed the up-regulating effect of LPS on non-vacuolized macrophages in the bovine mammary gland during the initial stage of the inflammatory response.

CD44 is a major cell-surface type I transmembrane receptor for hyaluronan, and is expressed by most cells, including leukocytes. This receptor is involved in the binding and metabolism of hyaluronan, which plays an important role in maintaining tissue integrity (Vivers et al., 2002). Ligation of CD44 with short fragments of hyaluronan can induce the production of pro-inflammatory cytokines (McKee et al., 1996). Inflammation is associated with the increased expression of cell surface CD44 on hematopoietic cells (Cichy and Pure, 2003). Sladek and Rysanek (2009) demonstrated that CD44 receptor is expressed during the inflammatory response in the bovine mammary gland caused by LPS. The effect of LPS CD44 expression is evident during the initiation of the inflammatory response. Resolution of the inflammatory response is accompanied by a high expression of surface macrophage CD44. This is could be related to the involvement of surface CD44 as a competent phagocytic receptor on macrophages in the processes leading to the restitution of injured tissues (Sladek and Rysanek, 2009).

Macrophages are long-lived cells which are able to persist in non-inflamed tissues for weeks (Bellingan et al., 1996; Sladek and Rysanek, 2010). During this period, macrophages need to retain their viability if they are to fully function. Some macrophages re-emigrate into the supramammary lymphatic nodes while other macrophages undergo necrosis (Lee et al., 1980; Sladek and Rysanek, 1999). Bovine mammary gland macrophages can also undergo apoptosis (Sladek and Rysanek, 2010). These authors observed that in a fresh population of monocyte-like resident macrophages, approximately 10% are apoptotic and almost 8% are necrotic. The relatively low number of apoptotic monocyte-like resident macrophages suggests that the majority of these cells survive through phagocytising necrotic epithelia and other cells in the mammary glands ducts (Sladek and Rysanek, 1999; Sladek and Rysanek, 2010). As a consequence of their scavenger function, monocyte-like resident macrophages change into a vacuolized form approximately 5 days following migration (Wardley et al., 1976). Sladek and Rysanek (2010) found that approximately 33% of vacuolized resident macrophages were undergoing apoptosis. They also observed in a fresh population of monocyte-like inflammatory macrophages that 10% were apoptotic and less than 3% were necrotic 24 hours following phosphate buffered saline treatment. In contrast, following LPS treatment there were only 5% apoptotic cells. They suggest that macrophage apoptosis is halted by inflammatory stimuli that prolong their survival. On the other hand, the proportion of apoptotic monocyte-like inflammatory macrophages was more than doubled during the resolution of the inflammatory responses caused by LPS. Induction of apoptosis in inflammatory macrophages is a physiological mechanism that seems to be helpful for the reduction of inflammatory stress and prevent the transition to a chronic inflammatory response (Sladek and Rysanek, 2010). In addition, the induction of macrophage apoptosis and subsequent secondary necrosis was found to be caused by bacterial exotoxin with a histotoxic effect (do Vale et al., 2007). Sladek and Rysanek (2010) also observed that apoptosis of vacuolized inflammatory macrophages was higher than in monocyte-like inflammatory macrophages.

Effect of LPS on Neutrophils

Neutrophils are the first wave of immune defence by the mammary gland against bacteria. They are produced in the bone marrow, enter the peripheral blood and migrate into the lumen of the mammary gland where they phagocytise bacterial pathogens (Paape et al., 2003). The granules of neutrophils contain enzymes that kill pathogens (Bainton, 1975; Paape et al., 2003). When neutrophils undergo necrosis they release their dangerous content to the extracellular space and damage the mammary gland tissue (Capuco et al., 1986; Jaeschke et al., 2012). Therefore, apoptosis is a very important the process in these cells. Apoptotic neutrophils are removed from the mammary gland by macrophages. Neutrophil apoptosis is a protective mechanism that prevents mammary gland tissue damage (Sladek and Rysanek, 2001). Accumulation of persistent neutrophils in the mammary gland is typical for subclinical and chronic mastitis in dairy cows and may be caused by delayed apoptosis (Boutet et al., 2004).

LPS is known to affect the lifespan of mammary gland neutrophils (Langrova et al., 2008). There was a noticed inhibitory effect of LPS on spontaneous apoptosis of neutrophils *in vivo* (Watson et al., 1997) and *in vitro*

(Colotta et al., 1992; Watson et al., 1997). Contrary to that, bacteria *E. coli* induces apoptosis of neutrophils (Colamussi et al., 1999).

The immune system is capable of recognizing molecules of bacterial toxins by toll like receptors (TLR). TLR2 recognizes Gram-positive bacterial components and TLR4 recognizes LPS (Takeuchi et al., 2000). Both structural components have an affinity to CD14, a receptor that is expressed as a glycosylphosphatidylinositol-anchored cell surface molecule without a transmembrane domain. Engaging CD14 with LPS or apoptotic cells can result in either pro- or anti-inflammatory responses (Schutt, 1999). An inflammatory response of the mammary gland to LPS challenge is associated with an increased expression of CD14 receptors on neutrophils and macrophages (Paape et al., 1996; Sladek et al., 2002). Expression of CD14 depends on the stage of the inflammatory response of the mammary gland. Decreased expression of CD14 is observed in the initial phase of the inflammatory response (Paape et al., 1996), whereas increased expression of CD14 is found in the resolution of inflammation (Sladek et al., 2002). Moreover, the expression of CD14 on neutrophils highly correlates with apoptosis of neutrophils (Sladek and Rysanek, 2006). Association of LPS with LPS-binding protein and subsequent creation of a CD14-TLR4 complex can result in an induction of CD44 expression (Takeuchi et al., 1999). CD44 seems to be able to mediate neutrophil adhesion, but it does not affect migration within tissues (Khan et al., 2004). There is a coincidence in expression of CD14 and CD44 following induction of an inflammatory response with LPS. Expression of CD14 and CD44 is controlled by factors inducing an inflammatory response as well as by the mechanism of resolution (Langrova et al., 2008). CD14 is detected on apoptotic and on necrotic neutrophils, but also on non-apoptotic neutrophils. Almost 15% of non-apoptotic resident neutrophils are $CD14^+$, but this proportion decreases following *in vitro* cultivation. In non-apoptotic inflammatory neutrophils and blood neutrophils, there are less than 1% $CD14^+$ cells, but their proportion increases during *in vitro* cultivation. A decreased proportion of $CD14^+$ non-apoptotic resident neutrophils is related to an increase in the proportion of apoptotic cells during a 6-hour *in vitro* cultivation and their high CD14 positivity. Non-apoptotic $CD14^+$ resident neutrophils aged more quickly than inflammatory neutrophils, and thus became apoptotic. In resident neutrophils, more than 93% of apoptotic cells are positive for CD14. The expression of CD14 in inflammatory neutrophils is affected similarly as in blood neutrophils, in contrast to resident neutrophils (Sladek and Rysanek, 2011).

Effect of LPS on Lymphocytes

Lymphocytes are very important cells which recognize antigens through membrane receptors specific for invading bacteria (Sordillo et al., 1997). They are also necessary component of the mammary gland immune system (Hodgkinson et al., 2009; Denis et al., 2011). There are many bacterial pathogens that affect apoptosis of lymphocytes. Pathogens involved in lymphocyte apoptosis include Gram-positive or Gram-negative bacteria (Carrero and Unanue, 2006; Ullet and Anderson, 2006; Slama et al., 2009a; Slama and Kwak, 2011) and their components, especially such bacterial toxins as lipopolysaccharide (Slama et al., 2009b) which can modulate leukocyte apoptosis through the production of cytokines (Paape et al., 2003).

Milk from healthy cows contains mainly T cells (approximately 60% lymphocytes) and relatively few B cells (approximately 20% lymphocytes). The majority of T cells represent $CD8^+$ (e.g., cytotoxic T cells), while $CD4^+$ cells (e.g., T helper cells) are in a lower portion (Taylor et al., 1994; Soltys and Quinn, 1999). However, $CD4^+$ cells represent a higher proportion in infected mammary glands (Taylor et al., 1997).

LPS is known to modulate the cell death program of mammary gland lymphocytes. While Slama et al. (2009b) suggested that LPS delays apoptosis of bovine lymphocytes *in vitro*, Yokochi et al. (1996) had shown that administration of LPS may induce apoptosis of B memory lymphocytes and regulate B memory lymphocytes in an antigen-nonspecific manner. In another study, Slama et al. (2011a) reported that stimulation of the bovine mammary gland by LPS in an *in vivo* model resulted in a significant increase in the proportion of apoptotic lymphocytes. The portion of apoptotic lymphocytes peaked at 2 days following stimulation. Different results in the *in vivo* model could be caused by the complicated immunological characteristics of the mammary gland compared to the *in vitro* environment.

Negatively selected progenitor cells of T lymphocytes, called thymocytes, may undergo apoptosis as well (Cohen, 1991; Goldstein et al., 1991). Administration of LPS to mice induces DNA fragmentation within thymocytes in the cortex of the thymus (Zhang et al., 1994). The target cells in LPS-induced apoptosis of thymocytes are $CD4^+8^+$ immature thymocytes. LPS-induced thymocyte apoptosis is mediated by both glucocorticoids and TNF-α. These are direct effector molecules for LPS-induced thymocyte apoptosis and cooperate in the induction of thymocyte apoptosis (Kato et al., 1995). Nevertheless, simultaneous injection of anti-IFN-γ antibody with LPS prevents apoptosis of thymocytes. Pre-treatment of mice with IFN-γ increases LPS-induced apoptosis of thymocytes. Thymocyte apoptosis enhanced by IFN-γ occurs in the cortex of the thymus. Moreover, IFN-γ neither itself induces apoptosis of thymocytes nor does it increase the susceptibility of thymocytes to apoptosis. It has been suggested that IFN-γ may elevate LPS-induced apoptosis of thymocytes through increasing serum TNF-α and cortisol levels (Kato et al., 1997). This mechanism may prove useful in other animal species, including bovine. The study of lymphocyte progenitors will also be important to help understand the subsequent role of infectious events that result in changes in their cell cycle and cell death programs.

Acknowledgments

The study was prepared under the support from Grant no. QJ1310100 "Development and optimization methods for the determination of biogenic amines in response to increasing health security of silage," funded by the National Agency for Agricultural Research.

References

Bellingan GJ, Caldwell H, Howie SEM, Dransfield I, Haslett CH (1996). *In vivo* fate of the inflammatory macrophage during the resolution of inflammation. Inflammatory macrophages do not die locally, but emigrate to the draining lymph nodes. *J. Immunol.*, 157: 2577-2585.

Bainton DF (1975). Neutrophil granules. *Brit. J. Haematol.*, 29: 17-22.

Boutet P, Boulanger D, Gillet L, Vanderplasschen A, Closset R, Bureau F, Lekeux P (2004). Delayed neutrophil apoptosis in bovine subclinical mastitis. *J. Dairy Sci.,* 87: 4104-4114.

Capuco AV, Paape MJ, Nickerson SC (1986). *In vitro* study of polymorphonuclear leukocyte damage to mammary tissue of lactating cows. *Am. J. Vet. Res.*, 47: 663-669.

Carrero JA, Unanue ER (2006). Lymphocyte apoptosis as an immune subversion strategy of microbial pathogens. *Trends. Immunol.* 27: 497-503.

Chen TY, Lei MG, Suzuki T, Morrison DC (1992). Lipopolysaccharide receptors and signal transduction pathways in mononuclear phagocytes. *Curr. Top. Microbiol. Immunol.* 181: 169-188.

Cichy J, Pure E (2003). The liberation of CD44. *J. Cell Biol.*, 161: 839-843.

Cohen JJ (1991). Programmed cell death in the immune system. *Adv. Immunol.,* 50: 55-85.

Colamussi ML, White MR, Hartshosrn KL (1999). Influenza A virus accelerates neutrophil apoptosis and markedly potentiates apoptotic effect of bacteria. *Blood*, 93: 2395-2403.

Colotta F, Re F, Polentarutti N, Sozzani S, Mantovani A (1992). Modulation of granulocyte survival and programmed cell death by cytokines and bacterial products. *Blood*, 80: 2012-2020.

Concha C, Holmberg O, Astrom G (1986). Cells found in non-infected and staphylococcus-infected bovine mammary quarters and their ability to phagocytose fluorescent microspheres. *J. Vet. Med. B*, 33: 371-378.

Denis M, Lacy-Hulbert SJ, Buddle BM, Williamson JH, Wedlock DN (2011). *Streptococcus uberis*-specific T cells are present in mammary gland secretions of cows and can be activated to kill *S. uberis*. *Vet. Res. Commun.,* 35: 145-156.

Dentener MA, Bazil V, Von Asmuth EJ, Ceska M, Buurman WA (1993). Involvement of CD14 in lipopolysaccharide-induced tumor necrosis factor-alpha, IL-6 and IL-8 release by human monocytes and alveolar macrophages. *J. Immunol.*, 150: 2885-2891.

Do Vale A, Costa-Ramos C, Silva A, Silva DS, Gartner F, Dos Santos NM, Silva MT (2007). Systemic macrophage and neutrophil destruction by secondary necrosis induced by a bacterial exotoxin in a Gram-negative septicaemia. *Cell. Microbiol.* 9: 988-1003.

Goldstein P, Ojcius DM, Young JD (1991). Cell death mechanisms and the immune system. *Immunol. Rev.* 121: 29-65.

Grant RG, Finch JM (1996). Phagocytosis of *Streptococcus uberis* by bovine mammary gland macrophages. *Res. Vet. Sci.*, 62: 74-78.

Hill AW, Finch JM, Field TR, Leigh JA (1994). Immune modification of the pathogenesis of *Streptococcus uberis* mastitis in the dairy cow. *FEMS Immunol. Med. Microbiol.*, 8: 109-117.

Hodgkinson AJ, Carpenter EA, Smith CS, Molan PC, Prosser CG (2009). Effects on adhesion molecule expression and lymphocytes in the bovine mammary gland following intra-mammary immunisation. *Vet. Immunol. Immunopathol.*, 131: 110-116.

Jaeschke H, Williams CD, Ramachandran A, Bajt ML (2012). Acetaminophen hepatotoxicity and repair: the role of sterile inflammation and innate imunity. *Liver Int.,* 32: 8-20.

Jensen DL, Eberhart RJ (1975). Macrophages in bovine milk. *Am. J. Vet. Res.* 36: 619-624.

Kato Y, Morikawa A, Sugiyama T, Koide N, Jiang GZ, Takahashi K, Yokochi T (1995). Role of tumor necrosis factor-alpha and glucocorticoid on lipopolysaccharide (LPS)-induced apoptosis of thymocytes. *FEMS Immunol. Med. Microbiol.* 12: 195-204.

Kato Y, Morikawa A, Sugiyama T, Koide N, Jiang GZ, Lwin T, Yoshida T, Yokochi T (1997). Augmentation of lipopolysaccharide-induced thymocyte apoptosis by interferon-gamma. *Cell. Immunol.* 177: 103-108.

Khan AI, Kerfoot SM, Heit B, Liu L, Andonegui G, Ruffell B, Johnson P, Kubes P (2004). Role of CD44 and hyaluronan in neutrophil recruitment. *J. Immunol.*, 173: 7594-7601.

Kobayashi SD, Braughton KR, Whitney AR, Voyich JM, Schwan TG, Musser JM, DeLeo FR (2003). Bacterial pathogen modulate an apoptosis differentiation program in human neutrophils. *Proc. Nat. Acad. Sci. USA,* 100: 10948-10953.

Landmann R, Ludwig C, Obrist R, Obrecht JP (1991). Effect of cytokines and lipopolysaccharide on CD14 antigen expression in human monocytes and macrophages. *J. Cell. Biochem.* 47: 317-329.

Langrova T, Sladek Z, Rysanek D (2008). Expression of CD14 and CD44 on bovine polymorphonuclear leukocytes during resolution of mammary inflammatory response induced by muramyldipeptide and lipopolysaccharide. *Vet. Med. Czech*, 53: 1-11.

Lee CS, Wooding FB, Kemp P (1980). Identification, properties, and differential counts of cell populations using electron microscopy of dry cow's secretions, colostrum and milk from normal cows. *J. Dairy Res.*, 47: 39-50.

McKee CM, Penno MB, Cowman M, Burdick MD, Strieter RM, Bao C, Noble PW (1996). Hyaluronan (HA) fragments induce chemokine gene expression in alveolar macrophages. The role of HA size and CD44. *J. Clin. Invest*. 98: 2403-2413.

Miller RH, Paape MJ, Fulton LA (1991). Variation in milk somatic cells of heifers at first calving. *J. Dairy Sci.*, 74: 3782-3790.

Otterlei M, Sundan A, Skjak-Braek G, Ryan L, Smidsrod O, Espevik T (1993). Similar mechanisms of action of defined polysaccharides and lipopolysaccharides: characterization of binding and tumor necrosis factor-alpha induction. *Infect. Immunity*, 61: 1917-1925.

Paape MJ, Lilius EM, Wiitanen PA, Kontio MP, Miller RH (1996). Intramammary defence against infections induced by *Escherichia coli* in cows. *Am. J. Vet. Res.*, 57: 477-482.

Paape MJ, Bannerman DD, Zhao X, Lee JW (2003). The bovine neutrophil: Structure and function in blood and milk. *Vet. Res.*, 34: 597-627.

Pure E, Cuff CA (2001). A crucial role for CD44 in inflammation. *Trends Mol. Med.*, 7: 213-221.

Rysanek D, Babak V, Sladek Z, Toman M (2001). Variations among unbred heifers in the activities of polymorphonuclear leukocytes from the mammary gland and blood. *J. Vet. Med.* B, 48: 31-41.

Schutt C (1999). MOlecules in focus, CD14. *Int. J. Biochem. Cell Biol.* 31: 545-549.

Skladanka J, Nedelnik J, Adam V, Dolezal P, Moravcova H, Dohnal V (2011). Forage as a primary source of mycotoxins in animal diets. *J. Int. Environ. Res. Public Health,* 8: 37-50.

Skladanka J, Adam V, Zitka O, Krystofova O, Beklova M, Kizek R, Havlicek Z, Slama P, Nawrath A (2012). Investigation into the effect of molds in grasses on their content of low molecular mass thiols. *J. Int. Environ. Res. Public Health,* 9: 3789-3805.

Sladek Z, Rysanek D (1999). Ultrastructure of phagocytes from mammary glands of non-pregnant heifers. *Anat. Histol. Embryol.* 28: 291-297.

Sladek Z, Rysanek D (2000a). Morphology of apoptosis of polymorphonuclear leukocytes isolated from mammary glands of unbred heifers. *Vet. Med. Czech,* 45: 71-81.

Sladek Z, Rysanek D (2000b). Apoptosis of polymorphonuclear leukocytes of the juvenile bovine mammary glands during induced influx. *Vet. Res.* 31: 553-563.

Sladek Z, Rysanek D (2001). Neutrophil apoptosis during resolution of bovine mammary gland injury. *Res. Vet. Sci.*, 70: 41-46.

Sladek Z, Rysanek D, Faldyna M (2002). Activation of phagocytes during initiation and resolution of mammary gland injury induced by lipopolysaccharide in heifers. *Vet. Res.,* 33: 191-204.

Sladek Z, Rysanek D (2006). The role of CD14 during resolution of experimentally induced *Staphylococcus aureus* and *Streptococcus uberis* mastitis. *Comp. Immunol. Microbiol. Infect. Dis.*, 29: 243-262.

Sladek Z, Rysanek D (2008). Expression of macrophage CD14 receptor in the course of experimental inflammatory responses induced by lipopolysaccharide and muramyl dipeptide. *Vet. Med. Czech*, 53: 347-357.

Sladek Z, Rysanek D (2010). Apoptosis of resident and inflammatory macrophages before and during the inflammatory response of the virgin bovine mammary gland. *Acta Vet. Scand.*, 52: 12.

Sladek Z, Rysanek D (2011). Cell death and CD14 expression in resident and inflammatory polymorphonuclear leukocytes from virgin bovine mammary gland. *Res. Vet. Sci.* 90: 226-234.

Slama P, Sladek Z, Rysanek D, Langrova T (2009a). Effect of *Staphylococcus aureus* and *Streptococcus uberis* on apoptosis of bovine mammary gland lymphocytes. *Res. Vet. Sci.*, 87: 233-238.

Slama P, Sladek Z, Rysanek D (2009b). Lipopolysaccharide delays apoptosis of bovine lymphocytes. *FEBS J.*, 276: 223.

Slama P., Kwak JY (2011). Bacterial pathogens and apoptosis of lymphocytes. In Kwak JY, Han JY (eds) Cellular and genetic practices for translational medicine, *Research Signpost*, India, pp 89-105.

Slama P, Sladek Z, Rysanek D (2011a). Effect of different lymphocyte-bacteria ratios and bacterial toxins on apoptosis of bovine mammary gland lymphocytes. *Proc. ECOpole.*, 5: 109-113.

Slama P, Sladek Z, Slamova R, Pavlik A (2011b). Production of bovine IL-10 following stimulation with lipopolysaccharide and muramyl dipeptide. *FEBS J.*, 278: 304.

Slama P, Sladek Z, Slamova R, Pavlik A, Havlicek Z, Skladanka J, Watanabe A (2012). Production of bovine transforming growth factor beta 1 following stimulation with lipopolysaccharide. *FEBS J.*, 279: 459.

Soltys J, Quinn MT (1999). Selective recruitment of T-cell subsets to the udder during staphylococcal and streptococcal mastitis: analysis of lymphocyte subsets and adhesion molecule expression. *Infect. Immunity*, 67: 6293-6302.

Sordillo LM, Shafer-Weaver K, DeRosa D (1997). Immunobiology of the mammary gland. *J. Dairy Sci.*, 80: 1851-1865.

Takada H, Yokoyama S, Yang S (2002). Enhancement of endotoxin activity by muramyldipeptide. *J. Endotoxin Res.*, 8: 337-342.

Takeuchi O, Hoshino K, Kawai T, Sanjo H, Takada H, Ogawa T, Takada K, Akira S (1999). Differential roles of TLR2 and TLR4 in recognition of Gram-negative and Gram-positive bacterial cell wall components. *Immunity*, 11: 443-451.

Takeuchi O, Hoshino K, Akira S (2000). Cutting edge: TLR2-deficient and MyD88-deficient mice are highly susceptible to *Staphylococcus aureus* infection. *J. Immunol.*, 165: 5392-5396.

Taylor BC, Dellinger JD, Cullor JS, Stott JL (1994). Bovine milk lymphocytes display the phenotype of memory T cells and are predominantly $CD8^+$. *Cell. Immunol.* 156: 245-253.

Taylor BC, Keefe RG, Dellinger JD, Nakamura Y, Cullor JS, Sott JL (1997). T cell populations and cytokine expression in milk derived from normal and bacteria-infected bovine mammary glands. *Cell. Immunol.* 182: 68-76.

Ulevitch RJ, Tobias PS (1995). Receptor-dependent mechanisms of cell stimulation by bacterial endotoxin. *Res. Vet. Sci.*, 70: 41-46.

Ullet GC, Anderson EE (2006). Regulation of apoptosis by gram-positive bacteria: Mechanistic diversity and consequences for immunity. *Curr. Immunol. Rev.*, 2: 119-141.

Van Miert ASJ (1991). Acute phase response and non-cellular defence mechanisms. *Flem. Vet. J.,* 62: 69-91.

Vivers S, Dransfield I, Hart SP (2002). Role of macrophage CD44 in the disposal of inflammatory cells corpses. *Clin. Sci. London*, 103: 441-449.

Vogt L, Dippold L (2005). *Escherichia coli* O157:H7 outbreak associated with consumption of ground beef, June-July 2002. *Pub. Health Rep.,* 120: 174-178.

Wang JE, Jorgensen PF, Ellingsen EA, Almiof M, Thiemermann C, Foster SJ, Aasen AO, Solberg R (2001). Peptidoglycan primes for LPS-induced release of proinflammatory cytokines in whole human blood. *Shock*, 16: 178-182.

Wardley RC, Rouse BT, Babiuk LA (1976). The mammary gland of the ox: a convenient source for the repeated collection of neutrophils and macrophages. *J. Reticuloendothel. Soc.*, 19: 29-36.

Watson RWG, Redmont HP, Wang JH, Condron C, Bouchier-Hayes D (1996). Neutrophil undergo apoptosis following ingestion of *Escherichia coli*. *J. Immunol.*, 156: 3986-3992.

Weiss SJ (1989). Tissue destruction by neutrophils. *New Engl. J. Med.*, 320: 365-376.

Yokochi T, Kato Y, Sugiyama T, Koide N, Morikawa A, Jiang Z, Kawai M, Yoshida T, Fukada M, Takahashi K (1996). Lipopolysaccharide induces apoptotic cell death of B memory cells and regulates B cell memory in antigen-nonspecific manner. *FEMS Immunol. Med. Microb.*, 15: 1-8.

Zhang XM, Morikawa A, Takahashi K, Jiang GZ, Kato Y, Sugiyama T, Kakai M, Fukada M, Yokochi T (1994). Localization of apoptosis (programmed cell death) in mice by administration of lipopolysaccharide. *Microb. Immunol*. 38: 669-671.

Editor Contact Information

Dr. Edmund B. Rucker III,
Department of Biology
University of Kentucky
Lexington, KY 40506
Tel: 859-257-2175 Fax: 859-257-1807
Edmund.rucker@uky.edu

Index

A

α-lactalbumin (α-LA), 194
abuse, 158
accessibility, 22, 64, 72, 81, 83
accounting, 71
acetylation, 73, 74, 106
acid, viii, 46, 56, 59, 61, 87, 90, 91, 92, 110, 143, 151, 154, 168, 171, 203, 213
acidic, 2, 18, 80, 205
action potential, 83
AD, 31, 108
adaptability, 149
adaptation, 158
adenoma, 114
adenomatous polyposis coli, 83
adhesion, 66, 67, 79, 81, 95, 108, 143, 241, 244, 247
adhesions, 128
adipocyte, 114, 167
adipose, 1, 48, 121, 142, 146
adipose tissue, 121, 142, 146
adiposity, 69, 91
adrenal gland, 14
adult stem cells, 77, 100
adulthood, 13, 14, 22, 51, 89
adults, 87
adverse effects, 110, 138
aetiology, viii, 120
age, viii, 6, 17, 22, 46, 48, 53, 54, 57, 69, 74, 77, 88, 101, 109, 118, 119, 126, 137, 202
aggression, 123
aggressiveness, 114, 119
agonist, 155, 161
airways, 145
albumin, 194, 207
alertness, 159
algae, 195
allele, 13, 19, 86, 108, 181, 218
allergens, 145
alters, 42, 48, 54, 59, 60, 111, 112
alveolar macrophage, 166, 169, 190, 244, 245
alveoli, 7, 8, 17, 20, 143
amines, 89, 243
amino, 14, 50, 144, 155, 159, 170, 211, 215, 217, 232
amino acid, 144, 155, 159, 170, 211, 215, 217, 232
amino acids, 159, 211, 217, 232
Amphiregulin, 76, 103
anabolism, 149
anatomy, viii, 137, 138
androgen, 188
anemia, 19
angiogenesis, 69, 105, 127, 133, 134, 146
animal welfare, 147
antagonism, 194
antibiotic, 158, 159, 212

antibody, 38, 40, 177, 181, 242
antigen, 107, 133, 135, 145, 150, 194, 205, 215, 231, 232, 242, 245, 248
antigen-presenting cell, 145
antigen XE "antigen" -presenting cell XE "antigen-presenting cell" s, 145
anti-inflammatory drugs, 70, 98
antioxidant, 89, 210
APC, 108, 145, 146
apex, 172
apoptosis, vii, 2, 6, 8, 20, 21, 22, 24, 30, 31, 32, 53, 69, 83, 120, 134, 143, 165, 169, 205, 235, 236, 237, 239, 240, 241, 242, 243, 244, 245, 246, 247, 248
Apoptosis, 20, 23, 24, 237, 246, 247
arrests, 10
artery, 115
Asian countries, 91
Aspergillus, 237
aspiration, 122
assessment, 57, 110, 169, 186
astrocytes, 42
atmosphere, 35
ATP, 100
Atrazine, 50, 57
auditory nerve, 42
automobiles, 48
Autophagy, 8, 182, 184, 190, 191, 192
avoidance, 89
axons, 188

B

BAC, 176
Bacillus subtilis, 212
bacteria, ix, 144, 145, 146, 148, 149, 150, 151, 152, 153, 154, 156, 158, 159, 160, 162, 164, 174, 178, 181, 182, 184, 192, 194, 195, 196, 197, 201, 203, 204, 205, 208, 212, 213, 214, 216, 217, 226, 235, 236, 238, 240, 241, 242, 244, 247, 248
bacterial artificial chromosome, 176, 187
bacterial infection, 145, 162, 173, 202, 212, 225
bacterial pathogens, 181, 183, 189, 240, 242
bacteriostatic, 212, 214
bacterium, 151, 236
barriers, 82
basal lamina, 143
base, 73, 173, 176
base pair, 73
basement membrane, 7, 66, 67, 96, 106
B-cells, 203
Bcl-2, 21, 31, 32, 133
Bcl-x, 21, 31, 32
BD, 36, 58, 61
bedding, 195
beef, 90, 248
behaviors, 64
Belgium, 141, 167
beneficial effect, 119, 195, 213
benign, 80, 96, 105, 107, 114, 119, 120, 122, 123, 128, 134, 138
benign tumors, 114
bioavailability, 53
biochemistry, 110, 112
biological activity, 215, 217
biological behavior, 114, 126, 127, 131
biomarkers, 104, 110, 112, 208
biomolecules, 149
biopsy, 122
biosciences, 112
biotic, 162
birth weight, 86
bisphenol, viii, 46, 56, 57, 58, 59
blood, viii, ix, 53, 86, 115, 146, 161, 175, 199, 201, 203, 205, 206, 207, 209, 210, 212, 215, 217, 228, 236, 237, 239, 241, 246, 248
blood monocytes, 238
blood plasma, 210
blood supply, viii, 115
bloodstream, 143
body fluid, 213, 214, 215
body size, 117
body weight, 37, 49
BoLA allele, 218
bonds, 213
bone, 2, 6, 24, 44, 122, 123, 136, 217, 240
bone growth, 24

bone marrow, 240
bowel, 184
brain, 41, 42, 43, 44, 89, 109, 176
branching, 1, 3, 4, 6, 7, 8, 9, 10, 14, 15, 16, 27, 48, 49, 51, 52, 54, 66, 69, 76, 94, 95, 142, 164
Brazil, 198
breast carcinoma, 99, 105, 123, 162
breast milk, 47, 48, 51, 165, 166, 201
breastfeeding, 148, 150
breeding, 174, 195, 211, 213
Brno, 235
browser, 187
brucellosis, 201
buffalo, 198, 213, 220, 222, 228, 229, 231
Buffalo, 231, 232
building blocks, 73, 92
Butcher, 106

C

C/EBP, vii, 16, 17, 26, 28, 151, 168
calcium, 83, 92, 143, 199
cancer cells, 93
cancer progression, 96, 119
Canine, v, viii, 113, 114, 117, 121, 123, 131, 132, 135, 136, 138
Canine mammary tumours, 114, 136
capillary, 143
carbohydrates, 89, 149
carbon, 49, 72, 85, 89, 90
carcinogen, 46, 55, 111, 112
carcinogenesis, 46, 56, 58, 114, 119, 120, 123
carcinogenicity, 54
carcinoma, 54, 59, 76, 103, 105, 116, 122, 128, 129, 131, 132, 135, 136, 137, 172
cardiovascular disease, 86
carotene, 89, 93
carotenoids, 112
Carotenoids, 93
cartilage, 122, 123, 217
cascades, 8
casein, 19, 52, 69, 80, 83, 142, 199, 203, 224
catabolism, 154
cathepsin G, 205
cattle, 154, 160, 169, 173, 176, 177, 178, 183, 185, 186, 187, 193, 198, 217, 218, 219, 220, 224, 228, 229, 237
CCND2, 91
CD14, 24, 159, 166, 170, 238, 241, 244, 245, 246, 247
CD4, 126, 127, 145, 165, 166, 242
CD44, 75, 77, 78, 239, 241, 244, 245, 246, 248
CD8, 126, 127, 145, 165, 242, 248
CD8+, 127, 145, 165, 242, 248
cDNA, 165
cell biology, 95, 96, 97, 105, 108, 109
cell culture, 71, 75, 80, 82, 92, 93, 94, 168
cell cycle, 10, 47, 73, 82, 83, 108, 110, 120, 243
cell death, 6, 8, 17, 18, 20, 21, 30, 31, 32, 69, 142, 143, 146, 167, 169, 192, 235, 236, 242, 243, 244, 248, 249
cell differentiation, 18, 22, 28, 40, 57, 70, 97, 105, 138
cell division, 72, 88, 107
cell fate, 10, 17, 21, 26, 28, 42, 64, 75, 77, 98, 103
cell line, 17, 21, 22, 35, 68, 77, 83, 96, 97, 106, 109, 110, 123, 129, 138, 150
cell lines, 110, 123, 129
cell membranes, 194, 201, 207, 208
cell signaling, 18, 22
cell surface, 75, 239, 241
cellular immunity, 214
Central Europe, 230
cervical cancer, 90
challenges, 94, 96, 181, 191
changing environment, 237
cheese, 198, 205
chemical, viii, 46, 59, 72, 118, 193, 195, 196, 198, 204, 215, 228, 229, 232, 236
chemical characteristics, 228
chemical properties, 196
chemicals, viii, 45, 46, 48, 55
chemokine receptor, 155
chemokines, 146, 203

chemotaxis, 178, 188
chemotherapeutic agent, 128
chemotherapy, 24, 128, 130, 132, 133, 134
chicken, 26
childhood, 91
children, 58, 86
China, 33, 35, 38
chitosan, 164
chloral, 37
chlorine, 199
chondroitin sulfate, 188
chromosome, 80, 176, 179, 180, 218
chronic diseases, 87
CK18, 34, 38, 39, 40, 41, 42
classes, 92, 93, 189, 196, 215
classification, 99, 114, 122, 123, 132, 134, 139
cleft palate, 25
clinical application, 117, 120
clinical examination, 114, 122
clinical oncology, 103
clinical presentation, 125, 148
clinical symptoms, 148
clinical trials, 129, 130, 158
cloning, 26
closure, 59
clustering, 24
clusters, 52, 79, 80, 83
CNS, 148, 154, 162, 172
CO2, 35
coding, 83, 91, 100, 173
collaboration, 94
collagen, 68, 79, 80, 82, 105, 164, 172
colonization, 156
color, iv, 91, 111, 196
colostrum, 142, 203, 213, 214, 215, 217, 220, 221, 222, 228, 231, 232, 245
commercial, 48, 56, 58, 158, 198, 208, 230, 232
communication, 67, 81, 125, 148, 170, 216, 230
community, 126
compaction, 70
comparative analysis, 134
competition, 177, 184
competitors, 181
compilation, vii
complement, 149, 167, 214, 215
complex interactions, 115
complexity, 18, 129
composition, 79, 98, 154, 169, 193, 196, 198, 204, 220, 222, 223, 224, 225, 228, 229, 230
compounds, 48, 50, 57, 60, 93, 118, 147, 158, 160, 194, 211, 214, 232
conception, 109
Concise, 99
concordance, 15
condensation, 20
conductivity, 194, 210, 227
conference, 172
Congress, iv, 227
connective tissue, 1, 7, 66, 114, 143
consensus, 177
constituents, 142, 144, 164, 200
consumption, 89, 92, 118, 201, 204, 248
contaminant, 51
contamination, 201, 237
contingency, 189
control measures, 160
controlled studies, 128
controversial, 5
convention, 85, 115
cooperation, 106, 134
coordination, 81
corpus luteum, 10, 19
correlation, 89, 105, 133, 134, 136, 175, 202, 206, 207, 208, 209, 211, 213, 224
correlation coefficient, 202, 206, 207, 208, 209, 211, 213
cortex, 242
cortisol, 243
cost, 128, 152, 174, 175, 197, 199, 220, 221
Cox-2, 126, 129, 133, 136
CpG islands, 72
Cre/LoxP, 13, 22, 25
critical period, 55, 59
crops, 50
CSA, 37
CSF, 216

cues, 34, 66, 79, 80, 191
cultivation, 241
culture, 35, 43, 80, 81, 88, 92, 93, 94, 107, 111, 148, 149, 158
culture conditions, 80, 81
culture media, 149
cycles, 68, 76, 115
Cyclin D1, 9, 108
cyclooxygenase, 130, 131, 134
cyclophosphamide, 128
cytokines, ix, 145, 151, 154, 156, 161, 166, 216, 203, 216, 219, 238, 239, 242, 244, 245, 248
cytology, 122
cytometry, 75
cytoplasm, 182, 237
cytosine, 72, 100, 174, 180
cytoskeleton, 95
Czech Republic, 235

D

dairy industry, 147, 160, 173, 174, 179, 198, 199
damages, iv
danger, 147, 161
data analysis, 109
database, 89
DDT, viii, 46, 47, 55, 57, 58
DEA, 50
defects, 13, 14, 16, 17, 19, 20, 24, 25, 27, 29, 90
defence, 144, 145, 149, 151, 154, 167, 170, 171, 236, 238, 240, 246, 248
defense mechanisms, 216
deficiency, 15, 18, 24, 29, 86, 90, 191
degradation, 56, 184, 188, 208
Denmark, 130, 197
deposition, 79, 80
depth, 6, 149
deregulation, 77
derivatives, 106
dermis, 5
destruction, 215, 237, 244, 248
detectable, 9, 48
detection, 5, 13, 38, 39, 134, 135, 147, 161, 210, 219, 228
detergents, 213
developmental change, 45
developmental process, vii
deviation, 116
diabetes, 86, 89
diet, 64, 72, 74, 84, 85, 88, 89, 90, 91, 92, 93, 111, 118, 135, 138, 143, 154
dietary fat, 91, 92, 93, 111
dietary intake, 85
dietary supplementation, 90
diffusion, 82
digestion, 35, 189, 203
dimerization, 13, 18
dioxin, 52, 60
diploid, 86, 106
disclosure, 216
disease progression, 160
diseases, 33, 35, 42, 96, 110, 113, 144, 148, 152, 160, 161, 183, 194, 198, 201, 229
disequilibrium, 187
disorder, 184
distilled water, 38
distribution, 79, 81, 102, 106, 107, 130, 167, 199
divergence, 118
diversity, 72, 91, 95, 142, 203, 248
DNA, 8, 22, 64, 67, 70, 71, 72, 73, 77, 78, 79, 81, 85, 86, 87, 88, 89, 90, 91, 92, 96, 99, 100, 101, 103, 107, 108, 109, 110, 111, 120, 175, 177, 179, 181, 217, 242
DNA damage, 81, 107
DNA methylation, 64, 67, 70, 71, 72, 73, 77, 85, 86, 87, 88, 89, 91, 96, 99, 100, 101, 103, 108, 109, 110
DNA methyltransferase, 72, 73, 90
DNA repair, 71, 73, 90
DNase, 80
docetaxel, 137
dogs, vii, 113, 115, 116, 117, 118, 119, 122, 126, 127, 128, 129, 130, 131, 132, 133, 134, 136, 137, 138, 139
donors, 85
dopaminergic, 42

dosing, 52, 158
drainage, viii, 115, 116, 135, 138
drinking water, 53, 54
Drosophila, 29, 82, 83, 189, 190
drugs, 120, 129, 130
dynamism, 150

E

ECM, 2, 7, 8, 66, 69, 78, 79, 80, 81, 82, 84, 93, 143, 145, 146, 152
ECM, extracellular matrix, 2
economic losses, viii, 198, 219
ectoderm, 5, 114
eczema, 166
edema, 122
EGF, 120, 136, 192, 217
EGFR, 76, 120, 126, 127, 132
egg, 2
Egypt, 228
electric current, 210
electrical conductivity, ix, 201, 210, 222, 227, 230
electrodes, 210
electron, 245
electron microscopy, 245
ELISA, 151
elongation, 4, 7, 13, 14, 68
emboli, 122
embryogenesis, 9, 14, 19, 20, 84, 85, 86, 87, 89, 217
embryonic stem cells, 43, 44, 86, 87, 89, 104
employment, 161
encoding, 83, 164, 180
endocrine, 10, 22, 25, 43, 46, 47, 50, 51, 53, 56, 60, 119, 120, 229
endocrinology, 102
endoderm, 20
endothelial cells, 66, 146
energy, 91, 149, 154, 169, 203
engineering, 22, 158
England, 59, 198
environment (s), vii, 41, 47, 49, 50, 53, 64, 78, 79, 85, 86, 93, 115, 117, 149, 154, 160, 162, 166, 195, 212, 237
environmental effects, 89
environmental factors, 64, 66, 84, 85, 195, 230
environmental impact, 74, 93
Environmental Protection Agency, 45, 47, 55, 56, 57, 60
enzyme (s), 73, 83, 87, 90, 95, 97, 144, 149, 159, 194, 201, 205, 208, 213, 214, 222, 240
epidemiologic, 47, 48, 50, 51, 69, 92
epidemiologic studies, 47, 48, 51
epidemiology, 91, 103, 104, 110, 112, 131, 167
epidermis, 42, 112
epigenetic alterations, 77, 87, 88, 162
epigenetic modification, 70, 72, 74, 84, 88, 90, 108
epigenetic silencing, 71, 77
epigenetics, viii, 64, 72, 74, 78, 95, 99, 101, 104, 111
epithelia, 1, 4, 5, 7, 8, 9, 10, 13, 14, 17, 21, 41, 143, 144, 150, 151, 156, 163, 239
epithelial cells, vii, 6, 7, 8, 9, 13, 15, 16, 27, 28, 29, 30, 32, 34, 41, 67, 69, 75, 76, 77, 79, 80, 81, 82, 88, 91, 92, 95, 106, 107, 111, 121, 143, 146, 147, 150, 151, 164, 167, 168, 169, 170, 171, 174, 180, 182, 184, 192, 196, 201, 203, 205, 208, 210, 216, 217, 225
epithelial homeostasis, 100
epithelium, 4, 7, 19, 30, 31, 32, 34, 41, 49, 65, 66, 68, 69, 74, 76, 79, 80, 81, 82, 84, 87, 88, 92, 94, 95, 96, 97, 104, 106, 107, 120, 122, 136, 150, 151, 164, 207
epoxy resins, 53
ER, estrogen receptor, 2
ERE, estrogen responsive element, 2
erythroid cells, 21
ES cells, vii, 33, 34, 36, 39, 41
Escherichia coli, 34, 41, 149, 155, 167, 168, 169, 170, 171, 178, 195, 212, 213, 215, 216, 235, 236, 246, 248

estrogen, vii, 2, 6, 7, 13, 25, 26, 47, 58, 71, 76, 102, 103, 104, 111, 119, 120, 128, 134
etiology, 72, 114, 138, 148, 167, 210
euchromatin, 81, 83
eukaryote, 104
Europe, 204
European market, 204
European Parliament, 204
European Union (EU), 204
evidence, 2, 16, 64, 69, 72, 75, 77, 80, 82, 84, 86, 91, 98, 102, 117, 119, 125, 138, 183
evolution, 23, 29, 99, 163
excision, 27, 128
excretion, 142, 143
exons, 176, 218
exposure, viii, 46, 47, 48, 49, 50, 52, 53, 54, 55, 56, 57, 58, 59, 60, 61, 74, 76, 87, 88, 91, 92, 108, 151, 156, 169, 183, 191
extracellular matrix, viii, 2, 7, 66, 95, 96, 97, 104, 164
exudate, 159
EZH2, 73, 87, 101, 109

F

families, 173, 175, 176, 179, 180, 181, 183
family members, 16, 21, 178
famine, 86, 87, 109
farm size, 202
farmers, 198, 201
farms, 198, 208, 228
fat, 1, 3, 4, 6, 7, 9, 13, 17, 37, 40, 43, 51, 89, 91, 92, 97, 111, 118, 142, 190, 192, 199, 203
fat intake, 89, 91
Fata, 27, 95
fatty acids, 91, 92, 144, 164
female rat, 57, 58, 59
fermentation, 155
ferric ion, 210
fertilization, 85, 86
fetal development, 66, 68
fever, 196, 201
Fgf10, 5
fiber, 118
fibers, 153, 164
fibroadenoma, 114
fibroblast growth factor (FGF), 2, 5, 44
fibroblasts, 35, 66, 69, 76, 79, 83, 105, 187
Fibroblasts, 35
fibrosis, 79
first generation, 170
flame retardants, 48
flavor, 196
flexibility, 78, 108
flora, 154, 237
fluid, 143, 148, 210
fluorescence, 33, 34, 36, 38, 39
folate, 85, 90, 110
Folate, 90
folic acid, 87, 89, 90, 109, 110
food, 37, 50, 86, 88, 90, 91, 118, 147, 167, 236
Food and Drug Administration, 204
food industry, 167
food poisoning, 236
forebrain, viii, 173, 176, 187, 188
formation, vii, 4, 6, 18, 19, 23, 24, 47, 60, 64, 66, 69, 81, 82, 85, 88, 92, 117, 123, 142, 158, 188, 217, 237
fragments, 154, 239, 245
France, 95, 163, 230
free radicals, 212
fungi, 195, 212, 237, 238
Fusarium, 237
fusion, 158

G

gamete, 85
gametogenesis, 85, 87, 89
ganglion, 43
GAS, γ- interferon activation sites, 2
gastric mucosa, 216, 232
gastrointestinal tract, 214, 217
GATA3, 17, 69
gel, 181, 184

gene expression, 5, 6, 19, 24, 28, 30, 34, 41, 60, 67, 69, 71, 73, 77, 79, 81, 82, 84, 85, 96, 98, 99, 104, 105, 106, 109, 151, 168, 239, 245
gene promoter, 18, 73, 83
gene regulation, 100, 108, 191
gene silencing, 88, 111
gene transfer, 36
genes, vii, viii, 9, 14, 15, 17, 19, 22, 25, 64, 70, 71, 72, 73, 74, 77, 78, 80, 81, 83, 84, 86, 87, 88, 90, 91, 93, 94, 104, 107, 110, 120, 133, 151, 159, 161, 171, 173, 174, 175, 176, 177, 178, 179, 180, 182, 183, 184, 186, 190, 191, 194, 195, 218
genetic alteration, 114
genetic background, 150
genetic diversity, 152
genetic factors, 221
genetic marker, ix, 218
genetic mutations, 64, 88, 120
genetic traits, 149
genetics, 22, 26, 101, 103, 104, 109, 174
genome, viii, 81, 85, 86, 104, 117, 133, 173, 174, 175, 176, 180, 185, 187
genomic instability, 90
genomics, 64, 99, 101
genotype, 154, 155, 175, 179, 184, 218
genotyping, 175, 185, 227
germ cells, 85
germ line, 139
Germany, 35, 52
gestation, 4, 6, 17, 18, 22, 49, 79, 85
glucocorticoid, 89, 242, 245
glucocorticoid receptor, 89
glucose, 217
glutamine, 35, 231
glutathione, 93
GLV-1h68, 129
glycine, 173, 176, 177, 183
glycoproteins, 7
goat milk, 204, 208, 223, 229
grades, 90
grading, 132, 133
granules, 205, 212, 237, 240, 243
grasses, 246
groundwater, 56
growth, viii, 3, 6, 10, 13, 19, 22, 30, 34, 41, 43, 46, 48, 55, 59, 61, 66, 68, 69, 71, 76, 78, 79, 80, 82, 87, 106, 109, 114, 115, 119, 121, 126, 138, 142, 148, 149, 158, 159, 160, 163, 173, 180, 181, 191, 205, 207, 212, 216, 217, 220, 229
growth arrest, 80, 106
growth factor, viii, 22, 30, 61, 68, 76, 79, 109, 115, 120, 163, 173, 180, 181, 191, 217
growth hormone, 6, 20, 43, 46, 119, 138
growth rate, 30, 126
guidance, 178, 188
guidelines, 114, 222

H

hair, 10, 31, 142
hair follicle, 142
half-life, 47, 48, 49, 51, 52, 53, 58
haploid, 86
haptoglobin, 216
HDAC, 73
HE, 102, 105
health, vii, ix, 89, 108, 110, 111, 158, 171, 174, 185, 186, 194, 195, 201, 202, 203, 205, 210, 211, 212, 213, 219, 225, 227, 228, 229, 230, 232, 243
health status, 194, 195, 201, 202, 203, 205, 210, 211, 212, 229
heat shock protein, 164
height, 8
Helicobacter pylori, 215
hepatocytes, 44, 190
hepatotoxicity, 245
HER2/neu, 120
herbicide, 50, 58
heritability, 149, 194
heterochromatin, 73, 79, 80, 81, 86
heterogeneity, 101, 112, 125
high fat, 118
hippocampus, 89
histochemistry, 101
histogenesis, 123, 136

histology, 114, 122, 138
histone, 22, 64, 67, 70, 72, 73, 74, 78, 81, 83, 86, 87, 88, 89, 90, 92, 100, 101, 104, 106, 108, 110
histone deacetylase, 73
Histone modification, 70, 73, 101
history, 2, 69, 97
HIV, 165
HIV-1, 165
HM, 101, 105
HMT3522-S1 cells, 88
homeostasis, 64, 66, 74, 78, 82, 83, 85, 86, 92, 105, 146
hormonal control, 75, 77
hormones, 1, 6, 7, 9, 10, 12, 13, 14, 15, 16, 18, 19, 22, 44, 50, 61, 66, 68, 71, 76, 96, 98, 102, 103, 104, 114, 115, 119, 131, 136
horses, 197
host, 13, 37, 39, 42, 144, 148, 149, 150, 151, 153, 154, 155, 156, 158, 159, 161, 162, 164, 170, 173, 182, 183, 192, 195, 196, 203
housing, 13
human, 47, 53, 75, 80, 81, 83, 84, 86, 88, 92, 94, 95, 96, 97, 102, 103, 104, 105, 106, 107, 109, 110, 111, 112, 114, 117, 120, 123, 128, 129, 132, 133, 134, 135, 136, 137, 138, 148, 150, 152, 160, 176, 183, 187, 191, 195, 201, 204, 213, 215, 227, 244, 245, 248
human exposure, 53
human genome, 117, 187
human health, 195, 213
human milk, 227
human neutrophils, 245
humoral immunity, 215
Hunter, 23, 189
hydrogen, 214
hydrogen peroxide, 214
hydrolysis, 213
hypermethylation, 71, 90, 91, 111
hyperplasia, 21, 32, 54
hypertrophy, 7
hypothesis, 88, 119, 149, 155, 181, 182, 207

I

ideal, 5
identification, 15, 80, 93, 102, 126
identity, 144
IFN, 242
IGF I, 217
IL-1, 17, 28, 156, 161, 171, 178, 216, 238, 247
IL-13, 17, 28
IL-17, 162, 171
IL-8, 151, 152, 156, 159, 168, 169, 178, 183, 185, 191, 216, 244
ILAR, 25
illumination, 153
image, 107
image analysis, 107
images, 38, 172
imaging modalities, 122
immune function, 175, 185
immune reaction, 159, 203
immune response, 146, 148, 156, 168, 173, 178, 179, 185, 187, 195, 213, 218, 237, 238
immune system, 117, 145, 147, 152, 154, 159, 160, 162, 166, 195, 203, 216, 217, 223, 241, 242, 244
immunity, 22, 145, 149, 160, 162, 165, 166, 178, 184, 196, 215, 216, 221, 229, 248
immunization, 166, 171
immunobiology, 144
immunoglobulins, ix, 144, 213, 215, 220, 222, 223, 224, 225, 226, 232
immunohistochemistry, 76, 87, 123, 135
immunolocalization, 164
immunoprecipitation, 78, 177
immunosuppression, 145
implants, 37, 38, 41, 43
in transition, 129
in utero, 45, 49, 52, 53, 54, 59, 84, 86, 87
in vitro, viii, 9, 47, 52, 75, 88, 129, 149, 152, 154, 156, 158, 168, 171, 177, 191, 241, 242
in vitro environment, 242

in vivo, viii, 9, 16, 31, 32, 34, 41, 42, 52, 80, 94, 129, 148, 149, 150, 152, 153, 154, 156, 158, 160, 171, 177, 181, 184, 240, 242
incidence, viii, 51, 52, 54, 55, 57, 58, 59, 64, 71, 74, 89, 91, 92, 93, 95, 117, 118, 119, 131, 134, 135, 137, 139, 158, 179, 181, 184, 194, 196, 197, 199, 201, 218, 227, 228, 229, 231
independence, 119
India, 198, 247
individuals, 85, 87, 91, 218
inducer, 174, 183
induction, 16, 27, 84, 97, 153, 154, 178, 182, 192, 240, 241, 242, 246
industry, viii
ineffectiveness, 128
INF, 216
infancy, 166
infants, 2, 145
infection, viii, 144, 146, 148, 151, 153, 156, 158, 162, 164, 170, 171, 174, 176, 177, 178, 181, 182, 183, 185, 190, 194, 195, 196, 199, 203, 204, 205, 210, 212, 214, 216, 217, 222, 236, 238, 248
infectious agents, 107, 145
infertility, 13, 16, 19
inflammasome, 161
inflammation, 70, 146, 148, 150, 153, 154, 156, 157, 160, 161, 162, 171, 173, 184, 193, 195, 196, 197, 198, 201, 202, 203, 204, 208, 209, 211, 212, 215, 216, 228, 229, 236, 238, 241, 243, 245, 246
inflammatory cells, 66, 152, 158, 248
inflammatory disease, viii, 161
inflammatory mediators, 147, 150, 203, 236
inflammatory responses, 238, 240, 241, 247
infrastructure, 149
ingest, 205
ingestion, 203, 248
ingredients, 91, 214
inguinal, 5, 7, 36, 37, 38, 39, 40, 114, 115, 116, 152, 159
inhibition, 61, 169, 192
inhibitor, 5, 17, 120, 128, 129, 134, 160, 182, 183, 214
initiation, 4, 7, 17, 18, 23, 64, 69, 72, 74, 75, 82, 86, 119, 120, 162, 194, 211, 216, 222, 239, 246
injury (ies), iv, 33, 34, 195, 212, 217, 246
innate immunity, viii, 147, 150, 168, 174, 182, 183, 184, 185, 192, 212
inoculation, 157, 160
inoculum, 153
inositol, 83
insecticide, 47
insects, 237
insertion, 173, 176, 183
insulin, viii, 35, 120, 173, 180, 181, 189, 190, 191, 217
insulin signaling, 190
integration, viii, 34, 166
integrins, 66, 67, 69, 95, 164
integrity, 71, 81, 83, 239
interference, 83, 178
interferon, 2, 18, 165, 178, 245
interleukin-17, 165
interleukin-8, 169, 173, 190
internalization, 144, 164
intestine, 43
introns, 177
involution, vii, 1, 3, 4, 5, 6, 8, 16, 17, 20, 21, 22, 24, 28, 30, 31, 32, 66, 115, 142, 143, 147, 162, 163, 164, 167, 172, 184, 192
ionizing radiation, 72, 74, 118
ions, 83, 143, 196, 210, 212, 229
Iowa, 134, 223
ipsilateral, 116, 128
iron, 212
islands, 72
Israel, 233
Italy, 52, 139, 220, 221, 227, 232

J

JAK, Janus kinase, 2
Jak2, 18, 19, 28, 29
Japan, 173, 174, 175, 179

K

K^+, 209, 210
karyotype, 35
Ki67, 126
kidney, 83, 176
kill, 129, 165, 203, 240, 244
kinetics, 53, 171
Klebsiella pneumoniae, 183, 191, 195

L

labeling, 2, 8
lactate dehydrogenase, ix, 201, 205, 208, 221, 225, 227
lactation, vii, 1, 2, 3, 4, 7, 8, 13, 16, 18, 19, 20, 21, 24, 32, 41, 45, 66, 69, 79, 88, 115, 142, 147, 153, 159, 163, 167, 168, 169, 175, 179, 194, 197, 198, 199, 200, 202, 203, 205, 210, 211, 212, 215, 220, 221, 222, 223, 225, 227, 230
Lactation, 7, 28, 141, 223, 229
lactic acid, 194
lactoferrin (Lf), ix, 149, 164, 194, 211, 212, 213, 214, 216, 218, 219, 221, 222, 223, 224, 225, 227, 228, 231, 232
Lactoperoxidase (Lp), 214
lactose, ix, 143, 144, 194, 199, 201, 209, 210, 215
L-amino acid oxidase (LAO), 159
landscape, 64, 87, 100
larvae, 84
latency, 47, 54
later life, 89
lead, 64, 72, 74, 79, 159, 162, 198, 199, 237
Leahy, 191
leakage, 207
Lebanon, 63
Lef1, vii, 5, 10, 18
legislation, 204
lesions, 55, 57, 102, 121, 122, 123, 128, 130, 162
leukemia, 2, 20
LEUKOCYTES, 146, 201, 202, 203, 205, 216, 225, 235, 236, 237, 238, 245, 246, 247
liberation, 244
LIF, leukemia inhibitory factor, 2
life cycle, 97
life quality, 130
lifetime, 45, 46, 64, 71, 76, 84, 183
ligand, 2, 13, 14, 15, 16, 27, 159, 183
light, 37, 65, 66, 79, 90
linoleic acid, 92, 111
lipids, 7, 92, 93, 143, 149
lipolysis, 205
lipoproteins, 156
Listeria monocytogenes, 212
liver, 19, 21, 30, 90, 143
livestock, viii, 198, 237
localization, 15, 67, 82, 177
loci, 175, 185, 186, 187, 218
locus, 15, 29, 174
longevity, 117, 184, 189, 191
longitudinal study, 93
loss of appetite, 196
LTA, 151
luciferase, 180
lumen, 6, 7, 66, 67, 143, 147, 240
Luo, 103, 188
lycopene, 93, 112
lymph, viii, 46, 114, 115, 116, 120, 122, 123, 126, 130, 135, 142, 165, 166, 243
lymph node, 46, 114, 116, 120, 122, 123, 126, 130, 142, 165, 243
lymphatic system, 115, 144
lymphocytes, viii, ix, 107, 126, 127, 131, 144, 145, 146, 165, 201, 203, 236, 237, 242, 244, 247, 248
lymphoid, 31, 32, 112, 145
lymphoid tissue, 112, 145
lysine, 70, 73, 106
lysozyme (Lz), ix, 144, 149, 164, 194, 211, 213, 214, 220, 221, 225, 226, 227

M

machinery, 64, 80, 182
macromolecules, 82, 92

macrophage inflammatory protein, 147
macrophages, viii, ix, 8, 66, 126, 127, 136, 144, 146, 147, 152, 156, 166, 167, 190, 201, 203, 205, 216, 236, 237, 238, 239, 240, 241, 243, 244, 245, 247, 248
majority, 1, 4, 20, 34, 79, 88, 239, 242
malaria, 47
malignancy, 119, 123, 124, 125, 126
malignant tumors, 114
mammalian cells, 100
mammals, viii, 2, 3, 84, 100, 145, 148, 150, 154, 181, 182, 183, 212
management, viii, 98, 149
manipulation, 128
mapping, 174, 175, 186, 187
MAS, 195, 218
mass, 34, 121
mastectomy, 128, 138, 139
matrix, 8, 44, 69, 97, 105, 106, 143
matrix metalloproteinase, 8, 69
matter, iv, 79, 118
MB, 59, 100, 245
measurement(s), 47, 93, 214, 230
meat, 118
mechanical stress, 20
media, 167
medical, 103
medicine, 98, 99, 101, 103, 111, 114, 117, 128, 129, 148, 231, 247
Mediterranean, 220
membranes, 82
memory, 100, 165, 203, 242, 248
menopause, 77, 118
menstrual cycles, 66, 77
mesenchyme, 10, 122
messenger RNA, 181
messengers, 83
meta-analysis, 59, 98, 104
metabolism, 53, 86, 90, 102, 170, 203, 214, 217, 228, 232, 239
metabolites, 47, 50, 51, 58, 81, 83, 203, 237
metalloproteinase, 2
metastasis, 54, 58, 83, 97, 116, 120, 122, 123, 125, 128, 130, 136, 145, 146, 165, 166
Metastasis, 166
metastatic disease, 122, 130
methodology, 122
methyl group, 72
methylation, 22, 64, 67, 70, 71, 72, 73, 74, 77, 85, 86, 87, 88, 89, 90, 91, 96, 99, 100, 101, 103, 106, 108, 109, 110, 112
microfabrication, 94
microorganisms, 146, 195, 196, 208, 212, 214, 215, 237
microsatellites, 187
microscope, 36, 38
microscopy, 36, 79, 94
microspheres, 171, 244
microstructure, 94
migration, 51, 53, 68, 178, 183, 191, 217, 239, 241
Milk, 58, 142, 149, 154, 166, 167, 199, 207, 208, 219, 224, 229, 230, 232, 233, 242
milk quality, viii, 148, 194, 202, 205, 215, 224, 230
milk quantity, 174
mimicry, 112
Minimal inhibitory concentration (MIC) test, 158
MIP, 147, 156
Missouri, 131, 133
misuse, 158
mitochondria, 31
mitotic index, 126
MMP, metalloproteinase, 2
MMPs, 8, 69
MMTV-Cre, 17, 19, 21
MMTV-erbB2, 54, 58
models, viii, 5, 8, 10, 12, 13, 14, 15, 17, 18, 21, 22, 24, 26, 33, 45, 46, 54, 55, 60, 75, 80, 88, 93, 101, 112, 136, 145, 148, 149, 152, 153, 154, 155, 156, 157, 159, 160, 161, 162, 163
modifications, 64, 67, 70, 71, 72, 73, 74, 78, 79, 80, 81, 87, 88, 91, 92, 100, 101, 106
modules, 164
molds, 246
molecular biology, 100, 111, 112, 148, 152, 155

molecular mass, 246
molecular medicine, 100
molecular structure, 226
molecular weight, 211, 213, 215, 217
molecules, 3, 66, 82, 92, 93, 143, 144, 147, 154, 157, 158, 241, 242
monoclonal antibody, 38, 107, 228
monolayer, 80
Moon, 51, 59, 164
morphogenesis, 1, 4, 6, 15, 16, 18, 20, 23, 25, 27, 28, 69, 79, 88, 95, 97, 107, 108
morphology, 20, 71, 82, 105, 222
mortality, 52, 118
mortality rate, 118
Mouse embryonic fibroblast (MEF), 35
MR, 95, 244
MRI, 172
mRNA(s), 21, 28, 31, 120, 151, 152, 181, 184, 185, 190, 192
Msx, homeobox, msh-like, 2
mucin, 164
mucosa, 145
mucus, 232
multi-protein complexes, 161
mutagenesis, 112, 162
mutant, 8, 18, 25, 189
mutation(s), 5, 22, 29, 71, 74, 87, 99, 120, 127, 134, 139, 174, 176, 191
Mycobacterium tuberculosis, 182, 190
mycotoxins, 237, 246
myosin, 68

N

Na^+, 209, 210
National Academy of Sciences, 95, 96, 99, 102, 103, 106, 107, 108, 109, 168
National Health and Nutrition Examination Survey (NHANES), 47
National Institutes of Health, 94
necrosis, 169, 216, 236, 239, 240, 244
negative relation, 214
neonates, 9, 10, 141
Netherlands, 87, 199
neurons, 31, 42, 176, 188
neuroscience, 109
neutral, 205
neutrophils, viii, ix, 146, 152, 156, 167, 169, 183, 201, 203, 205, 212, 216, 236, 237, 238, 240, 241, 248
New Zealand, 204, 229
next generation, 85, 91
NHANES, 47
nitric oxide, 155, 156
nitric oxide synthase, 155, 156
nitrogen, 36, 207
nodes, 4, 116, 122, 239
nodules, 43, 161
normal development, viii, 22, 64, 68, 69, 74, 84
NOTCH, 69
nucleic acid, 83
nucleolus, 80
nucleoplasm, 79
nucleosome, 100, 101
nucleotides, 83
nucleus, 10, 14, 17, 18, 38, 66, 67, 71, 78, 79, 81, 82, 83, 84, 93, 96, 107, 108, 177
null, 9, 10, 13, 15, 20, 25, 29
nutrient, 83, 84, 85, 87, 88, 89, 90, 91, 93, 144, 149, 174, 182
nutrition, viii, 47, 64, 73, 84, 86, 89, 94, 95, 108, 111, 112, 147, 226, 228, 230, 231, 235
nutritional status, 86

O

obesity, 69, 87, 89, 111, 118, 130, 138
oncogenesis, 14, 83
opportunities, 77
optimization, 243
optimization method, 243
organ, vii, 1, 22, 24, 34, 66, 141
organelles, 92
organism, 13, 123, 213, 217
organize, 66
organochlorine compounds, 47
organs, 10, 25, 34, 94, 130, 144
osmotic pressure, 209

ovarian cancer, 57
ovariectomy, 139
ovaries, 61
overproduction, 161
oviduct, 26
ovulation, 13, 85
ox, 248
oxidation, 214
oxidative stress, 181, 189, 210
oxygen, 147, 205, 216

P

Pakistan, 200, 221, 224
parallel, 5, 68, 150
parasites, 212
parathyroid hormone, 2, 6
parenchyma, 8, 40, 105, 143
parity, 69, 227
participants, 47
partition, 47, 50
pasteurization, 214
pathogenesis, 152, 162, 169, 223, 244
pathogens, 145, 146, 148, 149, 150, 152, 154, 156, 158, 159, 160, 162, 167, 172, 181, 182, 184, 195, 214, 235, 236, 240, 243, 247
pathology, 97, 102, 134, 155, 169
pathophysiological, 155, 216
pathways, viii, 10, 13, 22, 23, 29, 46, 60, 71, 82, 87, 93, 142, 152, 154, 160, 162, 171, 185, 190, 244
pattern recognition, 151
PCNA, 47, 83, 108, 126, 133, 135
PCR, 151, 176, 177, 178, 180
penetrance, 9
penicillin, 35, 212, 222
Penicillium, 237
peptide(s), 2, 6, 10, 18, 144, 164, 167, 168, 203, 205, 217, 226
perinatal, 3
peripheral blood, 240
permeability, 207
permeation, 207
permission, iv
peroxide, 214
pesticide, 51, 52, 59
pH, 36, 38, 196, 210, 224
phage, 158
phagocytic cells, 8, 203
phagocytosis, 146, 184, 190, 215, 236
pharmaceutical, 169
pharmacology, 98
phenocopy, 13, 15
phenotype(s), viii, 5, 8, 9, 12, 13, 19, 21, 25, 41, 72, 79, 81, 82, 84, 96, 101, 105, 107, 108, 120, 129, 132, 165, 174, 175, 176, 248
Philadelphia, 131, 136
phosphate, 36, 240
phosphatidylserine, 146, 147, 169
phosphorylation, 30, 73, 83, 108
phylogenetic tree, 144
physical features, 84
physical properties, 105, 196
Physiological, 96, 221, 229
physiology, 150, 152, 222
PI3K, 182
pigs, 217
pituitary gland, 6
plants, 237
plasma levels, 191
plasma membrane, 159
plasticity, 72, 78, 84, 89
plastics, 53
platform, 158
plexus, 116
PM, 26, 57, 58, 60, 99, 102
Poland, 193, 198, 231
polarity, 66, 67, 69, 71, 81, 82, 83, 88, 90, 92, 94, 96, 100, 107, 111
polarization, 28, 82, 98
policy, 56
polybrominated diphenyl ethers, 58
polycarbonate, 53
polycarbonate plastics, 53
polycystic kidney disease, 21
polycystic kidneys, 31
polymerase, 176
polymerase chain reaction, 176

polymorphism(s), 175, 176, 180, 183, 184, 187, 189, 224, 232
polypeptide, 115, 211, 215, 217
polysaccharides, 213, 245
polyurethane, 48
polyurethane foam, 48
pools, 66
population, 42, 44, 51, 52, 80, 86, 90, 95, 99, 117, 131, 174, 186, 191, 195, 198, 203, 218, 237, 239
Portugal, 113
positive correlation, 194, 202, 203, 205, 208, 212, 214
positive relationship, 207, 215
postoperative outcome, 137
potassium, 210
PR, progesterone receptor, 2
pregnancy, vii, 1, 3, 4, 7, 9, 10, 13, 14, 15, 16, 18, 19, 20, 21, 24, 37, 39, 40, 45, 50, 51, 53, 55, 60, 66, 69, 75, 76, 88, 97, 111, 115, 142, 143
preparation, iv, 19, 94
preservation, 115
prevention, ix, 89, 91, 103, 104, 110, 111, 112, 145, 172, 199, 201, 203, 235
prevention of infection, 203
primary function, 2
principles, 72, 100
probability, 197, 217, 218
process control, 115
producers, 204
profitability, 198
progenitor cells, 19, 43, 64, 68, 71, 77, 78, 89, 91, 94, 242
progesterone, vii, 2, 6, 9, 26, 27, 28, 54, 76, 102, 103, 119, 128, 132, 136
prognosis, 99, 114, 120, 126, 127, 133, 135, 136, 139
programming, 88, 108, 109, 220, 221
pro-inflammatory, 145, 146, 147, 162, 216, 237, 239
prolactin, vii, 2, 10, 28, 29, 43, 76, 119, 120, 128, 136, 142, 163
proliferation, 1, 7, 8, 9, 16, 17, 20, 25, 28, 30, 47, 68, 69, 76, 77, 79, 83, 91, 92, 93, 105, 115, 120, 121, 126, 129, 132, 133, 144, 145, 146, 160, 163, 195
promoter, 15, 18, 21, 26, 36, 71, 72, 77, 80, 88, 111, 151, 177
propagation, 72
prophylactic, 129
prostate cancer, 105
protection, 69, 80, 91, 92, 145, 170
protective role, 97, 203
protein family, 21
protein-protein interactions, 107
proteins, 7, 21, 30, 32, 66, 68, 72, 73, 81, 82, 83, 87, 88, 96, 107, 109, 142, 144, 149, 166, 167, 199, 205, 207, 215, 216, 229, 238
proteoglycans, 7, 188
proteolysis, 205
proteomics, 161
Pseudomonas aeruginosa, 181
PThrP, parathyroid hormone related peptide, 2
pubertal development, 1, 5
puberty, viii, 1, 3, 4, 6, 7, 13, 15, 17, 45, 46, 48, 51, 59, 66, 68, 69, 74, 77, 85, 87, 88, 115, 142
Puberty, 6
public health, 90, 160
pumps, 53
pyelonephritis, 183, 191

Q

QTL, 174, 175, 176, 179, 180, 183, 185, 186, 187, 218
question mark, 157

R

radiation, 74, 99, 101
radical mastectomy, 128
radicals, 216
radiotherapy, 128
RANK, receptor activator of nuclear factor κβ, 2

RANKL, RANK ligand, 2
Rapamycin, 184, 192
RE, 25, 59
reactions, 90, 165, 237
reagents, 152
receptors, 6, 10, 12, 14, 22, 24, 25, 29, 67, 71, 76, 102, 103, 119, 120, 128, 132, 137, 147, 156, 159, 168, 177, 203, 235, 237, 238, 241, 242, 244
reciprocal interactions, 9, 96
reciprocity, 97
recognition, 1, 238, 247
recombination, 43
recommendations, iv
recovery, 42
recurrence, 125, 127, 128, 138
redistribution, 81
redundancy, 9
regeneration, 22, 34, 35, 42, 75
Registry, 134
regression, 22, 24, 143
relevance, 22, 162, 220
remission, 125
remodelling, 97
repair, 203, 216, 217, 245
repellent, 178, 188
replication, 73
reporters, 177
repression, 70, 73, 83
repressor, 10
reproduction, 22, 163
requirements, 204, 220
researchers, 5, 22, 118, 126, 129, 148, 150, 153, 155, 194
reserves, 149
residues, 73, 107, 174, 180, 215
resistance, viii, 160, 173, 174, 175, 179, 181, 182, 183, 184, 187, 188, 189, 190, 191, 194, 195, 207, 213, 216, 218, 221
resolution, 100, 237, 238, 240, 241, 243, 245, 246
response, ix, 1, 4, 7, 8, 9, 13, 14, 16, 19, 21, 24, 51, 56, 57, 58, 60, 66, 68, 80, 81, 84, 91, 92, 105, 107, 131, 134, 145, 150, 151, 152, 154, 156, 157, 158, 160, 165, 171, 173, 174, 176, 178, 182, 184, 185, 190, 203, 216, 235, 236, 239, 240, 241, 243, 245, 247, 248
restitution, 239
reticulum, 142
retinol, 112
RH, 245, 246
Rho GTPase, 79
rights, iv
risk factors, 69, 74, 98, 104, 105, 114, 228
RNA(s), 72, 83, 88, 100, 177, 178, 217
rodents, vii, 51, 54, 91, 92
room temperature, 38
root, 43
routes, 53
rural areas, 59
Russia, 53

S

safety, 49, 222, 231
saliva, 212
Salmonella, 190, 212, 214
Salmonella typhimurium, 190, 212
scarcity, 128
Schwerin, 186
science, 98, 100, 106, 107
scope, 13
secrete, 66, 67, 69, 79, 145, 174
secretion, 105, 115, 142, 143, 146, 152, 163, 169, 204, 210, 212, 215
security, 243
seeding, 35
selenium, 232
SEMA5A, 173, 174, 177, 178, 180, 183, 185
semen, 212
senescence, 57, 105
sensitivity, 50, 54, 168, 207, 212
sequencing, 117, 176, 181
serine, 108
serotonin, 20
serum, ix, 35, 38, 51, 52, 53, 76, 93, 112, 131, 156, 169, 194, 199, 201, 207, 215, 216, 223, 225, 229, 243

serum albumin, ix, 194, 201, 207, 223, 225, 229
services, iv
sex, 85, 137, 142
sexual development, 25
sexual dimorphism, 30
sham, 37, 153
shape, 78, 81, 106
sheep, vii, 197, 204, 210, 225, 226, 227, 228
shelf life, 205
Shigella dysenteria, 212
shock, 181
showing, 20, 47, 51, 92, 123, 156
siblings, 86
side effects, 129, 167
signal transduction, 29, 82, 108, 244
signaling pathway, vii, 6, 10, 18, 22, 31, 69, 77, 78, 79, 91, 97, 190, 191
signalling, 23, 28, 104, 123, 142, 146, 152, 156, 157, 160, 161, 162, 165, 188
signals, 6, 10, 29, 30, 66, 79, 81, 82, 145, 161, 216
signs, 71, 121, 122, 129, 204
single-nucleotide polymorphism, 218
sinuses, 143
siRNA, 177, 178, 179
skewness, 175
skin, 121, 142, 172, 195
small intestine, 236
smooth muscle, 7, 68
sodium, 35, 199
software, 4, 38, 157
solution, 35, 210
somatic cell, ix, 144, 148, 175, 185, 186, 187, 194, 196, 197, 201, 202, 203, 205, 207, 208, 216, 218, 219, 220, 221, 222, 223, 224, 225, 226, 227, 228, 229, 230, 231, 232, 245
South Africa, 214, 233
Soya, 91
species, vii, 2, 5, 43, 51, 56, 57, 92, 117, 144, 145, 147, 148, 149, 154, 158, 160, 162, 184, 196, 198, 204, 217, 219, 231, 243
sperm, 21
spindle, 68
Sprague-Dawley rats, 51, 52
Spring, 43, 97, 99, 102, 166
stability, 184, 193, 198
stabilization, 82
standardization, 165
staphylococci, 225
Staphylococcus aureus, 145, 155, 164, 165, 166, 167, 168, 170, 171, 181, 185, 192, 195, 212, 214, 216, 222, 227, 229, 246, 247, 248
starvation, 182, 190
stasis, 8, 20
STAT, signal transducers and activators of transcription, 2
STAT1, 18, 20
STAT3, 17, 18, 20, 24, 30
STAT5, 18, 19
state, 2, 7, 8, 22, 69, 70, 83, 85, 86, 109, 142, 143, 161, 198, 201, 216
states, 106, 137
stem cell differentiation, 77
stem cells, 34, 40, 42, 64, 65, 66, 68, 72, 74, 75, 76, 77, 78, 85, 87, 88, 93, 96, 98, 101, 102, 109, 143
sterile, 148, 245
steroids, 163
stimulation, 7, 14, 19, 61, 76, 145, 242, 247, 248
Streptococcus agalactiae, 174, 182, 195
Streptococcus dysgalactiae, 195
Streptococcus mutans, 212, 215
Streptococcus pyogenes, 182
Streptococcus uberis, 165, 168, 170, 195, 244, 246, 247
stress, 8, 89, 109, 202, 203, 216, 237, 240
stress response, 109
striatum, 41
stroma, 1, 7, 8, 46, 53, 65, 66, 69, 74, 79, 94, 104, 114, 143, 152
stromal cells, 6, 76, 150, 162
structural defects, 17
structure, 1, 3, 7, 10, 14, 19, 64, 67, 70, 71, 73, 78, 81, 83, 93, 97, 100, 104, 134, 142, 143, 144, 161, 215, 219, 228, 231

subgroups, 97
substrate, 189
sucrose, 38
supplementation, 16, 87, 89, 90, 92, 108, 109, 110
suppression, 120
surfactant, 49
surgical removal, vii, 134
survival, 19, 21, 32, 34, 36, 38, 39, 40, 41, 43, 125, 126, 127, 128, 131, 133, 137, 143, 182, 190, 195, 240, 244
survival rate, 40, 41, 126, 127, 131
survivors, 74, 101
susceptibility, viii, 54, 55, 56, 69, 74, 84, 87, 97, 109, 158, 166, 178, 179, 180, 182, 184, 185, 191, 194, 195, 218, 243
suspensions, 41
sweat, 114
Sweden, 131, 199, 230
swelling, 196
SWI/SNF, 106
Switzerland, 135
symptoms, viii, 196
syndrome, 148, 161
synergistic effect, 213
synthesis, 47, 217, 220

T

T cell, 145, 150, 165, 166, 171, 178, 242, 244, 248
T cell XE "T cell" s, 145, 165, 166, 178, 242, 244, 248
T lymphocytes, 165, 242
tamoxifen, 129, 138
Tamoxifen Citrate, 128
target, 9, 10, 14, 15, 17, 18, 22, 70, 73, 83, 149, 160, 161, 162, 174, 177, 182, 242
Tbx, T-box protein, 2
Tbx3, 6
T-cells, 127, 145, 146, 203
TEB, terminal end bud, 2
techniques, 123, 153, 155
technology, 22, 94, 161, 174, 232
TED, terminal end duct, 2
teeth, 10
telomere, 106
TEM, 102
temperature, 37, 38, 210
testing, 158
tetrachlorodibenzo-p-dioxin, 57, 58, 60
TGF, 20, 80, 147, 166, 217, 238
TGF-β, 20, 217
Th, T helper, 2
T-helper cell, 145
therapeutic agents, 161
therapeutic targets, 126, 160
therapeutics, 107
therapy, vii, 42, 71, 76, 103, 128, 129, 130, 133, 158, 161, 216, 219
threshold level, 204
thymus, 242
time frame, 147
TIN2, 80, 106
tissue, vii, 2, 5, 13, 15, 19, 21, 24, 29, 35, 38, 41, 45, 46, 53, 59, 64, 65, 66, 68, 69, 72, 73, 74, 78, 79, 81, 82, 84, 85, 86, 87, 88, 90, 91, 92, 93, 96, 97, 98, 102, 104, 105, 107, 111, 114, 115, 120, 122, 137, 138, 146, 148, 150, 152, 153, 157, 162, 167, 168, 183, 195, 203, 210, 216, 217, 236, 239, 240, 243
tissue remodelling, 24
TLR, 146, 155, 156, 160, 169, 178, 241
TLR2, 157, 170, 241, 247, 248
TLR4, 156, 157, 179, 241, 247
TNF, 147, 151, 155, 156, 159, 162, 169, 178, 183, 185, 216, 223, 238, 242
TNF-alpha, 169, 223
TNF-α, 151, 155, 156, 159, 162, 216, 242
tocopherols, 112
Toll like receptor (TLR), 146
tooth, 25
total energy, 91
toxicity, 159
toxin, 171
trade, 56
traits, 149, 150, 185, 186, 218, 224, 227, 229, 230
trajectory, 24, 45, 46, 54, 85

transcription, 2, 16, 17, 19, 22, 28, 30, 64, 70, 72, 73, 74, 77, 78, 83, 92, 93, 99, 106, 108, 151, 156, 161, 173, 176, 177, 180, 181, 183, 184, 189
transcription factors, 22, 72, 78, 106, 177, 189
transducer, 30
transfection, 36, 177
transferrin, 212
transformation, 110
transforming growth factor, 147, 217, 238, 247
transgene, 15
transitional cell carcinoma, 133
translation, 184, 192
translocation, 151, 217
transmission, 2, 83, 165
transplant, 123
transplantation, 16, 22, 34, 36, 37, 38, 39, 40, 41, 42
Transplantation, 13, 14, 34, 42, 44
transport, 143
treatment, viii, ix, 35, 38, 54, 58, 98, 99, 102, 103, 110, 128, 129, 131, 132, 135, 137, 152, 157, 160, 161, 162, 170, 174, 178, 182, 183, 185, 193, 198, 199, 219, 235, 240, 243
TRIF, 178
triggers, 157
trypsin, 35
tuberculosis, 182, 184, 190, 201
tumor, 47, 51, 54, 55, 57, 58, 60, 64, 71, 75, 79, 82, 83, 86, 92, 93, 94, 97, 98, 99, 101, 102, 105, 108, 110, 122, 123, 130, 131, 132, 133, 134, 135, 136, 138, 144, 146, 147, 154, 155, 162, 171, 173, 178, 190, 238, 244, 245, 246
tumor cells, 75, 154, 162
tumor development, 54, 79, 82, 144, 162
tumor growth, 105
tumor necrosis factor, 138, 147, 155, 171, 173, 178, 190, 238, 244, 245, 246
tumor progression, 162
tumorigenesis, 25, 26, 31, 102, 103, 111, 112
TUNEL, Terminal deoxynucleotidyl transferase dUTP nick end labeling, 2
typhoid, 47
tyrosine, 30, 164

U

ubiquitin, 214
UK, 131
ultrasound, 122
umbilical cord, 44
underlying mechanisms, 22, 89
uniform, 15
United Kingdom, 51, 227
United States (USA), 36, 42, 50, 56, 60, 87, 95, 96, 99, 102, 103, 106, 107, 108, 109, 110, 168, 187, 192, 223, 224, 231, 245
urea, 54
urinary bladder, 133, 134
urinary bladder cancer, 134
USDA, 175

V

vaccine, 166, 171
vagina, 116
vancomycin, 212
variables, 91, 114, 135
variations, 71, 82, 108, 126, 175
vector, 36
vegetables, 89, 90
versatility, 151
vertebrates, 9
vessels, 116, 122
vestibulocochlear nerve, 43
Vietnam, 51
viruses, 118, 195, 212
visualization, 71
vitamin A, 93
vitamin D, 89, 92, 93, 112
Vitamin D, 92, 111, 112
vitamins, 89
vulnerability, 89, 91
vulva, 132

W

WAP, whey acidic protein, 2
WAP-Cre, 18, 19, 20, 21
Washington, 56, 57, 134
water, 37, 51, 59, 195, 229
weight gain, 89, 111, 237
welfare, 160, 185
Western blot, 182
white blood cells, 203
wild animals, 134
wild type, 189
windows, 45, 48, 49, 50, 74, 84, 87, 88, 89, 91
Wisconsin, 51, 59
Wnt signaling, 10
Wnt10b, 5, 23
Wnt6, 5
World Health Organization, 97, 110, 114, 121, 122, 123, 134, 135
wound healing, 162

Y

yeast, 182, 189, 190
yield, 149, 174, 186, 194, 197, 205, 215, 218, 220, 223, 224, 227
young women, 57, 71

Z

zinc, viii, 173, 176, 177, 187, 188, 225
zygote, 85